MW00441962

	IIIa 13	IVa 14	Va 15	VIa 16	VIIa 17	He 4.002602 2
7	boron 5 **B** 10.811 2 3	carbon 6 **C** 12.011 2 4	nitrogen 7 **N** 14.0067 2 5	oxygen 8 **O** 15.9994 2 6	fluorine 9 **F** 18.9984032 2 7	neon 10 **Ne** 20.1797 2 8
6	aluminum 13 **Al** 26.981539 2 8 3	silicon 14 **Si** 28.0855 2 8 4	phosphorus 15 **P** 30.973762 2 8 5	sulfur 16 **S** 32.066 2 8 6	chlorine 17 **Cl** 35.4527 2 8 7	argon 15 **Ar** 39.948 2 8 8

10	Ib 11	IIb 12						
nickel 28 **Ni** 8.69 6 2	copper 29 **Cu** 63.546 2 8 18 1	zinc 30 **Zn** 65.38 2 8 18 2	gallium 31 **Ga** 69.723 2 8 18 3	germanium 32 **Ge** 72.59 2 8 18 4	arsenic 33 **As** 74.92159 2 8 18 5	selenium 34 **Se** 78.96 2 8 18 6	bromine 35 **Br** 79.904 2 8 18 7	krypton 36 **Kr** 83.80 2 8 18 8
palladium 46 **Pd** 06.42 3	silver 47 **Ag** 107.8682 2 8 18 18 1	cadmium 48 **Cd** 112.411 2 8 18 18 2	indium 49 **In** 114.82 2 8 18 18 3	tin 50 **Sn** 118.69 2 8 18 18 4	antimony 51 **Sb** 121.75 2 8 18 18 5	tellurium 52 **Te** 127.60 2 8 18 18 6	iodine 53 **I** 126.90447 2 8 18 18 7	xenon 54 **Xe** 131.29 2 8 18 18 8
platinum 78 **Pt** 05.08 2	gold 79 **Au** 196.96654 2 8 18 32 18 1	mercury 80 **Hg** 200.59 2 8 18 32 18 2	thallium 81 **Tl** 204.3833 2 8 18 32 18 3	lead 82 **Pb** 207.2 2 8 18 32 18 4	bismuth 83 **Bi** 208.98037 2 8 18 32 18 5	polonium 84 **Po** 209* 2 8 18 32 18 6	astatine 85 **At** 210* 2 8 18 32 18 7	radon 86 **Rn** 222* 2 8 18 32 18 8

❶ Alkali metals ❺ Actinide metals
❷ Alkaline earth metals ❻ Other metals
❸ Transition metals *** ❼ Nonmetals
❹ Lanthanide series ❽ Noble gases

*** Elements: 21-29 (scandium - copper), 39-47 (yttrium - silver), 57-79 (lanthanum - gold), and 89 (actinium) - on.

europium 63 **Eu** 1.965 8 2	gadolinium 64 **Gd** 157.25 2 8 18 25 9 2	terbium 65 **Tb** 158.92534 2 8 18 27 8 2	dysprosium 66 **Dy** 162.50 2 8 18 28 8 2	holmium 67 **Ho** 164.93032 2 8 18 29 8 2	erbium 68 **Er** 167.26 2 8 18 30 8 2	thulium 69 **Tm** 168.93421 2 8 18 31 8 2	ytterbium 70 **Yb** 173.04 2 8 18 32 8 2	lutetium 71 **Lu** 174.967 2 8 18 32 9 2
americium 95 **Am** 243* 8 8 2	curium 96 **Cm** 247* 2 8 18 32 25 9 2	berkelium 97 **Bk** 247* 2 8 18 32 27 8 2	californium 98 **Cf** 251* 2 8 18 32 28 8 2	einsteinium 99 **Es** 252* 2 8 18 32 29 8 2	fermium 100 **Fm** 257* 2 8 18 32 30 8 2	mendelevium 101 **Md** 258* 2 8 18 32 31 8 2	nobelium 102 **No** 259* 2 8 18 32 32 8 2	lawrencium 103 **Lr** 260* 2 8 18 32 32 9 2

Source: O'Brien & Gere Engineers, Inc., Syracuse, New York

RB
DFH
2

Calculation Methods
for Industrial Hygiene

Salvatore R. DiNardi

VAN NOSTRAND REINHOLD

I (T) P A Division of International Thomson Publishing Inc.

New York • Albany • Bonn • Boston • Detroit • London • Madrid • Melbourne
Mexico City • Paris • San Francisco • Singapore • Tokyo • Toronto

I(T)P ™ A division of International Thomson Publishing, Inc.
The ITP logo is a trademark under license

Printed in the United States of America

For more information, contact:

Van Nostrand Reinhold
115 Fifth Avenue
New York, NY 10003

Chapman & Hall GmbH
Pappelallee 3
69469 Weinheim
Germany

Chapman & Hall
2-6 Boundary Row
London
SE1 8HN
United Kingdom

International Thomson Publishing Asia
221 Henderson Road #05-10
Henderson Building
Singapore 0315

Thomas Nelson Australia
102 Dodds Street
South Melbourne, 3205
Victoria, Australia

International Thomson Publishing Japan
Hirakawacho Kyowa Building, 3F
2-2-1 Hirakawacho
Chiyoda-ku, 102 Tokyo
Japan

Nelson Canada
1120 Birchmount Road
Scarborough, Ontario
Canada M1K 5G4

International Thomson Editores
Campos Eliseos 385, Piso 7
Col. Polanco
11560 Mexico D.F. Mexico

3 4 5 6 7 8 9 10 QEB-FF 00 99 98 97

Library of Congress Cataloging-in-Publication Data

DiNardi, S. R. (Salvatore Robert)
    Calculation methods for industrial hygiene/S. R. DiNardi.
        p.   cm.
    Includes bibliographical references and index.
    ISBN 0-442-01821-5
    1. Industrial hygiene—Mathematics. 2. Industrial toxicology—
Mathematics. 3. Air—Pollution—Mathematics. 4. Chemistry,
Analytic. 5. Environmental chemistry. I. Title.
RC963.3.D56 1995
615.9'02'01541—dc20

94-40909
CIP

To:

Thomas and Mary DiNardi, for their life-long support and encouragement.

Peter Joseph and Christopher Thomas DiNardi, for loving me and sticking with me, and tolerating an occasionally ill-tempered father who was sometimes bewildered and distracted trying to work through a solution or derivation.

My sister Nancy, who says that she "forfeited all of her science and math genes so I could pursue a career in science." She is my most ardent supporter and the mother of my nieces Carla, Tana, Mari, and Regina and my nephew Thomas—but most importantly she loves me...unconditionally.

Joan Marie Culley, for her emotional support, which gave me the means to keep moving ahead. She made me understand the learning process and taught me critical thinking skills.

David Allison Fraser, with a very special tribute and thank you for inviting me to spend a sabbatical year at the University of North Carolina at Chapel Hill. That year launched my industrial hygiene career. It was truly the opportunity of a lifetime. I will never forget it. Dave passed away in November 1989, but the people who knew and loved him will never forget him.

Contents

Goals and Outcomes

The goal of this textbook is to educate users in basic physical chemical principles. These principles will be combined with critical thinking skills to solve quantitative problems in industrial hygiene, air pollution, and toxicology. After working through this textbook, users will be able to demonstrate these outcomes:

- Explain "Le Systeme Internationale," the SI system of metric units.
- Employ dimensional analysis in solving problems.
- Develop their computational skills on a rigorous scientific basis.
- Explain calculation techniques to each other, to practicing professionals, and to the public.
- Integrate basic physical chemical principles into the study of industrial hygiene, air pollution, and toxicology.
- Apply fundamental principles of the physical chemistry of gases, vapors, and particles related to air pollution, industrial hygiene, and toxicology to solve complex problems.
- Validate exposure assessments.
- Synthesize unique solutions to new problems.
- Justify the solutions to complex problems.
- Critique existing solutions to problems.
- Develop exposure assessment data.
- Evaluate exposure assessment data.
- Solve new problems using sound and fundamental scientific principles.
- Apply mathematical modeling techniques to calculate the concentrations of contaminants in air.
- Apply mathematical modeling techniques to predict worker exposure.

Preface

Something unusual happens when words are written down on paper—people believe them. This places an immense burden on an author, the burden of truth. The author carries this burden for life. The responsibility to say it clearly, concisely, and correctly is a Sisyphean task. Just as I think that what I have written is finally complete, a new view emerges. Like a rolling hill beyond a rolling hill, the task goes on forever. The joy of this book is that I have reached that last hill, and the view beyond it is magnificent. Sisyphus beat the stone. I have written this book not to teach the reader about industrial hygiene calculations, but to learn all there is to know about industrial hygiene calculations. The stone is starting to roll back!

The field of environmental health encompasses many science and engineering disciplines, including such specialities as industrial hygiene, air pollution, and toxicology as well as the more traditional disciplines of chemical, mechanical, and environmental engineering and the medical, chemical, and biological sciences. If the field of environmental health is to grow, develop, and continue to make great strides in the prevention, anticipation, recognition, evaluation, and control of health hazards in the environment, then those individuals trained in the discipline are compelled to communicate. As each of the supporting disciplines of environmental health has its own basic terminology and system of units, this communication may be difficult at times.

The goal of this book is to educate students and practicing professionals in basic principles of calculation techniques so they can start building at the same point of reference and begin to communicate with each other; hence the review of "Le Systeme Internationale," the SI system of metric units. These discussions must start at the same set of fundamental units, such as mass, length, and time. The relationship between the various units must be developed from fundamental principles. Developing an understanding of the fundamental physical chemistry of gases and vapors will enable the student to develop new methods based on sound fundamental scientific principles.

To facilitate communications among the myriad disciplines of environmental health, all users of this reference are encouraged at least to review the chapters on units and fundamentals of ideal gases. This will help them to understand new problems and experiments and new technology in the field.

Writing this book on quantitative methods in environmental health involves both a challenge and a letdown. The challenge is to explain the practical applications of physical chemistry in clearly understood terms. Most students who have survived a course in elementary physical chemistry have at their disposal all the knowledge that they need to solve these problems. The letdown is that they have not learned how to apply this knowledge to "real-world" problems.

Fully armed with this knowledge I entered the discipline of environmental health and, at first glance, assumed that these corrections and calculations were straightforward. After ten years of education in the chemical and physical sciences I can certify that they are. However, for students who wish to pursue a career in industrial hygiene, air pollution, and toxicology some of these methods appear to be more magic than science. I hope that this book addresses this issue and explains the magic by using scientific knowledge.

The beginning chapters start with fundamental concepts based on algebraic methods, not as a review but as a place to launch an attack on somewhat more esoteric problems. I wish to develop a problem-solving sixth sense in my students, and I believe that this can only happen when they are all building upon a common basic foundation. What may appear as an overemphasis on the ideal gas law is just that! Sure, many physical chemists may wish to dismiss the ideal gas equation in an attempt to get into the other interesting equations of state. I, however, have decided to beat it to exhaustion. This equation will be used to describe the behavior of gases and vapors in the environment, and this can be accomplished without apology. Calculations and measurements in the ambient, occupational, and indoor environment are in the parts per million (or milligram per cubic meter) and lower concentration ranges. This produces what the chemist considers as the indefinitely dilute solution. Under these conditions the ideal gas equation is an excellent descriptor. There is no need to apologize for using the ideal gas equation to describe such nonideal materials as water vapor, ethylene oxide, glycol ethers, and others ad infinitum. The list is not quite endless but is nearly so.

I assume that the entering student (a junior or senior undergraduate, beginning graduate student, or practicing professional) has a fundamental scientific background and will complete the material in this book in a one-semester course. I have tried to present a sufficient amount of background material to assist the neophyte and a sufficiently rigorous derivation of equations to provide insight to the experienced practitioner.

Selected chapters of this book make an excellent background for short courses and for continuing education programs for the professional wishing to learn industrial hygiene calculations. I recommend combining a review of temperature and pressure corrections to solve more difficult problems in industrial hygiene and industrial exhaust ventilation design. Several chapters will help the practicing professional to follow the correct approach to calibration procedures for air-moving devices and gas and vapor analyzers.

During my professional career, I have found many "quotable quotes" that are directly related to developing problem-solving and critical thinking skills in students and practicing professionals. I present them here without further comment:

- "The mass of men lead lives of quite desperation" (Henry David Thoreau).
- "I wished to live deliberately, to face only the essential facts of life, and see if I could not learn what it had to teach, and not, when I came to die, discover that I had not lived" (Henry David Thoreau).
- "Don't crack up. Bend your brain. See both sides. Cast off your mental chains" (Howard Jones).
- "Anyone who stops learning is old, whether at 21 or 80. Anyone who keeps learning stays young. The greatest thing in life is to keep your mind young" (Henry Ford).
- "For every complicated problem there is an answer that is short, simple and wrong" (H. L. Mencken).
- "The truth is always the strongest argument" (Sophocles).
- "We made the wrong mistakes" (Yogi Berra).
- "Patient observation and problem solving are the key that unlocks the wonders in the study of science" (S. R. DiNardi).
- "An expert is someone who has found all the mistakes in a very narrow field" (Niels Bohr as quoted by Edward Teller).
- "I was greatly surprised by the event, but I was not surprised by the surprise" (E. Teller).
- "A year can teach what a day cannot know" (R. W. Emerson).
- "Common sense is very uncommon" (Mark Twain).
- "Our greatest glory is not in falling, but in rising every time we fall" (unknown).
- "95% of baseball is pitching, the other 50% is hitting" (Yogi Berra).
- "It ain't what you don't know that makes you look like a fool; its what you do know that ain't so" (Appalachian Mountain proverb).

Acknowledgments

This book is the culmination of nearly twenty years of anguish and fun. The list of people who contributed to this work in mind, spirit, and text is very long, but I have tried not to exclude anyone. I owe a special thank you to:

- Harold Jacobsen, for his inspiration, encouragement, and infamous boy on the tricycle.
- Frances Sterrett and Howard Rosman, for their patient pedagogical style and unselfish sharing of their talent and their inspiration during the formative years of my career.
- Glenn Tisman and Walter Dilts, for staying up nights with me grinding out problems on the slide rule and never accepting an answer without intense questioning and always asking why. They pushed me to the furthest limits.
- David Fraser, John Hickey, Steve Guffey, and Parker Reist, for revealing the world of industrial hygiene, ventilation, and temperature and pressure effects.
- William Darity and Steve Gehlbach, for a laissez-faire administrative style that gave me the space to complete this.
- My labovisher rabbis Warren Litsky and Seth Goldsmith, for their encouragement through some difficult times.
- Thomas Hamilton, for critical thinking on exposure assessment, TLV-TWA, and break times.
- Claire Meissner, Sandy Orszulak, Ity Keedy, and Terry LaPointe, for their proficient and patient word-processing skills that produced the various drafts.
- The consulting clients who have provided problems that appear in this book.
- Ron Conrad, for spending seemingly endless hours discussing temperature and pressure effects on air sample volumes. We are still friends!
- The teaching assistants who discussed, argued, and cajoled me into thinking through and clarifying the concepts; the dozens of

students from the School of Public Health, Environmental Health Science Program at the University of Massachusetts at Amherst who suffered through various versions of this material; my graduate students who patiently and devoutly applied these concepts in classes and laboratories or buried them in the appendixes of their masters' dissertations; and the students in my Industrial Hygiene Laboratory and Quantitative Methods in Environmental Health courses for working through many problems and correcting and rewriting many of them. I thank Marc Abromovitz, Hamid Bekrani, Susan Brighenti, Lori Chamberlin, Jane (Clapprood) Pisani, Tom Cronin, Dirk Decker, Amy Gittleman, George Hynes, Susan McDonald, Maritza McLaughlin, Martha McManus, Marc Muranaka, Robert Murphy, David Nolan, John Ochs, Lawrence Park, Patty Parks, Dennis Pinski, Marc Rothney, Linda Secor, Linda Sicardi, Dawn Speranza, Douglas Smith, Christopher Steger, Mark Tartaglia, Theresa Tiernan, Al Vaz, Peter Waldron, and too many others to name.

- The hundreds of students whom I had the pleasure to teach in the continuing education offerings of Basic Industrial Hygiene, Calculation Techniques in Industrial Hygiene, and ABIH Certification Review courses at the University of Massachusetts at Amherst and the University of North Carolina at Chapel Hill.

- Bill and Polly Read and Steve and Karen Dimock, for helping me through the difficult times in my life so that I could reach this point.

- Janice Laura Pratte, for forcing me to clarify my career goals and keeping me on target early in my career.

- Dr. Reginald Jordan, whose hard work and long hours cannot be adequately described. Dr. Jordan devoted himself to a careful, critical, and constructive review of the final manuscript, and his efforts brought this project to a timely and successful conclusion. Also Wesley Van Pelt reviewed the final manuscript, and his comments and insights were very helpful. His review of Chapter 6 helped me resolve temperature and pressure effects on air sample volume.

- Constance Marsh MacDonald, for making this book readable.

Abbreviations and Symbols

cc or cm^3	cubic centimeter
cc/min	cubic centimeters per minute
cm	centimeter
f	fibers
f/cc or f/cm^3	fibers per cubic centimeter
ft	feet
g	gram(s)
h or hr	hour
LEL	Lower Explosive Limit
LFL	Lower Flammable Limit
l	liter(s)
liters per minute	l/min or lpm
m	milli- (1/1000 part of) or meter
mA	milliAmperes
mg	milligram
mg/m^3	milligrams per cubic meter
min	minute
ml	milliliter
ml/min	millimeters per minute
ng	nanogram
ng/m^3	nanograms per cubic meter
ppm	parts per million
ppb	parts per billion
ppt	parts per trillion
sec	second
μg	micrograms
μg/m^3	micrograms per cubic meter
C	ceiling value
MAC	Measured Air Concentration
PEL	Permissible Exposure Limit
STEL	Short Term Exposure Limit
TLV	Threshold Limit Value

TWA	Time Weighted Average Concentration
LOD	Limit of Detection
LOQ	Limit of Quantification
Q	volume flowrate
P	pressure
V	volume
n	number of moles
R	universal gas constant (0.08205 liter atmosphere/mole K)
T	thermodynamic temperature
t	time or temperature °C
°C	Celsius temperature
°F	Fahrenheit temperature
°R	Rankine temperature (thermodynamic English system)
K	Kelvin temperature (thermodynamic SI system)
NTP	Normal Temperature and Pressure (298.15 K, 1 atmosphere)
STP	Standard Temperature and Pressure (273.15 K, 1 atmosphere)
BTP	Body (Basal) Temperature and Pressure (310.15 K, 1 atmosphere)
ρ	density (mass per volume)
η	nano (10^{-9})
μ	micro (10^{-6})
Δ	change in

Subscripts:

A	impurity
B	diluent air volume, room volume, chamber volume, etc.
M/V	concentration in mass per volume
C	calibration
F	field
S	standard

1

Arithmetic and Algebra Review

Outcome Competencies   *After studying this chapter you will be able to:*

- *List examples of arithmetic processes.*
- *List examples of algebraic processes.*
- *Recall various arithmetic manipulations.*
- *Employ algebraic techniques to solve units problems.*
- *Apply algebraic techniques to dimensional analysis problems.*
- *Recognize that a hazard may not be controlled with dilution ventilation.*
- *Derive conversion factors from basic knowledge.*
- *Define a conversion factor.*
- *Describe significant figures.*

1. PURPOSE

Calculation techniques in industrial hygiene are based on the physical chemistry of gases and vapors. The first step is to review arithmetic, starting with simple fractions, and then algebra. The rules governing the manipulation of numbers, symbols, and fractions should be familiar to the reader. This chapter will not teach arithmetic and algebra to someone who is not familiar with basic mathematics; but it will provide a review, with an emphasis on the manipulation of units (mass, length, time, etc.).

2. FRACTIONS

A fraction is a ratio of whole numbers and is one or more of the equal or unequal portions of anything. The terms used to describe a fraction are the:

- Numerator: the number, integer, or digit on top.
- Denominator: the number, integer, or digit on the bottom.

Recall that an integer expresses a whole unit, and a fraction is a ratio of integers. An integer may be either a positive or a negative number. Also recall that the symbol $\equiv$ is used to indicate that the quantities on either side of the symbol are identical to each other. For example 24 hours/ 1 day $\equiv$ 1! More on this appears later in the chapter.

Multiplication

To multiply a fraction by an integer, multiply the numerator of the faction by the integer, and place the product over the same denominator. For example:

$$5(3/7) \equiv (5 \times 3)/7 = 15/7$$

To multiply a fraction by a fraction, multiply the numerators of the fraction, yielding a new numerator and multiply the denominators of the fractions, yielding a new denominator. For example:

$$(2/3)(5/7) \equiv (2 \times 5)/(3 \times 7) = 10/21$$

Division

The reciprocal of a number is one (1) divided by that number. To divide an integer by a fraction, multiply the integer by the reciprocal of the fraction:

$$(2)/(4/7) \equiv (2 \times 7)/(4) = 14/4$$

Factors

The factors of a number are all the numbers that when multiplied together produce the given number:

$$2 \times 3 \times 5 \times 9 = 2 \times 3 \times 5 \times 3 \times 3 = 270$$

The numbers 2, 3, 5, and 9 are a set of factors of 270. A multiple of a number contains that number as a factor. A common factor of two or more numbers is a factor of each.

Addition and Subtraction

Only similar fractions can be added or subtracted. Similar fractions contain a common or identical denominator. To add fractions, add the numerators and place the sum over the common denominator:

$$2/5 + 1/5 \equiv (2+1)/5 = 3/5$$

Dissimilar fractions must be transformed to a similar fraction by finding the lowest common multiple of the denominators. Divide the denominator of each fraction into the lowest common multiple to get the factor used to reduce the given fraction. The following example illustrates the rule:

$$2/3 + 4/7 + 5/9$$

The lowest common multiple is 63, that is, the lowest number into which all three denominators will go an even number of times:

$$2/3 \times 21/21 + 4/7 \times 9/9 + 5/9 \times 7/7 = 42/63 + 36/63 + 35/63 \equiv 113/63$$

Operations

The application of simple arithmetic operations is a powerful problem-solving technique. If the numerator and the denominator of a fraction are multiplied or divided by the same number, the value of the fraction is not changed. This rule is fundamental to handling complicated units conversion to solve nearly every problem in this book and throughout one's professional career. For example:

$$3/4 \equiv (3/4)(2/2) \equiv (3 \times 2)/(4 \times 2) = 6/8$$

If the same number is added to or subtracted from both the numerator and the denominator of a fraction, the value of the fraction changes. For example, $3/4$ is not the same as $(3+2)/(4+2)$, which equals $5/6$.

In the multiplication of a fraction by a whole number, steps are followed that may not be explicitly shown. For example:

$$5 \times 3/7 = 15/7$$

This could be expressed as follows:

$$5 \times 3/7 = (5 \times 3)/7 = 15/7$$

Similarly:

$$6(2/9) = (6 \times 2)/9 = (6 \times 2)/(3 \times 3) = (3 \times 2 \times 2)/(3 \times 3) = 4/3$$

Any number can be multiplied by any other number, but multiplication by 1 produces an identity:

$$100 \times 1 = 100$$

Here the multiplication does not change the value of the number. Later, it will be demonstrated that "1" can be written in many ways. For example, the ratio of identical units equals 1. For example:

$$(\text{a particular unit})/(\text{a particular unit}) \equiv 1$$

Any fraction, say 22/7, can be multiplied by 1:

$$22/7 \times 1 \equiv 22/7$$

Multiplication by "1" does not change the value of the fraction.

The fundamental mathematical operation that enables the manipulation of numbers in the numerator and denominator is division. For example:

$$2/6 \equiv (2 \times 1)/(3 \times 2) = (1 \times 1)/(1 \times 3) = (1/1)(1/3) = 1 \times (1/3) = 1/3$$

$$(99 \times 6)/(48 \times 11) \equiv (9 \times 11 \times 6)/(8 \times 6 \times 11) = (1/1)(1/1)(9/8) = 9/8$$

3. MANIPULATING UNITS AS NUMBERS

The application of the elementary mathematical principle of division may be expanded to include units (e.g., centimeters, grams, hours, etc.). The units (which are words) may be treated as "numbers." It is possible to perform similar mathematical operations by combining numbers with units. For example,

$$(3 \text{ apples}/4 \text{ apples}) \equiv 3/4 \times (\text{apples}/\text{apples})$$

Since the ratio (apples/apples) is identical to 1, we have:

$$(\text{apples}/\text{apples}) \equiv 1$$

$$(3 \text{ apples}/4 \text{ apples}) \equiv (3/4) \times 1 = 3/4$$

Similarly, since $(\text{cm}^2/\text{cm}^2)$ is identical to one:

$$(2 \text{ cm}^3)/(7 \text{ cm}^2) = (2 \text{ cm}^2 \times \text{cm})/(7 \text{ cm}^2) = 2 \text{ cm}/7$$

The parts of the ratio of the units can be divided one by the other, and the quotient is one. There are many other ratios, containing equally diverse units, that are routinely used. Most of the time one forgets this critical and essential fact. Some examples are:

$$60 \text{ minutes}/1 \text{ hour} \equiv 60 \text{ minutes}/60 \text{ minutes} \equiv 1$$

$$5280 \text{ feet}/1 \text{ mile} \equiv 5280 \text{ feet}/5280 \text{ feet} \equiv 1$$

$$1 \text{ cm}^3/1 \text{ ml} \equiv 1 \text{ cm}^3/1 \text{ cm}^3 \equiv 1$$

$$3 \text{ feet}/1 \text{ yard} \equiv 3 \text{ feet}/3 \text{ feet} \equiv 1$$

$$10^{-6} \text{ m}/\mu\text{m} \equiv 10^{-6} \text{ m}/10^{-6} \text{ m} \equiv 1$$

$$1000 \text{ ml}/1 \equiv 1000 \text{ ml}/1000 \text{ ml} \equiv 1$$

Careful inspection shows that the items selected in the above example are conversion factors.

4. DIMENSIONAL ANALYSIS

All problems in this book are solved by using dimensional analysis, which is an essential technique that facilitates solving problems. The learning of problem-solving skills is the biggest difficulty facing aspiring environmental health scientists, industrial hygienists, and toxicologists. To those unfamiliar with the technique it first seems unnecessarily complex and difficult, but succumbing to such an attitude can shipwreck a career. The heart of applying dimensional analysis techniques to solving problems is knowing the correct dimensions for the answer.

An example of dimensional analysis that is common to everyday life is the unit pricing found in many grocery stores. A shopper can purchase a one-pound box of pasta for forty-eight cents in one store, whereas a warehouse store sells a five-pound bag of the same pasta for two dollars and fifty cents. The shopper will analyze this problem almost without thinking about it. The solution calls for reducing the problem to the price per pound. The pound is selected without much thought because it is the unit common to both stores. A shopper will pay fifty cents a pound for pasta in the warehouse store or forty-eight cents a pound in the local grocery store. Implicit in the solution to this problem is knowing the unit price, which is expressed in dollars per pound ($/lb).

Another simple problem is to convert 15 minutes into hours. This is facilitated by knowing the conversion factor for minutes to hours. This conversion can be written in two ways (recall that a conversion factor has a value equal to one, so that multiplying by the conversion factor does not change the value of the original quantity):

$$1 \text{ hour}/60 \text{ minutes} \quad \text{or} \quad 60 \text{ minutes}/1 \text{ hour}$$

The solution to this problem must be in hours; so one approach is:

$$(15 \text{ minutes})(60 \text{ minutes}/1 \text{ hour}) = 900 \text{ minute}^2/\text{hour}$$

The solution is stentorian, in both the magnitude of the number and the dimensions; so try the other form of the conversion factor:

$$(15 \text{ minutes})(\text{hour}/60 \text{ minutes}) = 0.25 \text{ hour}$$

The following examples demonstrate the use of dimensional analysis.

Example 1

Peter and Christopher are riding their tricycles on a straight, level, safe road. The children can pedal their tricycles so that they can travel 2 miles each hour. How far can they pedal in 12 minutes?

Solution 1

The distance traveled is equal to the speed (rate of travel) × time: $D = R \times t$. We may write:

$$D = (2 \text{ miles}/\text{hour})12 \text{ minutes} = (24 \text{ miles minutes})/\text{hours}$$

How can this "solution" be made to produce a useful piece of information? After all, the boys' father is patiently waiting for them to join him for a picnic lunch.

$$(24 \text{ mile minutes}/\text{hour}) \times (1 \text{ hour}/60 \text{ minutes}) = 0.4 \text{ mile}$$

This will work out just fine, because the picnic site is only 0.25 mile away, and the hamburgers are nearly ready.

Example 2

During the 1987 Rose Bowl Parade (A World of Wonders), announcer Christy Brinkley said that "the Dr. Pepper float, moving at 2.5 miles per hour would require 80 years to travel around the world." Was she correct?

Solution 2

$$r = 3963.34 \text{ mi}, C = 2\pi r = 2\pi(3963.34 \text{ mi})/2.5 \text{ mph} = 1.1 \text{ years}$$

However if the float traveled west from Pasadena around the world, it would sink into the Pacific Ocean in 8 to 15 hours!

Now that this "powerful" technique is available, it may be used in everyday activities. For example, with the introduction of the metric system of units into commerce, many manufacturers are labeling products with information in both the English system and the metric system.

Example 3

Convert 4000 feet per minute (ft/min) to miles per hour (mph).

Solution 3

$$4000(\text{ft/min}) \times (60 \text{ min/hr}) \times (\text{mile/5280 ft}) = 45.45 \text{ mile/hr} = 45.5 \text{ mph}$$

Example 4

Convert 120 feet per minute (ft/min) to miles per hour (mph).

Solution 4

$$120(\text{ft/min}) \times (60 \text{ min/hr}) \times (\text{mile/5280 ft}) = 1.4 \text{ mile/hr} = 1.4 \text{ mph}.$$

Example 5

A survey of labels from grocery store shelves appears in Table 1-1. Are these labels correct? Recall: 28.35 g/oz; 3.785 l/gal; 3785 cm^3/gal; 2.205 lb/kg; 453.59 g/lb (see the Appendix).

This method can be useful with a variety of conversion calculations.

Solution 5

TABLE 1-1. A check on the weight (mass) and volume labels in a grocery store

Label information	Calculated conversion value	Note
A can of tomatoes	794 g or 28 oz = 28 oz(28.35 g/oz) = 793.8 g = 794 g	Yes
Tomato paste	170 g or 6 oz = 6 oz(28.35 g/oz) = 170.1 g = 170 g	Yes
Catsup	907 g or 32 oz = 32 oz(28.35 g/oz) = 907.2 g = 907 g	Yes
Peanut butter	454 g or 16 oz = 16 oz(28.35 g/oz) = 453.6 g = 454 g	Yes
Salt	737 g or 26 oz = 26 oz(28.35 g/oz) = 737.1 g	Yes
Parsley	70.9 g or 2.5 oz = 2.5 oz(28.35 g/oz) = 70.88 g = 70.9 g	Yes
Oregano	28.4 g or 1 oz = 1 oz(28.35 g/oz) = 28.35 g = 28.4 g	Yes
Olive oil	16 fl oz = 16 fl oz(gal/128 fl oz)(3.785 l/gal) = 0.473 l	Yes
White vinegar	32 fl oz = 32 fl oz(gal/128 fl oz) × (3.785 l/gal) = 0.946 l	Yes
Wine vinegar	32 fl oz = 32 fl oz(gal/128 fl oz) × (3.785 l/gal) = 0.946 l	Yes

Note: The entry in this column indicates if the label entry is correct.

5. SIGNIFICANT FIGURES

The following is an elementary review of some workable rules and procedures to manage significant figures. This section is a review only and does
not replace the rigorous treatment of this topic contained in a text on the
theory of measurements. It is based on Schaum's *Outline Series on College
Chemistry* (1958). (Note: The student must not confuse significant figures
with the ten to sixteen decimal places that appear on the display of scientific
and engineering calculators.)

A measurement of "4 centimeters" suggests 4 ± 1 centimeters. It does not
suggest 4.0, 4.00, 4.000, or 4.0000 centimeters or greater precision. Measurement is never exact; it is an approximate representation of the true
value. The numerical value of every observed measurement is an approximation. Physical measurements of mass, length, time, volume, and velocity
are not without variability or bias. In statistics, bias is a systematic error
inherent in a method or caused by some feature of the measurement
system. The degree of bias of any measurement is limited by the reliability
of the measuring instrument, which is never totally unbiased. Calibration of
an air sampling device reduces some of the bias in the technique. Laboratory quality control and quality assurance program analysts work diligently
to minimize bias in their analytical determinations. Even with all this
effort, bias is normal and expected in measurement.

Let the volume of air collected by an air sampler be 12.4 liters. By
convention, this means the volume was measured to the nearest tenth
of a liter, and its exact value lies between 12.3 and 12.5 liters. If the
volume measurement were exact to the nearest hundredth of a liter, the
industrial hygienist would record it as 12.40 liters. The value 12.4 liters
represents three significant figures $(1, 2, 4)$, whereas the value 12.40
represents four significant figures $(1, 2, 4, 0)$. A significant figure is one
that is reasonably correct and guarantees the certainty of the preceding
figures.

In the laboratory determination of nuisance dust, a membrane filter is
weighed on an analytical microbalance. A recorded mass of 5.3059 mg
means that the filter mass loading was determined to the nearest tenth of a
microgram. This mass represents five significant figures $(5, 3, 0, 5, 9)$. The
last digit (9), being reasonably correct, guarantees the certainty of the mass
loading to the first four digits (5.306 mg).

A soap bubble flow meter, fabricated from a 50 ml burette, has markings
0.1 ml apart, and the hundredths of a milliliter are estimated. A measured
volume of 31.43 ml represents four significant figures. The last figure (3) is
an estimate, and may be in error by one or two digits in either direction (± 1
or 2). The preceding three figures $(3, 1, 4)$ are completely certain. In industrial hygiene and air pollution measurements and in the elementary measurements of chemistry and physics, the last figure is estimated and is
considered as a significant figure.

Zeros

A recorded volume of 54 ml represents two significant figures (5, 4). If this volume were written as 0.054 liter, it still would contain only two significant figures. Zeros appearing as the first figures of a number are not significant figures, as they merely locate the decimal point. The values 0.0540 liter and 0.540 liter represent three significant figures (5, 4, and the last zero); the value 1.054 liters represents four significant figures (1, 0, 5, 4); and the value 1.0540 liters represent five significant figures (1, 0, 5, 4, 0). Similarly, the value 207.21 for the atomic weight of lead contains five significant figures.

The mass of an impurity collected on an air sampling filter is measured as 1100 mg. This implies 1100 ± 1 (1099 mg to 1101 mg). The last two zeros may have been used to locate the decimal point and do not indicate unequivocally the accuracy of the weighing. Weighed to the nearest hundred milligrams, the weight contains only two significant figures and may be written exponentially as 1.1×10^3 mg. Weighed to the nearest ten milligrams, it may be written as 1.10×10^3 mg, which indicates that the value is accurate to three significant figures. Because the zero is not needed to locate the decimal point, it must be a significant figure. If the object were weighed to the nearest milligram, the mass could be written as 1.100×10^3 mg (four figures, 1, 1, 0, 0, are all significant figures). Similarly, the statement that the velocity of light is 186,000 miles per second is accurate to three significant figures, as this value is accurate only to the nearest thousand miles per second; to avoid confusion, it may be written as 1.86×10^5 mi/sec. It is customary to place the decimal point after the first significant figure.

Rounding Off

A number is rounded off to the desired number of significant figures by dropping one or more digits on the right side of the number. When the first digit dropped is less than 5, the last digit retained should remain unchanged; when it is more than 5, 1 is added to the last digit retained. When it is exactly 5, 1 is added to the last digit retained if that digit is odd; otherwise it is dropped. Thus successive approximations to 3.14159 are 3.1416, 3.142, 3.14, 3.1, and 3. The following mass readings are rounded off to demonstrate the principles:

Mass reading	Rounded value
51.35	51.4
51.45	51.4
51.55	51.6
51.65	51.6
51.75	51.8
51.85	51.8
51.95	52.0

To avoid producing errors during multiple steps in a calculation (propagating errors), do not round off the intermediate solutions. When the calculation is complete, then the final answer can be rounded to the appropriate number of significant digits.

Addition and Subtraction

To avoid the propagation of round-off errors, the final answer should be rounded off after addition or subtraction, to retain only those digits in the least significant number. (Remember that the last significant figure is an estimate.)

Examples: Add the following quantities expressed in grams:

	(1)	(2)	(3)	(4)
	25.340	58.0	4.20	415.5
	5.465	0.0038	1.6523	3.64
	0.322	0.00001	0.015	0.238
	31.127 g	58.00381 g	5.8673 g	419.378 g

Answers:

= 31.1 g	= 58.0 g	= 5.9 g	= 419.4 g

Multiplication and Division

The answer should be rounded off to contain only as many significant figures as are contained in the least exact factor. For example, when multiplying $7.485 \times 8.61 = 64.4$, or when dividing $0.1342 \div 1.52 = 0.0883$, the answers are correct to three significant figures because the least exact factor has only three significant figures.

Consider the division $9.84 \div 9.3 = 1.06$, to three places. By the rule given above, the answer should be 1.1 (two significant figures). However, a difference of 1 in the last place of 9.3 (9.3 ± 0.1) results in an error of about 1%, whereas a difference of 1 in the last place of 1.1 (1.1 ± 0.1) yields as error of roughly 10%. Thus the answer 1.1 is of a much lower percentage accuracy than 9.3. The answer should be 1.06 because a difference of 1 in the last place of the least exact factor used in the calculation (9.3) yields a percent error about the same (1%) as a difference of 1 in the last place of 1.06 (1.06 ± 0.01). Similarly, $0.92 \times 1.13 = 1.04$. The rule for multiplication and division is this: A product of quotients shall contain no more significant digits than contained in the number with the *fewest* significant digits.

The 1958 edition of Schaum's *Outline Series on College Chemistry* gave some advice that most neophytes to the field of industrial hygiene would do well to remember:

In nearly all academic and commercial calculations, a precision of only two to four significant figures is required. Therefore, the student is advised to use an inexpensive 10-inch slide rule that is accurate to three significant figures, or the table of logarithms in the Appendix, which is accurate to four significant figures. The efficient use of a slide rule or log table will save very much time in calculations without sacrificing accuracy.

When using a scientific calculator with ten to sixteen decimal-place displays (*not* ten to sixteen significant digits), keep the above paragraph in mind. While no one uses slide rules any more, the guidance from 1958 still applies.

6. GEOMETRY REVIEW

This review is merely a tabulation of relevant equations used to calculate areas and volumes for several geometric shapes that may be found in industrial hygiene calculations. It is *not* intended to educate the reader about the subject of geometry. To learn geometry or to review the subject in depth, the reader must refer to a standard textbook on the subject.

Circumference of a circle	$C = \pi d = 2\pi r$
Perimeter of a square with side a	$P = 4a$
Perimeter of a rectangle with sides a and b	$P = 2a + 2b$
Perimeter of a triangle with sides a, b, and c	$P = a + b + c$
Area A of a circle with radius r ($d = 2r$)	$A = \pi d^2/4 = \pi r^2$
Area of a duct in square feet when d is in inches	$A = 0.005454 d^2$
Area A of a triangle with base b and height h	$A = 0.5bh$
Area A of a square with sides a	$A = a^2$
Area A of a rectangle with sides a and b	$A = ab$
Area A of an ellipse with major axis a and minor axis b	$A = \pi ab$
Area A of a trapezoid with parallel sides a and b and height h	$A = 0.5(a + b)h$
Area A of a duct in square feet when d is in inches	$A = \pi d^2/576$ $= 0.005454 d^2$
Volume V of a sphere with a radius r ($d = 2r$)	$V = 1.33\pi r^3$ $= 0.1667\pi d^3$
Volume V of a cube with sides a	$V = a^3$
Volume V of a rectangular solid (sides a and b and height c)	$V = abc$
Volume V of a cylinder with a radius r and height H	$V = \pi r^2 h$ $= \pi d^2 h/4$
Volume V of a pyramid	$V = 0.33$ (base area)(height)

BIBLIOGRAPHY

This chapter was inspired by several classic works in elementary calculation techniques. A comprehensive review of elementary mathematics is that of Warren K. Eglof, Ph.D., Head of the Department of Chemistry, Niagara University, Niagara, NY.

An invaluable source is Schaum, D., Beckman, C. D., and Rosenberg, J. L., *Theory and Problems of College Chemistry*, Fourth Edition, Schaum Publishing Company, New York (1958).

PROBLEM SET

Problem 1

Convert 10 ounces dry weight per 1000 cubic feet to milligrams per liter.

Solution 1

Given 10 oz per 1000 ft^3, convert this to mg/l.

$$\left(\frac{10 \text{ oz}}{1000 \text{ ft}^3}\right) = \frac{\left(\dfrac{10 \text{ oz}}{1000 \text{ ft}^3}\right)\left(\dfrac{28.35 \text{ g}}{\text{oz}}\right)\left(\dfrac{1000 \text{ mg}}{\text{g}}\right)}{\left(\dfrac{\text{ft}^3}{28.317\,\text{l}}\right)}$$

$$= 10 \text{ mg/l}$$

$$\left(10 \text{ oz}/1000 \text{ ft}^3\right) = 10 \text{ mg/l}$$

Problem 2

You have just completed a trip in your car. Just as you left home you filled up the fuel tank with the car on level ground. You could see the fuel level in the fuel tank's neck when it was full. When you returned from your trip of 465 miles, you refilled the tank, at the same gas pump that you used earlier. It took 18.2 gallons of fuel to refill the tank to its pretrip level. What was your fuel economy for this trip in miles per gallon and kilometers per liter?

Solution 2

465 miles/18.2 gal = 25.5 mpg

$$(25.5 \text{ mpg})\left(\frac{5280 \text{ ft}}{\text{mile}}\right)\left(\frac{12 \text{ in}}{\text{ft}}\right)\left(\frac{2.54 \text{ cm}}{\text{in}}\right)\left(\frac{\text{m}}{100 \text{ cm}}\right)\left(\frac{\text{km}}{1000 \text{ m}}\right)\left(\frac{\text{gal}}{3.785\,\text{l}}\right)$$

$$25.5 \text{ mpg} = 10.8 \text{ km/l}$$

Problem 3

The tomb of King Khufu (known as King Cheops by the Greeks) is called the Great Pyramid and is located at Giza on the Nile River outside Cairo, Egypt. The Great Pyramid was built about 2600 to 2500 B.C., with more than two million limestone blocks that each weighed about 2.3 metric tons. The Great Pyramid originally had the following dimensions:

$$\text{base side} = B = 440.046 \text{ cubits}; \text{ height} = H = 280.000 \text{ cubits}$$

If one cubit equals 52.35 centimeters, calculate the base and the height in meters and feet. Next, determine the ratio [2(base)/height] and wonder at the result. John Tailor, an Egyptologist in the mid-1800s, said it was extraterrestrial magic!

Solution 3

In meters:

$$B = (440.046 \text{ cubits})(52.35 \text{ cm/cubit})(1 \text{ meter}/100 \text{ cm}) = 230.364 \text{ meters}$$

$$H = (280 \text{ cubits})(52.35 \text{ cubits/cm})(1 \text{ meter}/100 \text{ cm}) = 146.58 \text{ meters}$$

In feet: $B = (23{,}036.4 \text{ cm})(1 \text{ in}/2.54 \text{ cm})(1 \text{ ft}/12 \text{ in}) = 755.8 \text{ ft}$

$H = (14{,}658.0 \text{ cm})(1 \text{ in}/2.54 \text{ cm})(1 \text{ ft}/12 \text{ in}) = 480.9 \text{ ft}$

Determine the ratio $A = 2B/H$:

$$2B/H = 2(440.046 \text{ cubits})/(280 \text{ cubits}) = 3.14!$$

Was this extraterrestrial magic or divine intervention, or did they scoop the Greeks by 2000 years? The Greeks are credited to have "discovered" the 3.14 relationship 2000 years after the pyramid was built.

Problem 4

If a loaf of bread costs 1400 lire in Italy, what is the equivalent cost in American money?

$$1 \text{ dollar} = 1120 \text{ lire} = \pounds 1120$$

Solution 4

$$(1400 \text{ lire}/1 \text{ loaf})(\text{US } \$1.00/\pounds 1120) = \$1.25/\text{loaf}$$

Problem 5

You are on a sightseeing tour of the Niagara Frontier and decide to cross over the Rainbow Bridge into Canada. Gasoline is sold in Niagara Falls, New York, for an average price of 95 cents per gallon. At the Canadian Falls gasoline sells for CAN $2.30 per imperial gallon. Should we fill up the tank before we cross over the border into Canada?

Solution 5

Assume: US $1.00 = CAN $1.25

1 Imperial gallon = 5 quarts (U.S.)

$$\text{CAN } \$2.38/\text{Imp gal} = \left(\frac{\text{CAN } \$2.38}{\text{Imp gal}}\right)\left(\frac{\text{US } \$1.00}{\text{CAN } \$1.25}\right)\left(\frac{\text{Imp gal}}{5 \text{ qt}}\right)\left(\frac{4 \text{ qt}}{\text{gal}}\right)$$

CAN $2.38/Imp gal = US $1.52/gal

Fill up on the American side.

Problem 6

The star Alpha Centaurus is 2.5 light years from the earth.

   A. What is the distance to Alpha Centaurus in miles?
   B. How many seconds does it take for the light to travel this distance?

Solution 6

A. What is the distance to Alpha Centaurus in miles?

Distance = Rate × Time

$$\text{Distance} = \left(\frac{186{,}283 \text{ miles}}{\text{sec}}\right)\left(\frac{60 \text{ sec}}{\text{min}}\right)\left(\frac{60 \text{ min}}{\text{hr}}\right)\left(\frac{24 \text{ hr}}{\text{day}}\right)\left(\frac{365.25 \text{ days}}{\text{yr}}\right)(2.5 \text{ yr})$$

Distance = 1.47×10^{13} miles

B. A light year is the distance that light travels in one year.

$$(2.5 \text{ light years}) = (2.5 \text{ lyr})\left(\frac{1 \text{ yr}}{1 \text{ lyr}}\right)\left(\frac{365.25 \text{ days}}{\text{yr}}\right)\left(\frac{24 \text{ hr}}{\text{day}}\right)\left(\frac{60 \text{ min}}{\text{hr}}\right)\left(\frac{60 \text{ sec}}{\text{min}}\right)$$

$$(2.5 \text{ light years}) = 78.9 \times 10^6 \text{ sec}$$

Problem 7

Given the information in Problem 6, and that the speed of light is 2.99730×10^8 meters per second (m/s), calculate the distance (in km) of the earth to the star.

Solution 7

$$(78.9 \times 10^6 \text{ s})(2.99730 \times 10^8 \text{ m/s}) = 2.4 \times 10^{16} \text{ km}$$

Problem 8

A cyclist decides to ride a bike across the United States, covering a distance of 5400 km. The average speed for an 8-hour day turns out to be 6.8 miles/hr. If the cyclist only has June and July to cover the distance, is there enough time?

Solution 8

1. (6.8 miles/1 hr)(8 hr/day) = 54.4 miles/day
2. (5400 km/trip)(1 mile/1.609 km) = 3356 miles
3. (3356 miles)/(54.4 miles/day) = 61.9 days = 62 days

There are only 61 days in June and July. The cyclist will have to pedal faster or go downhill all the way!

Problem 9

Sal's Pizzeria ordered one dozen 23 cm pizza pans but received one dozen 26 cm pizza pans. Sal was concerned that he could not use the larger pans because of the incremental cost to produce the larger pizza. Sal sells a large plain 16 inch pizza for $7.65. What price should Sal ask for the 23 cm and the 26 cm pizzas?

Solution 9

Area of the 23 cm (9.1 in) pan:

$$A = \pi D^2/4 = \left[\pi (23 \text{ cm})^2/4 \right] = 415.5 \text{ cm}^2 \text{ or}$$

$$A = \pi D^2/4 = \left[\pi (23 \text{ cm})^2/4 \right] \left[\text{in}^2/(2.54 \text{ cm})^2 \right] = 64.4 \text{ in}^2$$

Area of the 26 cm (10.2 in) pan:

$$A = \pi D^2/4 = \left[\pi (26 \text{ cm})^2/4 \right] = 530.9 \text{ cm}^2$$

$$A = \pi D^2/4 = \left[\pi (26 \text{ cm})^2/4 \right] \left[\text{in}^2/(2.54 \text{ cm})^2 \right] = 82.3 \text{ in}^2$$

Area of the 16 inch (40.6 cm) pizza

$$A = \pi D^2/4 = \pi(16 \text{ in})^2/4 = 201 \text{ in}^2$$

Sal sells a 16 inch diameter (201 in^2) pizza for \$7.65 or:

$$\$7.65/201 \text{ in}^2 = \$0.038/\text{in}^2$$

Comparing the two pans:

$$(\$0.038/\text{in}^2)(64.4 \text{ in}^2) = \$2.45$$

$$(\$0.038/\text{in}^2)(82.3 \text{ in}^2) = \$3.13$$

In his entrepreneurial spirit, Sal will exchange the 26 cm pan for the 23 cm pans and charge \$3.85 per pizza! This problem demonstrates that whether it is pizza pans or 25 mm versus 35 mm membrane filters for sampling asbestos or other aerosols, the problems are the same. (See Problem 10.)

Problem 10

The National Institute for Occupational Safety and Health recommended a modified air sampling method for asbestos. The filter size recommended in the new method (NIOSH #7400) is 25 mm. Previously a 35 mm filter was used (PC&AM 239). What is the percent change in filter areas?

Solution 10

Area of the 25 mm filter (NEW):

$$A = \pi D^2/4 = \left[\pi(25 \text{ cm})^2/4\right] = 490.074 \text{ mm}^2$$

Area of the 35 mm filter (OLD):

$$A = \pi D^2/4 = \left[\pi(35 \text{ cm})^2/4\right] = 962.113 \text{ mm}^2$$

Percent change:

$$\% \text{ change} = \{[\text{AREA}_{\text{NEW}} - \text{AREA}_{\text{OLD}}]/[\text{AREA}_{\text{OLD}}]\}100$$

$$\% \text{ change} = \{[490.074 \text{ mm}^2 - 962.074 \text{ mm}^2]/[962.113 \text{ mm}^2]\}100$$

$$\% \text{ change} = -49.1\%$$

Problem 11

A man gets into a tub (totally submerged) and displaces 0.25 m^3 of water. If 1 liter of displaced water is equivalent to 0.75 human pound, how much does the man weigh in grams?

Solution 11

Given: 28.32 l/ft^3
  2.54 cm/in
  453.59 g/lb
  1 m^3 = 1000 l

$$0.25 \text{ m}^3 = (0.25 \text{ m}^3)(1000 \text{ l/m}^3)(0.75 \text{ human lb/1 l})(453.59 \text{ g/lb})$$

$$= 85{,}048 \text{ g}$$

Problem 12

How many air filtration devices operating at 33.3 ft^3/sec each would be required to completely change the air in a room 10 m long by 20 m wide by 5 m high at least four times per hour? Assume uniform flow and sufficient makeup air.

Solution 12

(1) Convert dimensions from meters to feet:

$$(10 \text{ m})(100 \text{ cm/1 m})(1 \text{ in/2.54 cm})(12 \text{ in/ft}) = 32.8 \text{ ft}$$

$$(20 \text{ m})(100 \text{ cm/1 m})(1 \text{ in/2.54 cm})(12 \text{ in/ft}) = 65.6 \text{ ft}$$

$$(5 \text{ m})(100 \text{ cm/1 m})(1 \text{ in/2.54 cm})(12 \text{ in/ft}) = 16.4 \text{ ft}$$

(2) Calculate volume of room (air) in ft^3:

$$32.8 \text{ ft} \times 65.6 \text{ ft} \times 16.4 \text{ ft} = 35{,}297 \text{ ft}^3$$

(3) Correct flow of device from ft^3/sec to ft^3/min:

$$(33.3 \text{ ft}^3/\text{sec})(60 \text{ sec/1 min}) = 1998 \text{ ft}^3/\text{min}$$

(4) 4 air changes/hour = 1 air change/15 min
    Calculate volume of air one device can handle in 15 min:

$$(1998 \text{ ft}^3/\text{min})(15 \text{ min}) = 29{,}970 \text{ ft}^3$$

(5) Calculate minimum number of devices required:

$$(35{,}297 \text{ ft}^3/30{,}000 \text{ ft}^3) = 1.2 \text{ devices} \equiv 2 \text{ devices minimum}$$

Problem 13

On Sunday, December 17, 1989, *Parade* magazine ran an "Ask Marilyn" question from Max Travis, Nyack, New York:

> Some time ago, a very large section of an iceberg near New Zealand broke off. It was 26 miles long, 4 miles wide and a mile deep. How many one inch ice cubes would that ice make?

Marilyn Vos Savant, one of the "most intelligent people in the world," gave the following response:

> The figure is really stunning. A chunk of ice this size could be cut into 26,453,238,349,824,000 one inch cubes. And if you were to put six cubes in each glass, it would fill 4,408,873,058,304,000 glasses—enough for nearly 900,000 glasses of lemonade for every person on earth!

Was Marilyn Vos Savant correct? What was the world's population on December 17, 1989?

Problem 14

A home owner has a coal bin that measures 40 inches high by 48 inches wide by 40 inches deep. Can the home owner order 2 tons of coal and be assured that it will all fit in the coal bin?

Solution 14

density of anthracite coal = 2.6 g/cm^3

density = mass/per unit volume; $\rho = m/V$; $V = m/\rho$

$$V = (2 \text{ tons})\left(\frac{2000 \text{ lb}}{\text{ton}}\right)\left(\frac{\text{kg}}{2.2 \text{ lb}}\right)\left(\frac{1000 \text{ g}}{\text{kg}}\right)\left(\frac{\text{cm}^3}{2.6 \text{ g}}\right)\left[\frac{(\text{in})^3}{(2.54 \text{ cm})^3}\right]$$

$$= 42{,}674 \text{ in}^3$$

Two tons of coal ($\rho = 2.6$ g/cm^3) would occupy 42,674 cubic inches. This assumes that the coal is packed without void spaces. Obviously, the packing fraction depends on the size of the pieces of coal. Assume that the packing fraction is 0.56. The volume of the coal bin is:

$$V(\text{Bin}) = L \times W \times H = (40 \text{ in})(40 \text{ in})(48 \text{ in}) = 76,800 \text{ in}^3$$

As long as the packing fraction is less than 0.61, then the actual volume of the 2 tons of coal is:

$$\text{Actual volume} = \text{Calculated volume/Packing fraction}$$

$$= 46,6746 \text{ in}^3/0.61 = 76,515 \text{ in}^3$$

The 2 tons of coal will fit into the 40 inch by 40 inch by 48 inch coal bin if the packing fraction is 0.61 or larger.

Problem 15

This is a "back of the envelope" calculation related to wood burning and air quality. The average stove owner burns three cords of wood during the heating season. There are about 1000 stoves in use in the region. A standard cord of wood, when stacked neatly, measures 4 feet high, 4 feet wide, and 8 feet long, and 37% of this volume is void. Hard wood that is aged for six months in a dry enclosure retains a 20% moisture content and weighs 26 pounds per cubic foot. Calculate the total weight of wood burned in the region in kilograms and pounds.

Solution 15

$$\left(\frac{3 \text{ cords}}{\text{stove}}\right)\left(\frac{1000 \text{ stoves}}{\text{region}}\right)\left(\frac{4 \times 4 \times 8 \text{ ft}^3}{\text{cord}}\right)\left(\frac{0.63}{\text{actual volume}}\right)\left(\frac{0.8}{\text{dry weight}}\right)\left(\frac{26 \text{ lb}}{\text{ft}^3}\right)\left(\frac{\text{kg}}{2.2 \text{ lb}}\right)$$

$$= 2.29 \times 10^6 \text{ kg}$$

2.29×10^6 kg of wood is burned during each heating season.

5.03×10^6 pounds of wood is burned during each heating season.

Problem 16

In the April 1991 issue of *Super Ford* magazine, Frank Bohanan, Jr. of Professional Flow Technologies of Madison Heights, Illinois, presented data on the performance of the Pro-M^R mass air sensor versus a stock Ford mass air sensor. At 650 cfm the Ford OEM mass flow sensor had a pressure drop of 48 inches of water, and the Pro-M^R had a pressure drop of 7 inches of water. Bohanan reported a mass air flowrate of 1380 kg/hr at 650 cfm. What air density (in the English system) did Bohanan assume?

Solution 16

density $= \rho = m/v$

$m = 1380 \text{ kg/hr}$

$v = 650 \text{ ft}^3/\text{min}$

$\rho = \left[(1380 \text{ kg/hr})(1 \text{ hr}/60 \text{ min})(2.204 \text{ lb/kg})\right]/(650 \text{ ft}^3/\text{min})$

$\quad = 0.078 \text{ lb/ft}^3$

2

The SI System of Units

Outcome Competencies   *After studying this chapter you will be able to:*

- *Explain the SI system of units.*
- *List the SI base units.*
- *List the SI supplementary units.*
- *Compute SI derived units.*
- *Justify the rules for using the SI system.*
- *Validate the exceptions for the SI system's rules.*

1. PURPOSE

For people in technical societies to communicate and interact, they must be able to understand each other's standards. This includes such esoteric issues as social order and procedural activities in business meetings. To communicate in the critical areas of commerce, it is imperative that people understand the systems of weights and measures. To facilitate commercial activity, the Romans maintained a "keeper of measurement." This person would measure the volume of wine that was placed into a wine carafe and place a lead seal through a loop that the glass blower placed at that section of the carafe that just contained one liter. The seal certified the glass blower's one liter mark.

Societies have moved a long way from the Roman "system" to an internationally recognized system of weights, measures, units, and symbols.

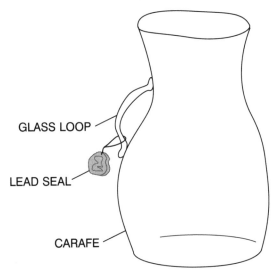

GLASS LOOP

LEAD SEAL

CARAFE

Figure 2-1. A classic wine carafe (not to scale) (Glenora Wine Cellars, Dundee, NY).

Le Systeme International d'Unites (SI system) was established to simplify the myriad of units currently in use throughout the world. Many students of science and engineering in the United States are familiar with the cgs, mks, and English system. The SI system is used in this text.

2. THE INTERNATIONAL SYSTEM OF UNITS

The SI system divides units into three categories: base units, supplementary units, and derived units, which are outlined in Tables 2-1 through 2-3.

The base units consist of seven well-defined and dimensionally independent quantities: length, mass, time, electric current, thermodynamic temperature, amount of a substance, and luminous intensity. The symbols and units for these quantities are listed in Table 2-1. The base units are considered the foundation of the SI system.

Supplementary units may be regarded as either base or derived units. They are listed in Table 2-2.

Derived units, listed in Table 2-3, arise from the fundamental laws and definitions of physics.

The choice of the symbol used to represent a unit is quite simple. If the unit is named after a person, to honor past research efforts, then it is capitalized (e.g., temperature, Kelvin; current, Ampere; etc.); otherwise a lowercase letter is used (e.g., meter, m; kilogram, kg). Punctuation is *never* used with a units symbol.

TABLE 2-1. The SI system: base units

Quantity	Unit	Symbol
Length	metre (U.S. meter)	m
Mass	kilogram	kg
Time	second	s
Electric current	Ampere	A
Thermodynamic temperature	Kelvin	K
Amount of substance	mole	mol
Luminous intensity	candela	cd

TABLE 2-2. The SI system: supplementary units

Quantity	Unit	Symbol
Plane angle	radian	rad
Solid angle	steradian	sr

These may be regarded as either base or derived units.

TABLE 2-3. The SI system: derived units

Quantity	Unit	Symbol	Formula
Frequency (of a periodic phenomenon)	Hertz	Hz	$1/s$
Force	Newton	N	$kg\,m/s^2$
Pressure, stress	Pascal	Pa	N/m^2
Energy, work, quantity of heat	Joule	J	Nm
Power, radiant flux	Watt	W	J/s
Quantity of electricity, electric charge	Coulomb	C	As
Electric potential, potential diff. emf	Volt	V	W/A
Capacitance	Farad	F	C/V
Conductance	Siemans	Sx	A/V
Magnetic flux	Weber	Wb	Vs
Magnetic flux density	Tesla	T	Wb/m^2
Inductance	Henry	H	Wb/A
Luminous flux	Lumen	lm	cdsr
Illuminance	Lux	lx	lx/m^2
Activity (radionuclides)	Becquerel	Bq	$1/s$
Absorbed dose	Gray	Gy	J/kg

3. COMPUTING DERIVED SI UNITS

Fundamental units in the SI system are the seven base units (Table 2-1), which are explicitly defined by the SI system. The laws and definitions of physics, mechanics, thermodynamics, or electricity and magnetism explicitly define the derived units (Table 2-3). An example is Newton's law of force:

$$\text{Force} = \text{Mass} \times \text{Acceleration: } F = ma = kg(m/sec^2)$$

The unit of force is the Newton (N). One Newton $= 1 \text{ kg m/s}^2$.

TABLE 2-4. The SI system, additional derived units

Quantity	Definition	Unit	Symbol	Formula
Force	(mass)(acceleration)	Newton	N	$kg\,m/s^2$
Pressure	force per area	Pascal	Pa	N/m^2
Energy	(force)(distance)	Joule	J	Nm
Density	mass per volume	kilogram per cubic meter	p	m/V
Area	(length)(length)	square meter	m^2	m^2
Volume	(length)(length)(length)	cubic meter	m^3	m^3
Velocity	distance per time	meter per second	v	m/s
Concentration	quantity per volume	mole per cubic meter	mol/m^3	mol/m^3

The symbol *mol* is used for kilogram mole; *mole* is used for gram mole.

Energy (E) or work (W) equals a force (F) moved through a distance (s). Energy is work, and the unit of work is given by the Joule (J).

$$\text{Energy} = \text{Force} \times \text{Distance: } E = W = Fs = kg(m/sec^2)(m) = Nm$$

$$1\,J = Nm = kgm^2/s^2$$

The pressure unit is named for Pascal (Pa). Pressure is equal to the force/unit area:

$$\text{Pressure} = \text{Force per area: } P = F/a = kg(m/sec^2)(m^2) = Nm^2$$

$$1\,Pa = 1\,N/m^2 = 1\,kg/s^2m$$

Additional derived SI units (Table 2-4) were approved at the General Conference on Weights and Measures (CGPM) (the French Conference Generale des Poids et Mesures) in 1975.

4. SOME GENERAL RULES ON USING THE SI SYSTEM

If a unit standard, or any standard, is to be generally applicable throughout the world, then all of the system's users must agree to follow a specific set

TABLE 2-5. Caveats on the use of the SI system of units

Do not use	Do use
micron	$1\,\mu m = 10^{-6}\,m$ (μm = micrometer)
millimicron	$1\,nm = 10^{-9}\,m$ (nm = nanometer)
Γ, mass	Γ (mass) = 1 μg
Λ, volume	Λ (volume) = 1 μl
standard atmosphere	mm Hg
centigrade	Celsius

of rules. These rules are included in the standard and eliminate ambiguous interpretation and poor past practices.

a. The following spelling of units will be allowed in the United States: e.g., meter for metre and liter for litre.

b. Periods are never used after a unit: e.g., g *not* g.; m *not* m.

c. Plurals are never used: e.g., 5.0 g *not* 5.0 gms or 5.0 gs.

d. The volume standard in the SI system is the cubic meter, m^3.

e. Liter is approved for one thousandth of a cubic meter and is restricted to the measure of gases and liquids, and no prefix other than milli or micro should be used, e.g., microliter is 10^{-6} l. Clinical laboratories use cl for a centiliter (10 ml) and dl for a deciliter (100 ml).

f. In volumes and areas, hecto, deka, deci, and centi are acceptable: i.e., square hectometers, cubic centimeters.

g. The SI unit for mass is the kilogram, kg.

h. With large masses it is acceptable to use Mg (megagram).

i. Metric ton = 1000 kg (used in commerce).

j. Use only one prefix in compound units: i.e., kJ/g *not* kJ/kg.

k. Omit the degree sign for the Kelvin scale, e.g., 50 K *not* 50°K.

l. Time is always in seconds (s), but can be changed to conform to real life: i.e., calendar years, minutes, hours, and days.

m. Group digits in threes about a decimal point or decimal comma: i.e., 129 346 723 *not* 129,346,723.

n. Numbers should fall between 0.1 and 1 000. For example:

vehicle velocity = 60 kilometers/hour, not 6 000 meters/hour

vehicle velocity = 60 km/h not 6 000 m/h

Table 2-5 lists warnings on the use of units that do not comply with the SI system. These units have resulted from the careless application of the cgs and mks systems. They are in essence a jargon that is usually understood by a small group of scientists within a discipline. With the adoption of the SI system, these units are no longer permitted to be used. This prohibition may appear to be rather drastic but it is the only way to bring order and sanity to the world of units.

5. EXCEPTIONS IN THE SI SYSTEM

There are some exceptions allowed in the SI system to accommodate many different interest groups. The American Chemical Society's *Journal of Analytical Chemistry* (January 1982) provided the list that appears as Table 2-6.

TABLE 2-6. Exceptions in the SI system

Quantity	Unit
Area	barn, 10^{-28} m^2
Concentration	molal = mole per kilogram
	m = mol/kg
	molar = mole per liter
	M = mole/l; not formal or normal
Conductance	mho, 1/Ohm
Density	gram per cubic centimeter, g/cm^3
Energy	electronvolt (eV); also keV, MeV
Length	angstrom (Å); 1×10^{-10} m/A
Plane angle	degree (°), minute ('), second ('')
Pressure	atmosphere (atm), mm Hg, bar
Radioactivity of radionuclides	disintegrations per second (dps)
Temperature	degree Celsius, °C, degree Kelvin, K
Time	minute (min), hour (h), day (d)
Volume	liter (l), milliliter (ml), microliter (μl)
Wavenumber	1 per centimeter (cm^{-1})
Kelvin	T = thermodynamic temperature
Absolute zero	$T° = -273.15°C$ (definition) = 0 K

American Chemical Society, *Journal of Analytical Chemistry* 54(1):157 (January 1982).

TABLE 2-7. SI system of multiplication factors: prefixes and suffixes

Multiplication factor	Prefix	Symbol
10^{18}	exa	E
10^{15}	peta	P
10^{12}	tera	T
10^{9}	giga	G
10^{6}	mega	M
10^{3}	kilo	k
10^{2}	hecto	h
10^{1}	deka	da
10^{-1}	deci	d
10^{-2}	centi	c
10^{-3}	milli	m
10^{-6}	micro	μ
10^{-9}	nano	n
10^{-12}	pico	p
10^{-15}	femto	f
10^{-18}	atto	a

Source: *Metric Practice Guide*, Vol. 14.02, ASTM, Philadelphia, PA.

6. PREFIXES AND SUFFIXES

The SI system also provides for the use of a standard set of prefixes and suffixes as presented in Table 2-7.

An example of the use of these multiplication factors is as follows:

$$12,300 \text{ mm} = 12.3 \text{ m}$$

$$12.3 \times 10^3 \text{ m} = 12.3 \text{ km}$$

7. CONCENTRATION

Mass concentration is given in units of mass per unit volume, for example, milligrams per cubic meter (mg/m^3) and micrograms per cubic meter ($\mu g/m^3$). This unit implies the mass of an impurity (gases, vapors, or particles) in the total volume of air. By definition:

$$1 \text{ ng/m}^3 = 10^{-9} \text{ kg (gas)/m}^3 \text{ (mixture)}$$

Volume concentration is given by ppm, parts of a pure gas in a million parts of the mixture. By definition:

$$1 \text{ ppm} = \left[10^{-6} \text{ m}^3 \text{ (gas)/m}^3 \text{ (mixture)} \right]$$

$$1 \text{ ppb} = \left[10^{-9} \text{ m}^3 \text{ (gas)/m}^3 \text{ (mixture)} \right]$$

$$1 \text{ ppt} = \left[10^{-12} \text{ m}^3 \text{ (gas)/m}^3 \text{ (mixture)} \right]$$

Chapter 5 covers this in much greater detail; if you do not understand this concept now, you will later.

Some Interesting Notes on Units

- The Japanese flute is called the Shocku Hatche. A hatche is 8/10 of a shocku, which is a unit of measure in Japanese and is equal to 22 inches. Therefore, Shocku Hatche music is played on a flute that is = 8/10 shocku in length, about 18 inches long.
- The science of analytical chemistry has advanced to the point where measurements as small as 10^{-15} gram (a femtogram) can be measured ("1 part per ???").

8. TEMPERATURE

Temperature is presented in more detail in Chapter 3; it is introduced in Table 2-8 for purposes of definition only.

TABLE 2-8. Temperature scales

Reference point	Fahrenheit scale (°F)	Celsius scale (°C)	Absolute Temperature	
			Kelvin scale (K)	Rankine scale (R)
Boiling point of water	212	100	373.15	671.67
Melting point or freezing point of water	32	0	273.15	491.67
(Absolute zero)	−459.67	−273.15	0	0

deg C = (deg F − 32)/1.8;   9 C = 5 F − 160
K = °C + 273.15;   R = °F + 459.67.

TABLE 2-9. Units commonly encountered in environmental health

Quantity	English	cgs	SI
Mass	slug	gram (g)	kilogram (kg)
Length	foot (ft)	centimeter (cm)	meter (m)
Time	second (sec)	second (s)	second (s)
Force	pounds (lb_M)	dyne (dyne)	Newton (N)
Pressure	lb_F/ft^2	$dyne/cm^2$	N/m^2

9. SUMMARY

In summary, Table 2-9 presents a range of base units plus force and pressure commonly encountered in air pollution, industrial hygiene, and environmental health.

BIBLIOGRAPHY

1. American Society for Testing and Materials, *Metric Practice Guide*, D-22 Committee Book of ASTM Standards, Vol. 14.02, Industrial Water, Atmospheric Analysis. ASTM, Philadelphia, PA (annual issue).
2. American Chemical Society, *Journal of Analytical Chemistry* 54(1):157 (January 1982).

PROBLEM SET
Problem 1

If Rapunzel's hair grows at 125 nm/min, what will its lifetime length be (in feet), barring any visits to a snip-happy hair salon? Disregard leap years. Lifetime is taken as 70 years.

Solution 1

$$\left(\frac{125 \text{ nm}}{\text{min}}\right)\left(\frac{10^{-9} \text{ m}}{\text{nm}}\right)\left(\frac{100 \text{ cm}}{\text{m}}\right)\left(\frac{1 \text{ in}}{2.54 \text{ cm}}\right)\left(\frac{1 \text{ ft}}{12 \text{ in}}\right)\left(\frac{60 \text{ min}}{\text{hr}}\right)\left(\frac{24 \text{ hr}}{\text{d}}\right)\left(\frac{365 \text{ d}}{\text{yr}}\right)(70 \text{ yr})$$

$= 15.1$ ft in a lifetime

Problem 2

Knowing that long scarves are popular this fall, a woman commissions you to make one. If she pays you \$9.00/yd of scarf completed and 5×10^4 stitches are needed for the scarf to be fashionably "in," how much money will you be paid if 10 stitches equal one centimeter?

Solution 2

$$(5 \times 10^4 \text{ stitches})\left(\frac{1 \text{ cm}}{10 \text{ stitches}}\right)\left(\frac{1 \text{ in}}{2.54 \text{ cm}}\right)\left(\frac{1 \text{ ft}}{12 \text{ in}}\right)\left(\frac{1 \text{ yd}}{3 \text{ ft}}\right)\left(\frac{\$9.00}{\text{yd}}\right)$$

$= \$492.13$ (Better look for a blue-light special!)

Problem 3

A king-size filter cigarette contains 16 mg tar (FTC method). Calculate the cumulative daily and lifetime mass of tar received by a 160 pound young adult male who smokes one pack of 20 cigarettes per day. Assuming that the 320 mg tar/day contains 1 mg of carcinogen, calculate the total lifetime carcinogen mass in a 40 year smoking lifetime (dose is mg of chemical delivered per kg of body mass).

Solution 3

$$\left(\frac{16 \text{ mg tar}}{1 \text{ cig}}\right)\left(\frac{20 \text{ cig}}{\text{pack}}\right)\left(\frac{1 \text{ pack}}{\text{day}}\right)$$

$$= \frac{320 \text{ mg tar}}{\text{day}} = \frac{116\,800 \text{ mg tar}}{\text{year}}$$

$$\left(\frac{1 \text{ mg carcinogen}}{\text{day}}\right)\left(\frac{365 \text{ days}}{\text{year}}\right)(40 \text{ years})$$

$$= \frac{14\,600 \text{ mg carcinogen}}{\text{lifetime}}$$

$$\left(\frac{1 \text{ mg carcinogen}}{\text{day}}\right)\left(\frac{365 \text{ days}}{\text{year}}\right)(40 \text{ years})\left(\frac{\text{g}}{1000 \text{ mg}}\right)\left(\frac{\text{lb}}{454 \text{ g}}\right)\left(\frac{16 \text{ oz}}{\text{lb}}\right)$$

$$= \frac{0.5 \text{ oz carcinogen}}{\text{lifetime}}$$

Problem 4

In the Commonwealth of Massachusetts, a body of water is considered unsafe for swimming if it contains more than 10 *Escherichia coli* per milliliter of water. If 800 kilograms of waste containing an average of 1,800 *E. coli* per gram were released into a previously pristine pond containing 250,000 gallons of water, should the pond be considered unsafe for swimming?

Solution 4

Assume the released waste is uniformly distributed throughout the pond

$$E.\ coli/\text{ml} = \frac{800\ \text{kg}}{(250{,}000\ \text{gal}\ H_2O)\left(\dfrac{1{,}800\ E.\ coli}{g}\right)\left(\dfrac{1{,}000\ g}{\text{kg}}\right)\left(\dfrac{\text{gal}}{3.785\ l}\right)\left(\dfrac{1}{1{,}000\ \text{ml}}\right)}$$

$$= (1.44 \times 10^9\ E.\ coli/9.96 \times 10^8\ \text{ml}) = 1.5\ E.\ coli/\text{ml}$$

The pond is "safe" if the released waste is uniformly distributed throughout the pond.

Problem 5

Your laboratory was asked to collect water samples for pathogenic protozoa (e.g., *Giardia lamblia*), and *Standard Methods for Water and Waste Water* (American Public Health Association, Washington, D.C.) requires the use of a limiting orifice with a flow rate of 6.3×10^{-5} m^3/s with an orifice pressure drop of 100 to 130 kPa. The supplier of the orifice only sells the limiting orifice based on a flowrate in gallons per minute at standard atmospheric pressure.

> **a.** What is the flowrate of an orifice rated a 6.3×10^{-5} m^3/s in gallons per minute?
> **b.** What is the pressure change requirements of 100 to 130 kPa in pounds per square inch?
> **c.** Minimum sample volume is 380 l. What sampling time is needed to collect the minimum volume?

Solution 5

a. $\left(\dfrac{6.3 \times 10^{-5}\ \text{m}^3}{s}\right)\left(\dfrac{1000\ l}{\text{m}^3}\right)\left(\dfrac{1\ \text{gal}}{3.785\ l}\right)\left(\dfrac{60\ s}{\text{min}}\right) = 0.9986$ gpm (gallons per minute)

b. $(130\ \text{kPa})\left(\dfrac{760\ \text{mm Hg}}{1.013 \times 10^5\ \text{Pa}}\right)\left(\dfrac{1000\ \text{Pa}}{\text{kPa}}\right)\left(\dfrac{14.7\ \text{psi}}{760\ \text{mm Hg}}\right) = 18.9$ psi

c. $\left(\dfrac{1\ \text{gal}}{\text{min}}\right)\left(\dfrac{3.785\ l}{\text{gal}}\right)(X) = 380$ l; solving for the time, X, in minutes gives $X = 100.4$ min

Note: $(100 \text{ kPa})\left(\dfrac{760 \text{ mm Hg}}{1.013 \times 10^5 \text{ Pa}}\right)\left(\dfrac{1000 \text{ Pa}}{\text{kPa}}\right)\left(\dfrac{14.7 \text{ psi}}{760 \text{ mm Hg}}\right) = 14.5 \text{ psi}$

Problem 6

Convert 8.314×10^7 ergs/mole K to liter atmospheres/mole K.

Solution 6

Recall:
  1 Joule/10^7 ergs
  1 Joule/Nm
  $N = \text{kg m/s}^2$

8.314×10^7 ergs/mole K

$$= \left(\frac{8.314 \times 10^7 \text{ ergs}}{\text{mole K}}\right)\left(\frac{\text{Joule}}{10^7 \text{ ergs}}\right)\left(\frac{\text{Nm}}{\text{Joule}}\right)(\text{Pa/N/m}^2)\left(\frac{1 \text{ atm}}{1.013 \times 10^5 \text{ Pa}}\right)\left(\frac{10^3 \text{ l}}{\text{m}^3}\right)$$

8.314×10^7 ergs/mole K $= 0.08205$ l atm/mole K

Problem 7

A certain species of wood produces 22,000,000 BTU per cord when burned. In a particular timber tract, 10 cords of this species can be harvested per acre. How many kilocalories (kcal) are contained in a woodlot measuring 20 m by 20 m?

Solution 7

Assume: 43,560 ft^2/acre; 2.540 cm/in; 252 cal/BTU; 20 m $\times$ 20 m = 400 m^2

$$(400 \text{ m}^2)\left(\frac{100^2 \text{ cm}^2}{\text{m}^2}\right)\left(\frac{1 \text{ in}^2}{2.54^2 \text{ cm}^2}\right)\left(\frac{1 \text{ ft}^2}{12^2 \text{ in}^2}\right)\left(\frac{\text{acre}}{43,560 \text{ ft}^2}\right)\cdots$$

$$\cdots\left(\frac{10 \text{ cord}}{1 \text{ acre}}\right)\left(\frac{22,000,000 \text{ BTU}}{1 \text{ cord}}\right)\left(\frac{252 \text{ cal}}{\text{BTU}}\right)\left(\frac{1 \text{ kcal}}{1000 \text{ cal}}\right)$$

$$= 5,479,809 \text{ kcal}$$

5,479,809 kcal of wood heat energy are contained in this woodlot.

Problem 8

Dioxin is emitted from a mass burn incinerator at a rate of 10,000 ag/s (attograms per second). How many micrograms of dioxin are produced in 1 year of continuous, around-the-clock incinerator operation?

Solution 8

$$\left(\frac{10 \text{ ag}}{\text{s}}\right)\left(\frac{60 \text{ s}}{\text{hr}}\right)\left(\frac{24 \text{ hr}}{\text{day}}\right)\left(\frac{365.25 \text{ day}}{\text{yr}}\right)\left(\frac{10^{-18} \text{ g}}{\text{ag}}\right)\left(\frac{1 \text{ } \mu\text{g}}{10^{-6} \text{ g}}\right) = 0.3 \text{ } \mu\text{g/yr}$$

Problem 9

From 1937 to 1970 asbestos fibers were counted by using impingers. The exposure limit was 5 million particles per cubic foot (mppcf). How does this compare with the current OSHA standard of 0.2 fiber per cubic centimeter (f/cc)?

Solution 9

$$(5 \times 10^6 \text{ particles/ft}^3)(1 \text{ fiber/1 particle})(\text{ft}^3)\left[\text{in}^3/(2.54 \text{ cm})^3\right]$$

$$= 177 \text{ f/cc}$$

$$= (177 \text{ f/cc})/(0.2 \text{ f/cc}) = 882.$$

This problem is for calculation purposes only; any attempt to justify this conversion scientifically will require information that is not available.

Problem 10

In a titration it was found that 36.46 ml of a base was necessary to neutralize 25 ml of 2.6 N acid. What is the normality of the base? (Recall that normality equals equivalents per liter or milliequivalents per milliliter.)

Solution 10

The number of equivalents of the acid must equal the number of equivalents of the base:

$$(\text{eq/liter acid})\text{liters acid} = (\text{eq/liter base})\text{liters base}$$

$$(36.46 \text{ ml base})(x) = (25 \text{ ml})(2.6 \text{ N acid})$$

$$x = 25 \text{ ml}(2.6 \text{ eq/l})/(36.46 \text{ ml}) = 1.78 \text{ eq/l} = 1.78 \text{ N}$$

Problem 11

On Saturday, February 10, 1990, Ronald V. Davis, President of the Greenwich, Connecticut–based Perrier Group of America, announced a total recall on all the bottled Perrier in America because it was contaminated with benzene. The recall resulted in the destruction of 72 million bottles of this famous French bottled water. The St. Petersburg, Florida *Times* story of Sunday, February 11, 1990, gave these details: "An entire class of people have just had their weekend ruined," said John Buckley a Republican consultant in Washington, D.C. A New York playwright said, "Oh, This is terrible! It's the end of an era. We'll all have to go back to Scotch!" The FDA reports that the level of benzene is two to four times the EPA standard for drinking water (5 ppb). The benzene concentration found in the bottled Perrier is reported to vary between 12 and 20 ppb. Perrier reports that the reason for the recall is that, "We're in the integrity business, selling purity and quality."

How much benzene did Perrier pour down the drain when they disposed of 72 million bottles of the contaminated product?

Solution 11

Calculate the volume of Perrier destroyed:

$$(72 \text{ million bottles})(10 \text{ oz/bottle})(1 \text{ gal}/128 \text{ oz})(3.785 \text{ l/gal})$$

$$72 \text{ million bottles} = 21.3 \times 10^6 \text{ l Perrier}$$

Calculate the volume of benzene in the Perrier destroyed; to complete this calculation assume that the benzene concentration is the mean of the reported concentration range of 12 ppb to 20 ppb, or 16 ppb:

$$(21.3 \times 10^6 \text{ l Perrier})(0.016 \text{ l benzene}/10^6 \text{ l Perrier}) = 0.34 \text{ l benzene}$$

3

BEHAVIOR OF GASES AND VAPORS

Outcome Competencies   *After studying this chapter you will be able to:*

- *Define various temperature scales (°F, °R, °C, and K).*
- *Define the standard atmosphere.*
- *Explain Boyle's, Charles' and Gay-Lussac's laws.*
- *Develop the equation of state for an ideal gas.*
- *Compute the molar gas constants for different unit systems.*
- *Define the chemical terms used to describe gases and vapors.*
- *Explain Dalton's law of partial pressures.*
- *Evaluate the composition of dry air.*
- *Calculate the apparent molecular weight of dry air.*
- *Define gas density and specific gravity.*
- *Derive the ideal gas equation in terms of density.*
- *Reconstruct the density correction factor for elevation.*
- *Justify the use of the ideal gas equation for all gases and vapors.*

1. PURPOSE

This chapter is a review of the basic physical chemistry and thermodynamics of gases and vapors. One of the fascinations of the ever growing science of industrial hygiene is the work of pioneers who labored at the very edge of the unknown. To reach the frontier now one must pass over a wide well-traveled road. The history of industrial hygiene is rich with pioneers who have followed this highway. An often overlooked lane along this broad highway is that of physical chemistry. The work of these pioneers is reviewed in the study of gases and vapors.

The development of the ideal gas equation is based on chemical thermodynamics. Knowledge of the physical chemistry of gases and vapors is essential to an understanding of the basic concepts of industrial hygiene, air pollution, and environmental health. Important concepts of temperature and pressure effects on gas and vapor volume are introduced here and developed more fully in Chapter 6.

2. TEMPERATURE

Temperature is defined as that property of a body which determines the flow of heat. Heat will flow from a warm body to a cold body. For example, place your hand, palm down, on the surface of a table in a room, and your hand begins to feel cool. The table's surface temperature is less than your hand's temperature; your hand is losing heat to the cooler surface of the table. Now suppose that the table has a dark color and is located in bright sunlight. When you place your hand, palm down, on this surface, your hand will feel "warm," maybe "hot." This occurs because the table's surface temperature is higher than that of your hand; so heat is flowing from the warmer body (table surface) to the cooler body (hand). Temperature is an intrinsic quantity that cannot be defined in the usual units of mass, length, and time.

There are several types of temperature scales in general use. These scales depend on the freezing and boiling points of water as boundary markers for the scale. In a conventional laboratory thermometer, the boundary points are conveniently selected to relate to the known properties of water. On the Celsius scale, the freezing point of water is assigned a value of 0 and the boiling a value of 100; the distance between these two points is divided into 100 equal increments, with each increment labeled as a Celsius degree (Table 3-1). On the Kelvin scale, the freezing point of water is assigned a value of 273.15 K and the boiling point a value of 373.15 K; the distance between these two points is divided into 100 equal increments, and each increment is labeled as a Kelvin degree (Table 3-1). On the Fahrenheit scale, the freezing point of water is assigned a valve of 32 and the boiling point a value of 212; the distance between these two points is divided into 180 equal increments, and each increment is labeled as a Fahrenheit degree (Table 3-1).

It is important to make a distinction between the actual temperature (°C and °F) and a temperature increment (Fahrenheit degree and Celsius degree). This distinction enables the derivation of a relationship between the two temperature scales. For example, a temperature of 100°C is the same as a temperature of 212°F. A temperature difference of 100 Celsius degrees is equal to a temperature difference of 180 Fahrenheit degrees.

TABLE 3-1. A comparison of temperature scales

Temperature scale	Celsius °C	Kelvin K	Fahrenheit °F	Rankine °R
Boiling point of water	+100	+373.15	+212	+671.67
	⎡100 equal divisions⎤		⎡180 equal divisions⎤	
Freezing point of water	0	273.15	+32	+491.67
Absolute zero	−273.15	—0	−459.67	—0

Note: K = °C + 273.15; R = °F + 459.67.
The ""°"" symbol is not used for the Kelvin temperature scale.
Recall: 9(°C) = 5(°F) − 160, can be solved for either °C or °F.

Setting up an equation gives:

$$100 \text{ C degrees} = 180 \text{ F degrees}$$

$$1 \text{ C degree} = 1.8 \text{ F degrees}$$

$$1 \text{ F degree} = 0.555 \text{ C degrees}$$

Instead of trying to memorize an equation, it is possible to derive a conversion between the temperature scales.

Example 1

What is the Celsius temperature corresponding to 72°F? Since 72°F is 40 F degrees above the freezing point of water:

72°F = 40 F degrees above the freezing point of water

72°F = 40(0.555) C degrees above the freezing point of water

72°F = 22.2 C degrees above the freezing point of water on the Celsius

scale, that is, 22.2 + 0.0 or 22.2°C

To convert between the Celsius and Fahrenheit scales the following relationships should prove to be very useful:

$$°C = 0.555(°F - 32) \qquad °F = (1.8°C + 32)$$

- Given 98.6°F, find the corresponding Celsius temperature:

$$°C = 0.555[98.6°F - 32] = 37°C$$

- Given 120°C, find the corresponding Fahrenheit temperature:

$$°F = [1.8(120°C) + 32] = 248°F$$

The Kelvin/Rankine relationship is:

$$T_{\text{Kelvin}} = (T_{\text{Rankine}})/1.8$$

An Interesting Note on Temperature   A cricket can be used to measure the temperature of its surroundings, using the following relationship:

$$\text{number of chirps}/14 \text{ seconds} + 40 \approx °F$$

3. STANDARD ATMOSPHERE

Standard atmospheric pressure is described in many ways by the myriad of disciplines within the environmental health field. Because each discipline has its own favorite set of units to describe standard atmospheric pressure, it is necessary to become conversant with many of these definitions. Some of the more commonly used units of pressure are given in Table 3-2.

4. INTRODUCTION TO IDEAL GASES

The study of ideal gases is an area of chemistry and physics that may serve as a review of the history of science. Without this historical perspective, this study is without a foundation and difficult to connect to the other basic scientific knowledge that we possess. A study of ideal gases cannot be considered complete without a review of the work of Boyle, Charles, Gay-Lussac, and Dalton, to name a few.

TABLE 3-2. The standard atmosphere

Numerical value	Unit	Notes
1.013×10^5	Pascals (Pa)	1
1.0	atmosphere (atm)	2
101.325	kiloPascals (kPa)	—
1.013	bars (B)	2
1,013	millibars (mB)	3
29.921	inches of mercury (in Hg)	4
760.0	millimeters of mercury (mm Hg)	1
76.00	centimeters of mercury (cm Hg)	—
0.76	meters of mercury (m Hg)	—
14.7	pounds per square inch (psi)	—
406.14	inches of water (in H_2O)	5

1. The SI system standard definition of pressure.
2. An acceptable exception in the SI system.
3. Used in meteorology.
4. The English system standard for pressure.
5. Based on the density of mercury, 13.5340 g/cm^3 or 13534.0 kg/m^3 at 1.01325×10^5 Pa, 25°C (Appendix).

Boyle's Law

Robert Boyle about 1662 stated what has come to be known as Boyle's law: The volume of any definite quantity of gas at constant temperature varies inversely as the pressure on the gas.

$$V = K_1/P$$

K_1 is function of temperature and is constant at a given T.

The behavior of ideal gases predicted by Boyle's Law is demonstrated in Figure 3-1. The family of curves are hyperbolas where K varies with temperature. These curves are commonly called isotherms or lines of constant temperature. In the plot of pressure versus volume given in the figure, one can graphically observe Boyle's law, $PV = K$.

In general:

$$P_1V_1 = K_1 \quad \text{and} \quad P_2V_2 = K_2$$

$$K_1 = K_2 = K$$

$$P_1V_1 = P_2V_2 = K$$

This equation is the mathematical formula for a hyperbola. The family of curves plotted in Figure 3-1 demonstrates the hyperbolic relationship.

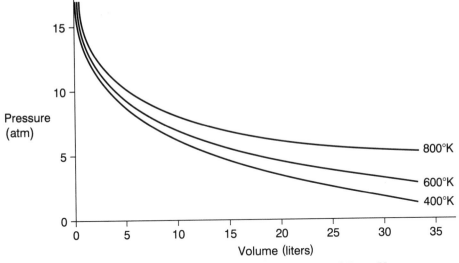

Figure 3-1. Boyle's law plots. Isothermal plots of P vs. V.

5. CHARLES' OR GAY-LUSSAC'S LAW

Charles observed that hydrogen (H_2), carbon dioxide (CO_2), oxygen (O_2), and air all expanded by an equal amount when heated from 0°C to 80°C at a constant pressure. Gay-Lussac (1802) found that all gases increase in volume for each one degree Celsius rise in temperature, and this increase is equal to approximately $1/273.15$ of the volume of the gas at 0°C. Using the observations of Gay-Lussac, it is possible to define a new temperature scale based on the decreases in volume with temperature T:

$$V/V_0 = T/T_0$$

$$V = (T/T_0)V_0$$

$$V = V_0 + [(273.15 + t)/273.15]V_0$$

where:

$T = (T_0 = t)$
$T_0 = 273.15$, and $t =$ temperature in °C
$V_0 =$ gas volume at a temperature of 0°C
$V =$ gas volume at a temperature of t°C

The "new temperature" (T) is the thermodynamic or Kelvin temperature scale. If these temperatures and volumes are labeled with 1 and 2, the following equation results:

$$V_2/V_1 = T_2/T_1$$

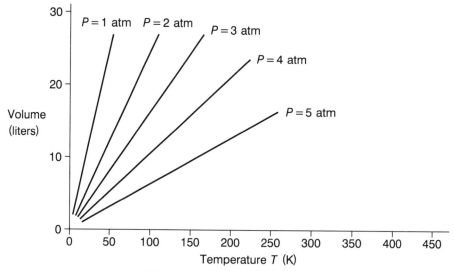

Figure 3-2. Charles' law plots.

This equation can be solved for V_2:

$$V_2 = V_1 T_2 / T_1$$

$$V_2 = K_2 T$$

K_2 is determined by pressure, the nature and the amount of the gas, and the volume (Charles' or Gay-Lussac's law of volumes). Figure 3-2 demonstrates the Charles'/Gay-Lussac's law of volumes. Note that $V_2 = K_2 T$ is a straight line when the pressure is constant. The plot of Figure 3-2 indicates that when a gas approaches absolute zero, the gas volume goes to zero. In the real world, the gas becomes a liquid first and then a solid long before it disappears at absolute zero (0 K). The straight lines in Figure 3-2 represent lines of constant pressure (isobars).

Reviewing the gas laws, we have:

- Boyle's law:

$$P_1 V_1 = P_2 V_2 = K$$

which may also be written:

$$V_X = V_1 P_1 / P_X$$

- Charles' (Gay-Lussac) law:

$$V_2 = K_2 T$$

which may also be written:

$$V_2 = V_X T_X / T_2$$

Substituting V_X in the equation for V_2 yields:

$$V_2 = V_1 P_1 T_2 / P_2 T_1$$

On rearranging this gives:

$$P_1 V_2 / T_2 = P_1 V_1 / T_1 = K \text{ (constant)}$$

which may also be written as:

$$PV = KT$$

This is known as the combined gas law.

The numerical value of K is determined by the number of moles of gas and is independent of the specific kind of gas. If the quantity (moles) of a gas is increased at constant P and T, then V must increase. The increase in quantity of the gas also increases the K value; actually:

$$K = nR$$

where R is the universal gas constant. The combined gas law becomes:

$$PV = nRT$$

usually known as the ideal gas law. This form of the gas law, also known as an equation of state, will be used throughout this book. It is a reliable predictor of the behavior of gases and vapors at or near standard atmospheric pressure and temperature and the dilute concentrations encountered in industrial hygiene and air pollution. An array of R values can be found in Table 3-3.

TABLE 3-3. Values of the molar gas constant R, the units for P, V, and T and the number of moles used to generate these values

R value and typical units	Units for pressure	Units for molar gas volume	Unit for moles	Absolute temp., degrees
0.08205 (l atm)/(mole K)	1 atm	22.41 l	mole	273.15 K
0.08205 (l atm)/(mole K)	1 atm	24.45 l	mole	298.15 K
82.056 (ml atm)/(mole K)	1 atm	22 413.6 ml	mole	273.15 K
62.363 (l mm Hg)/(mole K)	760 mm Hg	22.4136 l	mole	273.15 K
1.9872 (cal)/(mole K)	101 325 Pa	0.022414 m^3	mole	273.15 K
8.3144 (J)/(mole K)	101 325 Pa	0.022414 m^3	mole	273.15 K
8314.4 (J)/(mole K)	101 325 Pa	0.022414 m^3	mol	273.15 K
0.7302 (ft^3 atm)/(lb mole R)	1 atm	359 ft^3	lb mole	491.67 R
10.73 (ft^3 lb)/(in^2 lb mole R)	14.7 lb/in^2	359 ft^3	lb mole	491.67 R
555.0 (ft^3 mm Hg)/(lb mole R)	760 mm Hg	359 ft^3	lb mole	491.67 R
1544 (lb$_F$)/(lb mole R)	29.921 in Hg	359 ft^3	lb mole	491.67 R
21.85 (ft^3 in Hg)/(lb mole R)	29.921 in Hg	359 ft^3	lb mole	491.67 R

J = N m; degree K = °C + 273.15; degree R = °F + 459.67

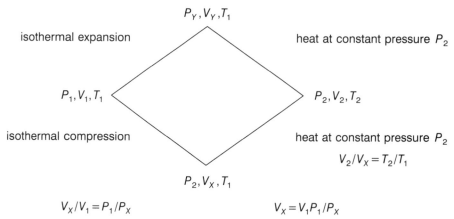

Figure 3-3. The expansion and compression of an ideal gas.

Figure 3-3 demonstrates the results of an expansion and a compression of an ideal gas. The pressure, volume, and temperature relationships that occur through these cycles may be predicted by using Boyle's and Charles' laws. Boyle's law at constant temperature may be used to predict the changes in volume from V_1 and V_Y (an isothermal compression from V_1 to V_Y):

$$V_Y = Y_1(P_1/P_Y)$$

Boyle's law can be used to predict changes in volume from V_1 to V_X:

$$V_X = V_1(P_1/P_X)$$

6. EQUATIONS OF STATE FOR IDEAL GASES

An equation of state relates the pressure, the volume, and the temperature of a gas to one another. Classical physical chemistry textbooks outline many forms of equations of state. In developing equations of state for a pure substance, it is assumed that the absolute or thermodynamic temperature (T) is the dependent variable and a function of the pressure (P) and the volume (V), which are the independent variables; that is, $T = f(P, V)$. Knowing two of the three variables, it is possible to solve for the third variable.

The ideal gas law is a simplified form of an equation of state and is given by the equation:

$$PV = nRT$$

where:

> P = pressure of the gas
> V = the volume of the gas
> n = number of moles of gas present
> R = universal gas constant
> T = absolute or thermodynamic temperature of the gas.

At infinite pressure, this equations predicts that the gas volume goes to zero, ignoring the volume of the gas molecules (this situation is not of concern at dilute concentrations and near atmospheric pressure). In describing an ideal gas, or a vapor that is reasonably expected to behave as an ideal gas, it is assumed that:

1. The gas is not near its condensation temperature.
2. The vapor is not near its boiling temperature.
3. The gas/vapor is not at an elevated pressure.

These assumptions are based on the fact that the intermolecular attractive forces between the gases molecules are negligible. This condition is satisfied with "infinitely dilute solutions" or gases and vapors at low concentrations (less than 1% in air).

There are many other equations of state, including that of van der Waals.

$$\left(P + \frac{n^2}{V^2} \right)(V - nb) = nRT$$

The ideal gas equation will be used exclusively throughout this book; but other equations can be used, and the related equations then can be derived.

Before calculations involving the ideal gas law are introduced, a review of several terms and definitions from physical chemistry may be helpful (see Table 3-3).

7. DEFINITIONS

Atomic weight is the relative mass of the atom on the basis of carbon 12 ($^{12}C \equiv 12$).

Gram molecular weight is the sum of the individual atomic weights of all the atoms in a molecule (express mass in units of grams, g).

Kilogram molecular weight is the sum of the individual atomic weights of all the atoms in a molecule (express mass in units of kilograms, kg).

Example 2

Calculate the kilogram molecular weight of carbon monoxide.

- Atomic weight of carbon in kilograms is 12.001 kg/mol.
- Atomic weight of oxygen in kilograms is 16.000 kg/mol.
- The sum of atomic weights in kilograms of the individual atoms in the molecule is equal to the kilogram molecular weight 28.001 kg/mol.

Example 3

Calculate the gram molecular weight of carbon monoxide.

- Atomic weight of carbon in grams is 12.001 g/mole.
- Atomic weight of carbon in grams is 16.000 g/mole.
- The sum of atomic weights in grams of the individual atoms in the molecule is equal to the gram molecular weight, 28.001 g/mole.

Molecular volume is the volume occupied by one molecular weight of a gas (either kilogram molecular weight or gram molecular weight).
Avogadro's number is the number of molecules (6.02×10^{23} molecules/mole) contained in one gram molecular weight or one gram molecular volume; for example

$$28.001 \text{ g CO} = 6.02 \times 10^{23} \text{ molecules CO}$$

One mole is the amount of substance represented by one molecular weight or one molecular volume.
One kilogram mole is the amount of substance represented by one kilogram molecular weight or one kilogram molecular volume (mol).
One gram mole is the amount of substance represented by one gram molecular weight or one gram molecular volume (mole).
Equation of state is an equation that relates the pressure P, volume V, and thermodynamic temperature T of an amount of substance n.
Ideal gas law is an equation of state—a relationship between the pressure, volume, and thermodynamic temperature of a gas. Air is not ideal, but it will be assumed in this book that gases, vapors, and air behave as ideal gases. This will be discussed later in Chapter 4.

$PV = nRT$, where P = pressure, V = volume, n = number of moles
  T = absolute temperature (°C + 273.15 = K)
  R = universal gas constant (0.08205 l atm/mole K) (Table 3-3).

Example 4

Given one mole of an ideal gas at a temperature of 0°C (32°F), and at a pressure of 1 atmosphere, calculate the volume that this gas will occupy. Solve the ideal gas equation for volume:

$$\frac{V}{n} = \frac{RT}{P} = \frac{(0.08205\ \text{l atm/mole K})(273.15\ \text{K})}{1\ \text{atm}}$$

$$= 22.4\ \text{l/mole} = 22.4\ \text{m}^3/\text{mol}$$

22.4 l/mole is the molecular volume at 273.15 K.

Example 5

Given one mole of an ideal gas at a temperature of 25°C, and a pressure of 1 atmosphere, calculate the volume occupied by the gas. Solving the ideal gas equation for volume yields:

$$V = \frac{nRT}{P} = \frac{(1\ \text{mole})(0.08205\ \text{l atm/mole K})(298.15\ \text{K})}{1\ \text{atm}}$$

$$= 24.45\ \text{l/mole} = 24.45\ \text{m}^3/\text{mol}\ (\text{the molecular volume at 298.15 K})$$

8. DALTON'S LAW

Dalton's law of partial pressure states that at constant temperature the total pressure exerted by a mixture of gases in a definite volume is equal to the sum of the individual pressures that each gas would exert if it occupied the same total volume above.

$$P_T = P_1 + P_2 \cdots + P_i = \sum_i P_i$$

In other words, the total pressure of a mixture of gases is equal to the sum of the partial pressures of the individual components of the mixture.

Assume that there are four rigid flasks and that each flask is 1 liter in volume. Flask 1 contains sulfur hexafluoride at 75 mm Hg pressure, flask 2 contains nitrogen at 120 mm Hg pressure, flask 3 contains methane at 45 mm Hg pressure, and flask 4 contains carbon monoxide at 60 mm Hg. Next, combine all four of these flasks into a one liter rigid flask to prepare a calibration gas mixture. What will the final pressure be after combining the contents of the four individual flasks into the one liter flask? Dalton's law of partial pressure is used to calculate total pressure, P_T:

$$P_T = \sum_i P_i = P_{SF_6} + P_{N_2} + P_{CH_4} + P_{CO}$$

$$P_T = 75\ \text{mm Hg} + 120\ \text{mm Hg} + 45\ \text{mm Hg} + 60\ \text{mm Hg} = 300\ \text{mm Hg}$$

Dalton's law will be applied to calibrating air sampling systems in Chapter 4.

TABLE 3-4. Approximate composition of dry air by volume

Component	Symbol	Percent concentration	ppm concentration	Notes
Nitrogen	N_2	78.084	780 840.	$\pm 0.004\%$
Oxygen	O_2	20.9476	209 476.	—
Argon	Ar	0.934	9 340.	$\pm 0.001\%$
Carbon dioxide	CO_2	0.0314	314.	—
Neon	Ne	0.001818	18.18	± 0.04 ppm
Helium	He	0.000524	5.24	± 0.004 ppm
Methane	CH_4	0.0002	2.	—
Sulfur dioxide	SO_2	0 to 0.0001	0 to 1	—
Hydrogen	H_2	0.00005	0.5	—
Krypton	Kr	0.0002	2.	1
Xenon	Xe	0.0002	2.	1
Ozone	O_3	0.0002	2.	1

Source: *ASHRAE Handbook of Fundamentals* (1993), p. 6.1, based on the atomic weight of carbon of 12.0000. ASHRAE also reports that the molecular weight of dry air is 28.9645 g/mole (28.9645 kg/mole) based on the carbon 12 scale.

Note 1: ASHRAE reports the sum of the volume contribution of these components as 0.0002%.

9. THE COMPOSITION OF AIR

The air that surrounds us and that we breathe is a dynamic mixture of many components (see Table 3-4). The bulk of the air in the environment is composed of nitrogen and oxygen with various other trace gases mixed in it. The mixture is dynamic in several respects. The moisture content or water vapor, the temperature, the pressure, and the trace gas constituents all can and do vary over time and in space.

10. MOIST AIR

ASHRAE defines moist air as: "A binary (or two component) mixture of dry air and water vapor. The amount of water vapor varies from zero (dry air) to a maximum which depends on temperature and pressure." The moisture content of air changes as a function of local weather conditions, which cause changes in the relative humidity. The relative humidity is an indication of the saturation of moisture in air. Air is a mixture or a solution, and as with all solutions the various components display varying degrees of solubility. If a particular air mass moves into a region where the relative humidity is 60%, this means that the air contains 60% of the total water vapor that it can possibly hold. If the relative humidity increases to a point where the air is fully saturated, water vapor can literally rain out of the air. If the air is at a given relative humidity at a particular temperature and pressure, and the temperature changes to a lower temperature, the dew point is reached and the relative humidity level increases.

This behavior explains the phenomenon of morning ground fog in many regions of the country. An air mass has a given amount of water vapor, and the air mass cools in the evening because of the earth's cooling as it radiates infrared energy out into space to warm the surrounding night sky. The resulting radiational cooling lowers the air temperature, and the water vapor that is present reaches the dew point, as cooler air can hold less water vapor then warmer air. The result is ground fog.

11. STANDARD AIR

To avoid dealing with a dynamic mixture of air and water vapor, and the complexities that this entails, it is convenient to define a mixture called "standard air," or "standard dry air," that contains a fixed amount of each of the common trace gases and NO water vapor. Atmospheric air may contain several hundred components, including gases, vapors, liquids, and aerosols. These components vary from the percent concentration range $(C_\%)$ to the parts per billion concentration range (C_{ppb}). Because water vapor in this mixture varies over time and space, it is convenient to describe an atmosphere devoid of water vapor (so-called dry air). The ASHRAE standard definition of dry air is given in Table 3-5. To avoid confusion with various definitions of standard air, the ASHRAE definition will be used throughout this book. The established definition of standard air is arbitrary in the values assigned to the trace constituents; however, that will have very little effect on the various parameters that can be derived once this definition is clarified.

The temperature, volume, and pressure behavior of standard air is described adequately by the ideal gas equation. In moving around the ambient environment, the temperature and the pressure of the air may change rather dramatically. By convention the reference atmospheric pressure is selected at sea level. The mean or average sea level is associated with low

TABLE 3-5. Standard conditions for various disciplines (dry air only)

Disciplines	Temperature standard	Absolute temperature	Pressure standard
Industrial hygiene NTP	25°C	298.15 K	101 325 Pa, 1 atm
Industrial ventilation	70°F, 21.1°C	529.67°R	29.921 inches Hg
Air pollution NTP	25°C	298.15 K	101 325 Pa, 1 atm
ASHRAE	15°C, 59.0°F	288.15 K	101 325 Pa, 1 atm
Chemistry/physics STP	0°C	273.15 K	760 mm Hg, 1 atm

tide—but how low? The temperature standard varies among various disciplines. In industrial hygiene, the usual standard temperature is 25°C (298.15 K). Table 3-5 lists temperature standards for various disciplines.

It is assumed that air behaves as an ideal gas. Although this assumption may introduce a small error, it does enable the calculation of the concentration of air contaminants in the workplace and the ambient environment.

12. THE APPARENT MOLECULAR WEIGHT OF AIR

One of the peculiar outcomes of selecting a standard definition of air is that it is possible to describe this mixture as though it was a single gas such as helium or nitrogen. All gases including air have a set of unique physical and chemical properties. If the composition of air is "defined," it is possible to calculate its molecular weight. To maintain the sanity of physical chemists and thermodynamics, this calculated entity is labeled the "apparent molecular weight." This caution is necessary because a gas that is composed of a single molecule (e.g., helium, nitrogen, etc.) can have a molecular weight, but mixtures normally are not described by a molecular weight. Although it is most common to describe mixtures in terms of the concentration of the

TABLE 3-6. Calculation of the apparent molecular weight of dry air

Component	Atomic symbol	Molecular weight (M_i)	Concentration percent (%)	Volume fraction (B_i)	$M_i B_i$
Nitrogen	N_2	28.01	78.084	0.78084	21.87132
Oxygen	O_2	32.00	20.9476	0.209476	6.70232
Argon	Ar	39.948	0.934	9.34×10^{-3}	0.373116
Carbon dioxide	CO_2	44.00	0.0314	3.14×10^{-4}	1.3816×10^{-2}
Neon	Ne	20.183	0.001818	1.818×10^{-5}	3.67×10^{-4}
Helium	He	4.0026	0.000524	5.24×10^{-6}	2.097×10^{-5}
Methane	CH_4	16.04	0.0002	2.0×10^{-6}	3.208×10^{-5}
Sulfur dioxide	SO_2	64.06	0 to 0.0001	0.1×10^{-6}	6.406×10^{-5}
Hydrogen	H_2	2.0159	0.00005	5.0×10^{-7}	1.008×10^{-6}
Krypton*	Kr	83.80	6.67×10^{-5}	6.67×10^{-7}	5.589×10^{-5}
Xenon*	Xe	131.30	6.67×10^{-5}	6.67×10^{-7}	8.757×10^{-5}
Ozone*	O_3	48.00	6.67×10^{-5}	6.67×10^{-7}	3.202×10^{-5}
			99.9998921	$\Sigma M_i B_i$ =	28.962

The values in this table are from the ASHRAE *Handbook of Fundamentals* (1993) and are based on the atomic weight of carbon of 12.0000. ASHRAE reports the sum of the volume contribution of Kr, Xe, and O_3 as 0.0002. For this problem the composition has been divided by 3, assuming an equal volume contribution from each component. The ASHRAE value for the molecular weight of air is 28.9645. M_i is equal to the molecular weight of the ith component; B_i is equal to the volume fraction of the ith component (Public Health Service, *Handbook of Air Pollution*, USDHEW-PHS, Pub. No. 999-AP-44, p. 13.11).

TABLE 3-7. Common units used to express density

Measurement system	Unit value
centimeter/gram/second (cgs)	g/cm^3
Systeme Internationale (SI)	kg/m^3
English	lb_M/ft^3

constituents, air is an unusual exception to this rule. Defining the constituents eliminates air's annoying dynamic properties.

It is possible to consider air to be a gas made up of "air molecules." The molecular weight of this mixture will be a weighted average of the molecular weights of the individual components. Each component will exert its molecular weight (M_i) weighted by its volume fraction (B_i). The volume fraction is the decimal equivalent of the percent of a constituent in the mixture. For example nitrogen's percentage in air is 78.084%; so its volume fraction is 0.78084. Table 3-6 details the calculation of the apparent molecular weight of dry air.

13. DENSITY

The density of a material (solid, liquid, gas, or vapor) is given by the relationship between the mass of the material and the volume the mass occupies. The units commonly used to express density in the metric and English systems are listed in Table 3-7.

Carefully weight out 13.5340 grams of liquid mercury at 25°C, into a calibrated flask. The observed volume occupied by this mass of mercury is equal to 1.0 cm³. One gram of liquid mercury would occupy 0.0739 cm³. This volume can be calculated from the reciprocal of the density, which is 13.5340 g/cm³ at 25°C. The densities of selected materials used in air pollution and industrial hygiene are given in Table 3-8.

The equation for density may be obtained directly from the definition:

$$density = mass/volume$$

$$\rho = m/v$$

This relationship holds for all the physical states of a material: a gas (vapor), liquid, or solid. The density of a gas (vapor) also will be equal to the mass of the gas (vapor) divided by the volume that this mass occupies.

TABLE 3-8. Density and specific gravity of working fluids at selected temperatures and one atmosphere

Material	Density (g/ml)		Density (kg/m³)	
	273.15	298.15 K	273.15 K	298.15 K
Water	0.99987	0.99707	999.87	9970.7
Mercury	13.5955	13.5340	13595.5	13534.0
Air	0.00129 (1)	0.001185 (2)	1.2922	1.1185
Acetylene tetrabromide	2.960		2960.0	
Carbon tetrachloride	1.600 (20°C)		1600.0	
Glycerine	1.260 (0°C)		1260.0	
Alpha-chloronaphthalene	1.194		1194.0	
Ethyl chloroacetate	1.159		1159.0	
Toluene	0.866 (4°C)		866.0	
Kerosene	0.82		820	
Ethyl alcohol	0.789 (20°C)		789.0	
Red gage oil	0.826		826.	
Yellow gage oil	0.826		826.	
Blue gage oil	1.910		1910.	
Violet gage oil	1.000		1000.	

ρ_{H_2O} at 4°C = 1.00000 g/ml = 1000 kg/m³.
ρ_{H_2O} at 25°C = 0.99707 g/ml = 9970.7 kg/m³.
Note 1: a calculated value.
Note 2: *Handbook of Chemistry and Physics*, ed. Weast, R. C., 70th Edition, CRC Press, Inc., Boca Raton, FL (1989), p. F-3.
Density of air = $[(0.001293)/(1 + 0.00367t)](H/76)$.
Where: t = °C, H = centimeters of mercury (Note 2).

14. GAS DENSITY

The definition of density may be used in the ideal gas equation to calculate the density of a gas assumed to be ideal:

$$PV = nRT = mRT/M \qquad (1)$$

where:

m = mass
M = molecular weight

and P_1, V_1, R_1, and T_1 have their usual meaning. Solving equation (1) for $m/V = \rho$ gives equation (2):

$$m/V = PM/RT = \rho \qquad (2)$$

where ρ is the density of interest. This relationship can be written for a mixture (mix) of gases as:

$$\rho_{mix} = P_{mix} M_{mix}/RT_{mix} \qquad (3)$$

Recall the ideal gas relationship for the ith component in a mixture:

$$P_i V_{\text{mix}} = n_i RT_{\text{mix}} = m_i RT_{\text{mix}}/M_{\text{mix}} \tag{4}$$

Rearranging equation (4) gives:

$$M_i/V_{\text{mix}} = P_i M_{\text{mix}}/RT_{\text{mix}} = \rho_i \tag{5}$$

where ρ_i is the gas density of the ith component.

Equations (3) and (5) permit the calculation of the density of a mixture of gases (e.g., air) and of a component of the mixture, respectively.

Example 6

Calculate the density of air in mg/cm^3 and kg/m^3 at standard industrial hygiene conditions.

Solution 6

To calculate the density of air, use equation (3) with several conditions specified:

Temperature $= 25°C = 298.15$ K;
pressure $= 1$ atm or 1.0135×10^5 Pa, dry air;
$M_{\text{air}} = 28.96$ g/mole

A. $\rho_{\text{air}} = P_{\text{air}} M_{\text{air}}/RT_{\text{air}}$

$$\rho_{\text{air}} = \frac{(1 \text{ atm})(28.9622 \text{ g/mole})}{(0.08205 \text{ l atm/mole K})(298.15 \text{ K})} = 1.18391 \text{ g/l}$$

$$\rho_{\text{air}} = \left(\frac{1.18391 \text{ g}}{1}\right)\left(\frac{10^3 \text{ mg}}{\text{g}}\right)\left(\frac{1}{10^3 \text{ cm}^3}\right) = 1.18391 \text{ mg/cm}^3$$

$\left(\rho_{\text{air}} \text{ Handbook value } 1.185 \text{ mg/cm}^3\right)$

B. $\rho_{\text{air}} = \left(\dfrac{1.185 \text{ mg}}{\text{cm}^3}\right)\left(\dfrac{1000 \text{ cm}^3}{1}\right)\left(\dfrac{1000 \text{ l}}{\text{m}^3}\right)\left(\dfrac{\text{g}}{1000 \text{ mg}}\right)\left(\dfrac{\text{kg}}{1000 \text{ g}}\right) = 1.185 \text{ kg/m}^3$

Example 7

Calculate the density of dry air in units of mass/volume or lb$_{\text{M}}$/ft^3 at 70°F, the industrial ventilation design standard.

Solution 7

$$\rho_{air} = P_{air} M_{air}/R T_{air} = \rho_{air}$$

$$\rho_{air} = \frac{(14.659 \text{ lb}_F/\text{in}^2)(28.9622 \text{ lb}/\text{lb mole})(144 \text{ in}^2)}{(1544 \text{ lb}_F/\text{lb mole } R)(529.6 \text{ } R)(\text{ft}^2)}$$

$$\rho_{air} = 0.074939 \text{ lb}_M/\text{ft}^3$$

Alternative: If you are unable to pull the value of $R = 1544 \text{ lb}_F/\text{lb mole } R$ from the air, it is possible to convert the solution to Example 6 to the desired units. Recalculate ρ_{air} in example 6 at 70°F(21.11°C):

$$\rho_{air} = \frac{(1 \text{ atm})(28.9622 \text{ g}/\text{mole})}{(0.08205 \text{ l atm}/\text{mole K})(273.15 + 21.1)\text{K}}$$

$$\rho_{air} = 1.1995 \text{ g}/\text{l}(\text{mg}/\text{cm}^3)$$

$$\rho_{air} = (1.1995 \text{ g})\left(\frac{28.32 \text{ l}}{\text{ft}^3}\right)\left(\frac{\text{lb}_M}{454.59 \text{ g}}\right) = 0.0749 \text{ lb}_M/\text{ft}$$

Example 8

Calculate the density of standard air at 200°C and 0.70 atm.

Solution 8

$$PV = nRT = mRT/M \qquad m/V = PM/RT = \rho$$

$$\rho = \frac{(0.70 \text{ atm})(28.96 \text{ g}/\text{mole})}{\left(\dfrac{0.08205 \text{ l atm}}{\text{mole K}}\right)(473.15 \text{ K})}$$

$$= 0.55 \text{ g}/\text{l}$$

15. SPECIFIC GRAVITY

Specific gravity (SG) is the ratio of the density of a substance to that of a reference material. In the case of a liquid the reference material is water, and for a gaseous substance the reference material is air at 25°C.

SG of a liquid $= (\rho \text{ of liquid})/(\rho \text{ of water})$
SG of a gas $= (\rho \text{ of gas})/(\rho \text{ of air})$

To calculate the specific gravity of mercury, a liquid at 25°C, the value of the density of mercury and water must be obtained from the literature (see Appendix). The density of mercury at 25°C is 13.5340 g/ml or 135340 kg/m^3. The density of water at 25°C is 0.99707 g/ml.

SG of a liquid = (ρ of liquid)/(ρ of water)

$$SG_{Hg} = \frac{\rho_{Hg}}{\rho_{H_2O}} = \frac{(13.5340 \text{ g/ml})}{(0.99707 \text{ g/ml})} = 13.57377 = 13.5738$$

Example 9

Calculate the specific gravity of mercury, which is a liquid at 4°C.

Solution 9

The density of mercury (CRC *Handbook*) at 4°C is 13.5856 g/ml.

SG of a liquid = (ρ of liquid)/(ρ of water)
$SG_{Hg} = (\rho_{Hg})/(\rho_{H_2O}) = (13.5856 \text{ g/ml})/(1.00000 \text{ g/ml}) = 13.5856$

Example 10

Given the SG for mercury of 13.57377 calculate the density of mercury in the English system. (Hint: 7.62 gallons/cubic foot.)

Solution 10

SG of a liquid = (ρ of liquid)/(ρ of water) = (X/0.99707 g/ml) = 13.57377
= 13.573.

$$\rho_{Hg} = 13.5462 \text{ g/ml at } 20°C \qquad \rho_{Hg} = 13.5438 \text{ g/ml at } 21°C$$
$$\rho_{Hg} = 13.5413 \text{ g/ml at } 22°C \qquad \rho_{Hg} = 13.5389 \text{ g/ml at } 23°C$$
$$\rho_{Hg} = 13.5364 \text{ g/ml at } 24°C \qquad \rho_{Hg} = 13.5340 \text{ g/ml at } 25°C$$

$$\left(\frac{13.534 \text{ g}}{\text{ml}}\right)\left(\frac{\text{kg}}{1000 \text{ g}}\right)\left(\frac{2.205 \text{ lb}}{\text{kg}}\right)\left(\frac{1000 \text{ ml}}{\text{l}}\right)\left(\frac{3.785 \text{ l}}{\text{gal}}\right)\left(\frac{7.62 \text{ gal}}{\text{ft}^3}\right) = \rho_{Hg}$$

$$\rho_{Hg} = 13.534 \text{ g/ml} = 860.76 \text{ lb/ft}^3$$

BIBLIOGRAPHY

1. *ASHRAE Handbook of Fundamentals* (1993), p. 6.1.
2. Public Health Service, *Handbook of Air Pollution*, USDHEW-PHS (Pub. No. 999-AP-44), p. 13.11.
3. *Handbook of Chemistry and Physics*, ed. Weast, R. C., 70th Edition. CRC Press, Boca Raton, FL (1989), p. F-3.

Detailed background information on the physical chemistry of gases and vapors is found in any textbook on elementary physical chemistry, college physics, or thermodynamics. The list is too long to include here. The reader is urged to review one of these classical texts for reference purposes:

1. Benson, S. W., *The Foundations of Chemical Thermodynamics*. McGraw-Hill, New York (1960).
2. Bent, Henry, *The Second Law*. Oxford University Press, New York (1965).
3. Castellan, G. W., *Physical Chemistry*. Addison-Wesley, Reading, MA (1964).
4. Daniels, F. and Alberty, R. A., *Physical Chemistry*, Second Edition. John Wiley & Sons, New York (1961).
5. Hill, Terrell L., *An Introduction to Statistical Thermodynamics*. Addison-Wesley, Reading, MA (1960).
6. Lewis, Newton and Randall, Merle, revised by K. S. Pitzer and L. Brewer, *Thermodynamics*. McGraw-Hill, New York (1961).
7. Maron, S. H. and Prutton, C. F., *Principles of Physical Chemistry*, Fourth Edition. The Macmillan Company, New York (1965).
8. Moore, Walter J., *Physical Chemistry*, Third Edition. Prentice-Hall, Englewood Cliffs, NJ (1962).
9. Sears, Francis W., *Mechanics, Heat, and Sound*. Addison-Wesley, Reading, MA (1958).

PROBLEM SET
Problem 1

Given the following data, compute the tire pressure of a car at the end of a trip from Brownsville, Texas, to Los Alamos, New Mexico.

	Brownsville	**Los Alamos**
Elevation	Sea level 0 feet	6000 feet
Atmosphere pressure	760 mm Hg	610 mm Hg
Tire temperature	27°C	67°C
Tire pressure	26 psi	???

Solution 1

The ideal gas relationship $PV = nRT$ can be written at various combinations of P, T, V as:

$$P_1 V_1 / T_1 = P_2 V_2 / T_2$$

Let condition 1 be in Brownsville and condition 2 be in Los Alamos.

$$P_1 = P_{G1} + P_{ATM1} \qquad T_1 = (27 + 273.15)\ \text{K} = 300.15\ \text{K}$$
$$P_2 = P_{G2} + P_{ATM2} \qquad T_2 = (67 + 273.15)\ \text{K} = 340.15\ \text{K}$$

Calculate P_{G2}:

$$(P_{G1} + P_{ATM1})V_1/T_1 = (P_{G2} + P_{ATM2})V_2/T_2$$

$$P_{G2} = (P_{G1} + P_{ATM1})(V_1/V_2)(T_2/T_1) - (P_{ATM2})$$

$$P_{G1} = 26 \text{ psi} \qquad P_{ATM1} = (760/760)(14.7 \text{ psi}) = 14.7 \text{ psi}$$
$$P_{G2} = x \qquad P_{ATM2} = (610/760)(14.7 \text{ psi}) = 11.8 \text{ psi}$$

Unless the tire's size changes dramatically (e.g., the tire expands like a balloon), it is safe to say that $V_1 = V_2$; therefore:

$$P_{G2} = (P_{G1} + P_{ATM1})(V_1/V_2)(T_2/T_1) - (P_{ATM2})$$

$$P_{G2} = (26 + 14.7)(340.15/300.15) \text{ psi} - 11.8 \text{ psi} =$$

$$P_{G2} = (46.1 - 11.8) \text{ psi} = 34.3 \text{ psi}$$

Problem 2

Ethyl alcohol has a molecular weight of 46.07 and a liquid density of 0.785 g/ml at 25°C. Calculate the volume occupied by one gram molecular weight of ethanol at 25°C and 760 mm Hg.

Solution 2

Given: m = 1 gram molecular weight; MW = 46.07 g/mole; $\rho = 0.785$ g/ml at NTP ethyl alcohol is a liquid (B.P. = 78°C); $1/\rho = 1.27$ ml/g. Assume one molecular weight of ethanol:

$$(46.07 \text{ g/mole})(1.27 \text{ ml/g}) = 58.5 \text{ ml/mole}$$

Problem 3

Calculate the pressure exerted by a 0.76 meter column of mercury, in Pascals.

Solution 3

A column of mercury 0.76 meter high is one atmosphere. Calculate the pressure exerted by this column. First the mass of mercury present must be determined. Assume that the column has a cross-sectional area of 1 m² in diameter. The volume of the column can be calculated:

$$V = hA = (0.76\text{m})(1\text{m}^2) = 0.76\text{m}^3$$

Given this volume and the density of mercury, it is possible to calculate the mass of mercury present in the column. Assume that the column of mercury is at a standard temperature of 298.15 K. This reading may have to be corrected for the temperature expansion of the glass column that contains it (Chapter 4). The gravity correction to the column of mercury also can be applied (Chapter 4). The density of mercury at 298.15 K is 13 534.0 kg/m^3 (Table 3-8).

Recall the definition of density: $\rho = m/v$. Then:

$$m = \rho v = (13\,534.0 \text{ kg/m}^3)(0.76 \text{ m}^3) = 10\,285.84 \text{ kg}$$

The definition of pressure as force per unit area, where force is given by Newton's law, is:

$$\text{Force} = (\text{Mass})(\text{Acceleration}) = ma$$

$$F = ma = (10\,285.84 \text{ kg})(9.807 \text{ m/s}^2) = 100\,873.2 \text{ kg m/s}^2$$

Recall that kg m/s^2 is a Newton (N). Therefore the force exerted by the mercury column is:

$$F = 100\,873.2 \text{ N}$$

Since pressure is force per unit area and the area is in m^2:

$$P = F/A = 100\,873.2 \text{ N/m}^2$$

$$P = 100\,873.2 \text{ Pa.}$$

This compares to the standard atmosphere in the SI system of 101 325 Pa. It is 0.4% low, but perhaps a temperature and gravity correction will improve this value (see Chapter 6).

Problem 4

Jane G. Student plans to fly to Destin, Florida, for a vacation during winter break. She plans to carry an inflated balloon with her and use it to measure the atmospheric pressure in the airline cabin. Make whatever assumptions you wish, including her getting past airport security and her choice of balloons, and produce an equation that can predict the relationship between the circumference of any balloon of diameter d and the pressure in an airline cabin. Commercial airline cabins are pressurized to 8000 feet above sea level.

Solution 4

Before Ms. Student boards the airplane, she will inflate the balloon only about halfway. This is essential. If the balloon is filled to capacity, its elasticity might prevent it from inflating farther as the air cabin pressure decreases. If the balloon were filled to near bursting at sea level, it could very well rupture and make an unpleasant sound at 8000 feet.

Recall that the volume of a sphere is given by:

$$V = (4/3)\pi r^3$$

$$r = D/2$$

$$r^3 = D^3/8$$

$$V = \pi D^3/6$$

Recall that the relationship between P, V, and T is:

$$P_1 V_1/T_1 = P_2 V_2/T_1 = \cdots \quad P_i V_i/T_i$$

Let 1 = at sea level condition = SL.
Let 2 = at 8000 foot elevation = EL.

$$P_{SL} V_{SL}/T_{SL} = P_{EL} V_{EL}/T_{EL}$$

$$V_{SL} = \pi D_{SL}^{3}/6$$

$$V_{EL} = \pi D_{EL}^{3}/6$$

$$P_{SL}\left(\pi D_{SL}^{3}/6\right)/T_{SL} = P_{EL}\left(\pi D_{EL}^{3}/6\right)T_{EL}$$

Assume a constant air temperature in the airline cabin at sea level (SL) and elevation (EL). Therefore:

$$T_{SL} = T_{EL}$$

Since $\pi/6$ occurs on both sides of the equation, the PV relationship becomes:

$$P_{SL} D_{SL}^{3} = P_{EL} D_{EL}^{3}$$

$$D_{EL} = (P_{SL}/P_{EL})^{1/3} D_{SL}$$

4

PRESSURE MEASUREMENTS

Outcome Competencies   *After studying this chapter you will be able to:*

- *Explain pressure and pressure measurements.*
- *Develop pressure corrections for moisture, altitude, and static pressure.*
- *Operate manometers and barometers to measure pressure.*
- *Evaluate pressure measuring devices.*
- *Evaluate Dalton's law of partial pressure.*

1. INTRODUCTION TO PRESSURE MEASUREMENTS

The pressure difference between gases in a calibration system and that of the laboratory, or between a ventilation system and its surroundings, is measured with a manometer. The atmospheric (barometric) pressure surrounding a system is measured with a barometer. The pressure difference at which these systems operate affects the volumetric flowrate moving through them. Flowrate measurements are important in all environmental quality measurements. When an air contaminant is monitored in any microenvironment (ambient, traditional and nontraditional workplaces, and indoor residential and nonresidential microenvironments), the concentration usually is expressed as a mass concentration (e.g., mass of pollutant per unit volume of air). For example:

- Measurement of respirable suspended particles in the workplace is reported in mg/m^3 (milligrams per cubic meter).

TABLE 4-1. Standard atmosphere pressure

$1.013\,25 \times 10^5$	Pascals (Pa)
101.325	kiloPascals (kPa)
29.921	inches of mercury (in Hg)
760.0	millimeters of mercury (mm Hg)
76.00	centimeters of mercury (cm Hg)
0.76	meters of mercury (mm Hg)
14.695	pounds per square inch (psi)
406.14	inches of water (in H_2O)
1.013	bars (bars)
1.0	atmospheres (atm)

- The ambient air quality standard for inhalable particles is reported in $\mu g/m^3$ (micrograms per cubic meter).
- Researchers report the concentration of highly toxic organics in air as low as fg/m^3 (femptograms per cubic meter).
- The concentration of asbestos in the air of a school building is reported as less than 0.02 f/cc (fiber/cubic centimeters).

To correctly report the volume of air sampled, use the pressure–volume relationship to correct the sampled volume to a standard condition (usually 1.0 atmosphere). Because pressure has a profound impact on the volume sampled, it must be analyzed and understood. Correcting the volume of air sampled also is essential because occupational exposure limits are normalized to a set of standard conditions. When one is comparing an individual's exposure to a health standard, the exposure and the standard must both be at the same set of conditions (760 mm Hg and 25°C). (See Table 4-1.)

2. PRESSURE

The pressure–volume (P–V) relationship is essential to predict the actual volumetric flowrate through a system. The pressure–volume relationship is the familiar ideal gas relationship, $PV = nRT$. Pressure is defined as the force exerted per unit area: $P = \text{force/unit area} = F/A$. The units of pressure are expressed as:

Newton per square meter: $N/m^2 = $ Pascal (Pa) (SI system)
millimeters of mercury: mm Hg or atmospheres (atm) (SI system, alternate)
pounds per square foot: lb/ft^2 (English system)
pounds per inch square: lb/in^2 (English system)

In the cgs system pressure is reported in dynes per square centimeter, $dyne/cm^2$. However, this system is now obsolete and will not be discussed further.

3. WORKING FLUIDS

Pressure also is indicated by the height of a working fluid in a barometer or a manometer. The pressure exerted by a column of liquid can be calculated from the barometric equation:

$$P = \rho gh$$

The most commonly used working fluid for a barometer is mercury. Other fluids can be used but are not as convenient. There are many working fluids used in a manometer (see Table 3-8).

Working fluids are selected to give reasonable changes in h (Δh) for a given pressure. The height that the working fluid will reach in a manometer or barometer is calculated from:

$$P = \rho gh$$

$$h = P/\rho g$$

where:

P = pressure
ρ = density of the working fluid
g = acceleration due to gravity
h = height of the working fluid

Because the specific gravity of mercury is more than 13 times greater than that of water the height of mercury in a barometer is more than 13 times less than it would be if water were the working fluid. The high specific gravity of mercury is an advantage, as it produces a column of mercury that is about 30 inches high as compared to a column of water that would be nearly 40 feet high if water were the working fluid. Besides, it is difficult to read a water barometer after the liquid freezes! If antifreeze is added, then a density correction for the water and antifreeze mixture must be applied.

The purpose of using a working fluid with a specific gravity 13 times greater than that of water is to produce a shorter column (e.g., 29.921 inches of Hg compared to 406.1 inches of H_2O). Similarly, gauge oil with SG of 0.826 will amplify the liquid height observed in a manometer when compared to water (e.g., 491.7 inches gauge oil vs. 406.1 inches of water). This feature is very useful when pressure readings less than one inch of water are being indicated by a manometer.

The conversion from pressure in inches of mercury to pressure in inches of water (as indicated by a manometer) is direct. The conversion is based on calculating the equivalent height of a column of mercury by adjusting that height to the specific gravity of the working fluid at the prevailing temperature. At 25°C the specific gravity of mercury is:

$$SG = (\text{density of mercury at } 25°C)/(\text{density of water at } 25°C)$$

ρ mercury at $25°C = 13.5340$ g/cc
ρ water at $25°C = 0.99707$ g/cc
760 mm Hg $= 76.00$ cm Hg $= 29.921$ in Hg

$$(29.921 \text{ in Hg})(13.5738 \text{ SG of Hg}) = 406.141 \text{ in water} = 406.1 \text{ in water}$$

Example 1

Assume that two barometers are used side by side to measure atmospheric pressure (P_{ATM}). The first barometer uses mercury as the working fluid, and the other uses water as the working fluid. Calculate the height of the water column if it is selected as the barometric working fluid and the barometric pressure is (A) 29.921 inches of mercury and (B) 760.0 mm mercury.

Solution 1A

For the mercury barometer:

$$P_{ATM1} = \rho_{Hg} g h_{Hg}$$

For the water barometer:

$$P_{ATM2} = \rho_{H_2O} g h_{H_2O}$$

Since both devices are measuring the same atmospheric pressure:

$$P_{ATM1} = P_{ATM2} = P_{ATM}$$

$$\rho_{Hg} g h_{Hg} = \rho_{H_2O} g h_{H_2O}$$

Solve for the height of the column of water, h_{H_2O}, since the acceleration due to gravity is the same on both sides of the equation:

$$\rho_{Hg} h_{Hg} = \rho_{H_2O} h_{H_2O}$$

Solving for the height of the water column:

$$h_{H_2O} = (\rho_{Hg} h_{Hg})/\rho_{H_2O}$$

Recall that specific gravity at a given temperature is:

$$SG = \rho_{FLUID}/\rho_{WATER}$$

$$SG = \rho_{Hg}/\rho_{H_2O}$$

$$h_{H_2O} = SG(h_{Hg})$$

(at 25°C)

$$\rho_{H_2O} = 0.99707 \text{ g/cm}^3$$

$$\rho_{Hg} = 13.5340 \text{ g/cm}^3$$

$$SG = \rho_{Hg}/\rho_{H_2O} = 13.5340 \text{ g/cm}^3/0.99707 \text{ g/cm}^3 = 13.5738$$

$$h_{H_2O} = SG(h_{Hg}) = (13.5738)(29.921 \text{ in Hg}) = 406.141 \text{ in H}_2O$$

Solution 1B

$$h_{H_2O} = SG(h_{Hg})$$

(at 25°C)

$$\rho_{H_2O} = 0.99707 \text{ g/cm}^3$$

$$\rho_{Hg} = 13.5340 \text{ g/cm}^3$$

$$SG = \rho_{Hg}/\rho_{H_2O} = 13.5340 \text{ g/cm}^3/0.99707 \text{ g/cm}^3 = 13.5738$$

$$h_{H_2O} = SG(h_{Hg}) = (13.5738)(760.0 \text{ mm Hg}) = 10\,316.6 \text{ mm H}_2O$$

$$h_{H_2O} = (10\,316.6 \text{ mm H}_2O)(\text{in}/25.4 \text{ mm}) = 406.144 \text{ in H}_2O \text{ at } 25°C$$

Example 2

Calculate the height of liquid in a barometer using red gauge oil as the working fluid (SG = 0.826). The atmospheric pressure is 29.01 in Hg, and the temperature is 25°C. The barometer is located on the beach in Sagaponack, New York.

Solution 2

For Hg: $P_{\text{ATM1}} = \rho_{\text{Hg}} g h_{\text{Hg}}$, $h_{\text{Hg}} = 29.01$ in Hg (given)
For oil: $P_{\text{ATM2}} = \rho_{\text{OIL}} g h_{\text{OIL}}$, h_{OIL} must be calculated
Since $P_{\text{ATM1}} = P_{\text{ATM2}} = P_{\text{ATM}}$:

$$P_{\text{Hg}} g h_{\text{Hg}} = \rho_{\text{OIL}} g h_{\text{OIL}}$$

Recall: $\text{SG} = \rho_{\text{FLUID}}/\rho_{\text{WATER}} = \rho_{\text{OIL}}/\rho_{\text{WATER}}$

Therefore to compute the density of a fluid given the specific gravity, solve the equation for ρ_{FLUID} as ρ_{OIL}:

$$\rho_{\text{OIL}} = \text{SG}(\rho_{\text{H}_2\text{O}})$$

Given that the temperature is 25°C, $\rho_{\text{H}_2\text{O}} = 0.99707$ g/cc and $\rho_{\text{Hg}} = 13.534$ g/cc. Therefore:

$$\rho_{\text{OIL}} = 0.826(0.99707 \text{ g/cc}) = 0.824 \text{ g/cc}$$

$$h_{\text{OIL}} = \rho_{\text{Hg}} h_{\text{Hg}}/\rho_{\text{OIL}}$$

$$h_{\text{OIL}} = [(13.5340 \text{ g/cc})(29.01 \text{ in Hg})]/(0.824 \text{ g/cc})$$

$$h_{\text{OIL}} = 476.5 \text{ inches of oil column}$$

Note: If the barometer were water-filled, the water column height would be 392.62 inches of water column at a P_{ATM} of 29.01 inches of mercury.

Example 3

During a calibration session the wet test meter being calibrated operates at a meter static pressure, P_{SP}, of -2.5 inches of water. Calculate the wet test meter's operating static pressure in mm Hg.

Solution 3

P_{SP} from the meter manometer $= -2.5$ inches of H_2O. Therefore:

$$P_{\text{SP}} = (-2.5 \text{ in water})(760 \text{ mm Hg}/406.141 \text{ in water}) = -4.68 \text{ mm Hg}$$

This calculation shows conversion between the various pressure units. Several atmospheric pressure standards are given in Table 4-1.

4. PRESSURE MEASUREMENT

Most air sampling methods rely on active sampling with pumps, which may move air with volumetric flowrates from cubic centimeters per minute (cm^3/min) to those as large as cubic feet per minute (cfm). Regardless of the device used to sample the air, the flowrate through the air monitor or sampling train must be calibrated against a recognized air volume flowrate measurement standard, and this requires that the system operating static pressure be known.

Regardless of the analytical techniques used or the contaminants being measured the volume of air collected must be accurately known. The volume can be determined accurately only if the operating temperature, vapor pressure, and static pressure in the system are known. The vapor pressure of the liquid (e.g., water) used in the system varies with temperature and will affect the dry air volume. The static pressure in the system is the difference between the absolute pressure in the system and the surrounding atmospheric pressure. The volume of air collected is affected by the pressure operating on the air sampling system. All pressure measuring methods have the same basic principles in common, and these will be used to correct the volumetric flowrate through the air sampling system.

Air sampling trains all contain common elements that perform similar functions. They all consist of a sampling device, a flow or volume indicator, and a pump (see Figure 4-1).

Volume or flowrate calibration of an air sampling train can be accomplished by using many techniques. The most definitive method of flowrate calibration requires the use of a primary standard volume flowrate measuring device (reference volume). Traceability to the National Institute of Standards and Technology (NIST) is achieved through the use of various standard methods.

One example of a traceable primary standard for volume is a soap bubble flow meter. This device is calibrated by measuring the mass of liquid displaced from the meter at a known temperature and density. The volume of the meter then can be calculated by using the definition of density ($v = m/\rho$). The mass of water displaced is measured by using an NIST traceable calibrated laboratory balance. A spirometer is a primary standard. The spirometer bell volume displaced is measured by using NIST traceable measuring instruments (steel tape, calipers, and thickness micrometers). A

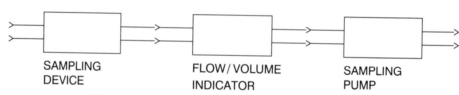

Figure 4-1. Flow diagram for an air sampling train.

Pitot tube and inclined manometer are a primary standard for measuring velocity.

Devices using wet test meters, dry gas meters and rotameters, or other variable area orifice meters, the measurement of the pressure drop across an orifice plate, and a critical orifice are examples of secondary volume flowrate standard measuring devices. They are considered secondary standards because they are calibrated with a primary standard volume-measuring device. A secondary standard is one step removed from the NIST primary standard because it depends on an indirect measurement of volume.

Several volume-measuring devices are available in an industrial hygiene laboratory. They are commonly used in the laboratory to calibrate air sampling pumps or to meter the flow of gases and vapors in various measurement and calibration situations. This discussion does not represent the universe of calibration or metering techniques or those devices available for measurements in the laboratory or the field.

The use and the calibration of all air sampling devices require a complete and detailed understanding of the effects of pressure changes on the volume flowrate as the gas moves through the system. The static pressure difference is measured with a manometer. The volume flowrate also depends on the ambient pressure measured with a barometer.

There are several methods commonly used to measure the relevant pressures for air sampling or ventilation system evaluations. The following sections describe the principles of operation of a Fortin-type barometer. Measuring a pressure difference using a liquid-filled manometer is described later in this chapter.

5. INTRODUCTION TO BAROMETERS

Barometric pressures are important in all aspects of air sampling and analysis. As the barometric pressure increases or decreases, a change occurs in the volume occupied by a sampled gas or vapor. Such changes in volume follow the ideal gas equation. The details of temperature and pressure corrections are described in Chapter 6.

6. PRINCIPLE OF OPERATION

A Fortin-type mercury barometer consists of a long glass tube, closed at one end, evacuated, filled with mercury, and inverted. The open end is submerged in a reservoir of mercury called the cistern. The mercury level in the cistern is adjustable. The column of mercury is supported in the glass tube by the atmospheric pressure acting on the mercury in the cistern. The height of the column of mercury is a measure of atmospheric pressure. Air must never be allowed to enter the barometer tube. Air in the barometer tube could cause a separation of the mercury column, causing a barometric reading to be biased high. Air could rise to the top of the column of mercury, depressing it and causing a barometric reading to be biased low. Pressure changes due to weather changes are relatively small (usually well below ± 1.0 inch of mercury) and must be measured accurately. During periods of fair weather, the barometric pressure may not change for several days. With the arrival of foul weather, however, the barometric pressure will drop markedly. Long scales are necessary to allow for different pressure levels at different elevations. When the pressure increases, the cistern level will be depressed, and mercury will rise in the glass barometer tube; when pressure falls, the opposite occurs.

7. READING BAROMETRIC PRESSURE WITH THE BAROMETER

The change in the level of the small-diameter glass barometer tube will be greater than that of the large-diameter cistern. When a reading is taken, the mercury level in the cistern is first set to the white zero pointer, and then the height of the mercury column is measured against a scale. Accuracy in setting each level is of equal importance; any setting error is directly reflected in the resulting measurement.

When the barometer is placed in a new location, the scales, brass barrel, mercury column and cistern, and glass tube must come to thermal equilibrium with the surrounding atmosphere before any measurements are attempted. The equilibrium process may take up to 24 hours. A barometer measures the local station pressure at the elevation where it is installed. This is not directly comparable to the reported "barometric pressure," which is always referenced to sea level. The barometer reading must now be corrected for temperature, gravity, and elevation (CRC Handbook).

8. INTRODUCTION TO MANOMETERS

A manometer is simply a tube, open at both ends, containing a working fluid, which is used to measure pressure difference. This pressure difference is also known as the static pressure. Some examples of static pressure measurement are:

- Between a ventilation system and the environment surrounding the system or room.
- Within an air sampling system to allow a pressure correction to the volume flowrate.
- Inside/outside a building to determine the pressure differential on a structure, etc.

The static pressure in the system, "the pressure differential," is measured at a point perpendicular to the fluid flow using a manometer. On the pressure side of a system, the system static pressure is always positive, that is, $\Delta P > O, (P_{SP} > 0)$. The placement of manometers to be used for measuring pressure differential (a negative pressure relative to the ambient) is then used to correct the volume flowrate in an air sampling system. This is depicted in Figure 4-2. Under a negative pressure differential relative to the ambient, a manometer will always indicate that the pressure in a system is less than atmospheric pressure ($< P_{ATM}$). In Figure 4-2, manometer M_1 is located on the fan inlet end of a ventilation system. This end of the system is operating at a negative static pressure as indicated by the displacement of the working fluid in manometer M_1. As the system is operating below atmospheric pressure, the ambient barometric pressure forces the working fluid in M_1 toward the lower pressure present in the system inlet to the fan. In Figure 4-2, manometer M_2 is located on the fan outlet end of the ventilation system. This end of the system is operating at a positive static pressure as indicated by the displacement of the working fluid in manometer M_2. Because the system is operating above atmospheric pressure, the higher pressure present in the system outlet duct forces the air out of the stack and the working fluid in M_2 toward the lower pressure present in the ambient environment.

Air flows from a zone of high pressure, P_{ATM}, to a zone of low pressure, P_{DUCT}, through the fan to the outlet duct. Because the outlet duct is at a pressure higher than the atmospheric pressure, the air will continue to flow from a zone of higher to lower pressure (i.e., from the room, through the duct to the fan, and out the stack).

As another example of the behavior of the working fluid in a manometer, review the apparatus flow diagram for the calibration of an air sampling

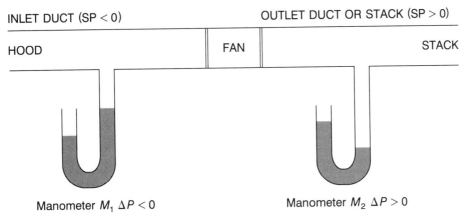

INLET DUCT (SP < 0)

OUTLET DUCT OR STACK (SP > 0)

HOOD   FAN   STACK

Manometer M_1 $\Delta P < 0$ Manometer M_2 $\Delta P > 0$

Figure 4-2. Measuring static pressures in a ventilation system.

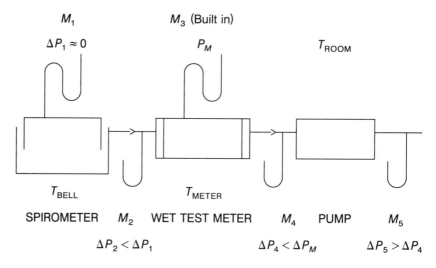

Manometers M_1, M_2, M_4, M_5 are optional. P_{ATM} is required.

Figure 4-3. Flow diagram for the calibration of an air sampling device.

device (Figure 4-3). To achieve a reliable calibration of the volumetric flowrate, the static pressure throughout the system must be measured or determined. Measuring this pressure permits correction of the volumetric flowrate from calibration conditions to normal conditions (1.0 atm or 760 mm Hg).

In the flow diagram of Figure 4-3:

- M_1 shows static pressure difference between the room and the spirometer. Ideally, $P_1 \approx 0$ and is then ignored. M_1 is *optional*.
- M_2 is upstream from the inlet to the wet test meter and measures the SP between the wet test meter and the room. M_2 is *optional*.
- M_3 shows static pressure difference between the wet test meter and the room. This is the static pressure at which the wet test meter is operating. It is built into the meter and is *required*.
- P_M is used to provide the static pressure correction to the measured atmospheric pressure.
- M_4 is downstream of the wet test meter and measures the entire static pressure loss in the system. M_4 *is optional*.
- M_5 shows the static pressure that the pump must work against at the outlet. This is the only manometer in the set that would indicate a positive static pressure. It is *optional*.

Recall that when the pressure differential is measured at a point perpendicular to the fluid flow, it is called the static pressure of the system. On the pressure side of a system, the system static pressure is always positive, that is, $\Delta P > 0$ ($P_{SP} > 0$). A $P < 0$ ($P_{SP} < 0$) implies that the pressure inside the system is less than P_{ATM}; the manometer is deflected toward the point of measurement in the system. The absolute pressure in the system, also called the actual pressure, P_{ACTUAL}, is calculated from: $P_{ACTUAL} = P_{ATM} + P_{SP}$ (note the sign of P_{SP}).

In air sampling systems and calibration procedures, it is essential for upstream and downstream pressure differences to be low enough that the pressure correction can be ignored. Chapter 6 discusses the criteria used to determine if pressure (and temperature) differences will cause unacceptable changes in volume. Both of these situations occur during an air sampling campaign, and both must be treated as described in Chapter 6.

In Figure 4-3, M_3 indicates the static pressure difference between the device being calibrated and the room. This reading is essential if one is to apply a pressure correction to the flowrate in the system. If M_3 reads less than a few inches of water static pressure, it is acceptable to ignore the pressure corrections because the static pressure differential is too small. The measurement of ΔP_3 will enable the correction of the volume flowrate of gas moving through the system at a standard pressure (1.0 atm or 760 mm Hg). If ΔP_3 is large enough, greater than -0.5 inch of mercury, then the system is moving a smaller volume flowrate than at a standard condition when $P_3 \approx 0$.

9. DALTON'S LAW

Dalton's law of partial pressure was introduced in Chapter 3. Recall:

$$P_T = P_1 + P_2 \cdots \Sigma_i P_i$$

In other words, the total pressure of a mixture of gases is equal to the sum of the partial pressures of the individual components of the mixture. In this chapter, Dalton's law is applied to the calibration of air sampling systems.

In the calibration and ventilations system discussed thus far the pressures that are measured are the input values used to correct the system's pressure to standard conditions. Note that the volume flowrate at normal conditions is a derived number because the air in a system may not be dry air (it may be a saturated air and water mixture), and the pressure in the laboratory will not, in general, be numerically equal to the standard pressure. The conditions that exist in the wet test meter will be normalized or corrected to NTP. (Dry air is assumed.) The dry air in the system is exerting its own dry air partial pressure, P_{DRY}, which can be calculated from the following equation.

$$P_{DRY} = P_D = P_{ATM} + P_{SP} - P_{VP}$$

where:

P_{DRY} = partial pressure dry air exerts in the system

P_{ATM} = atmospheric pressure measured in the laboratory during calibration

P_{SP} = static pressure at which the device being calibrated is operating

P_{VP} = vapor pressure that the water in either device is exerting

See a table of vapor pressures versus temperature.

10. ABSOLUTE PRESSURE

Absolute pressure is *never* less than zero. The absolute pressure in a system can approach zero, but for the pressure to be negative it would first have to pass through zero, which is like absolute temperature on a thermodynamic scale. It is possible to approach but not to reach absolute zero pressure. As the pressure approaches zero, the energy required to lower the pressure (i.e., move to the negative side of the coordinate axis) approaches infinity.

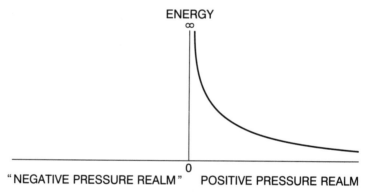

Figure 4-4. A schematic plot of pressure vs. energy.

Absolute pressure is obtained by algebraically adding gauge pressure or static pressure difference to the atmospheric or barometric pressure.

$$\text{Absolute pressure} = P_{\text{ABS}} = P_{\text{ATM}} + \Delta P_2$$
$$\text{Absolute pressure} = P_{\text{ABS}} = P_{\text{ATM}} + \text{SP}$$

that is, pounds per square inch absolute (psia).

BIBLIOGRAPHY

1. *Handbook of Chemistry and Physics*, ed. Weast, R. C., 70th edition. CRC Press, Inc., Boca Raton, FL (1989), p. E-37.

5

Gas and Vapor Concentration in Air

Outcome Competencies   *After studying this chapter you will be able to:*

- *Compute the concentration of gases in air.*
- *Compute the concentration of vapors in air.*
- *Define air at standard conditions (SI and English systems).*
- *Quote the limitations to standard air.*
- *Calculate the concentration of a gas in various containers.*
- *Calculate the concentration of a vapor resulting from a liquid spill.*
- *Validate the calibration of a continuous analyzer.*

1. INTRODUCTION

Education in basic chemistry emphasizes the study of concentrations of liquid solutions. Standard definitions used to describe the components of a liquid solution are given below:

Solution: a mixture of one or more components composed of a solvent and a solute.

Solute: the minor constituent of a solution; the impurity in a solution, for example, sodium chloride in a salt solution, sulfur dioxide in an air solution.

Solvent: the major constituent of a solution, for example, water in aqueous solution, air in a gaseous solution.

In liquid solutions, concentrations may be expressed in moles (mole: gram molecular weight) per liter or equivalents per liter. As the solutions become more dilute, approaching the infinitely dilute solution, millimoles or milliequivalents per liter units are more appropriate. The ratio of moles (mass) of solute (impurity) per volume of solvent is called molar solution; the ratio of moles (mass) of solute per mass of solvent is called molal solution. The concentration of a liquid solution is the ratio of an impurity (mass of solute or moles of solute) to the volume of pure solvent (usually but not always water). The logic used to describe liquid solutions may be expanded to gaseous solutions. For gaseous solutions (in air) the solute is the impurity and the solvent is air (also known as the diluent gas).

Concentration of gases and vapors in air can be expressed in several ways. These expressions are analogous to the methods used to express the concentration of liquid solutions, and some are more commonly used than others. Concentration is either mass- or volume-based, and can be expressed on a mass basis by the following relationships:

1. Percent of an impurity (solute) in a known mass of air (solvent), or mass fraction of an impurity (solute) in a known mass of air (solvent).
2. Mass of dissolved substance per definite mass of one of the constituents.
3. Mass of dissolved substance (solute) per total mass of the solution.
4. Number of moles of a substance in the total number of moles (mole fraction).
5. Moles of dissolved substance per 1000 grams of solvent (molal solution).

As these concentrations are based on the mass of impurity per mass of air (solvent), they are independent of temperature. Concentration also can be expressed on a volume basis by the following relationships:

1. Fractional volume (V_A) of the dissolved substance per total volume. The total volume is the volume of the solvent plus solute ($V_T = V_{solvent} + V_{solute}$); $C = (V_A/V_T)$ as a decimal fraction is not commonly used.
2. Fractional volume (V_A) of the dissolved substance per total volume. The total volume is the volume of the solvent plus solute ($V_T = V_{solvent} + V_{solute}$); $C = (V_A/V_T)10^2 = C_\%$ as a percent is commonly used, as discussed below.
3. Volume of impurity (solute) per volume of solvent (more on this later); $C = (V_A/V_B)10^2 = C_\%$ as a percent can only be used if and only if $V_A \ll V_B$.
4. Molarity or the number of moles of dissolved substance per liter of solution; $C = (moles_A/V_T)$ is not commonly used in air and industrial hygiene.

The effects of temperature and pressure on liquid solution are small and can be ignored. As the temperature and the pressure on a gaseous solution change, the volume of the solute varies at the same rate as the volume of the solvent. The equation for concentration is independent of temperature and pressure if the concentration is expressed on a volume per volume basis (e.g., ppm, ppb, etc.).

A general equation for the concentration of a contaminant (A) in a volume (B) in a static system of total volume V_T can be calculated as a decimal fraction:

$$V_T = (V_A + V_B)$$

A general equation for the concentration of a contaminant (A) in a volume (B) in a static system of total volume V_T can be calculated as a percent (%):

$$C_\% = [V_A/(V_A + V_B)]10^2$$

Percent means parts per hundred parts. Concentrations of contaminants in air rarely approach the percent level. The PEL for carbon dioxide in a dry ice plant is 1.0%. Parts per million (ppm) concentration is the range most commonly encountered in industrial hygiene. Expressing parts per million concentration is analogous to percent. Percent concentration is based on the parts of impurity per hundred parts of air plus impurity, as a decimal fraction; when the decimal fraction is multiplied by 100, a percent results. When a decimal fraction is very small, say 0.000001, it is convenient to multiply the fraction by a million (10^6). Such multiplication yields:

$[0.000001)10^1 = $ a decimal
$[0.000001)10^2 = 0.0001$ parts per hundred (%)
$[0.000001)10^6 = 1.0$ parts per million (ppm)

The use of parts per million (ppm) eliminates the need to track all the leading zeros preceding the digit "1"; report the value as 1 ppm.

There is an obvious relationship between the exponent "6" in parts per million (ppm) and the exponent "2" in percent (%). In the general case where there are i impurities present, an expression for concentration can be written as:

$$C_{\text{PPM}, A} = (V_A/\Sigma_i V_i)10^6$$

This is sometimes a difficult concept to grasp on first reading. Parts per million concentration is not something that is familiar to all; so it is summarized here for the reader's convenience. Consider the definition of percent (%), which is the volume or mass of a constituent substance A

TABLE 5-1. Equivalence between percent (%)
and parts per million (ppm)

percent (%)	parts per million (ppm)
100.0	1 000 000
10.0	100 000
1.0	10 000
0.1	1 000
0.01	100
0.001	10
0.0001	1

divided by the total volume or mass of the constituents present B:

$$C_\% = [V_A/(V_A + V_B)]10^2 \text{ (percent on a volume basis)}$$

$$C_\% = [m_A/(m_A + m_B)]10^2 \text{ (percent on a mass basis)}$$

$$C_{PPM} = [V_A/(V_A + V_B)]10^6 \text{ (parts per million on a volume basis)}$$

$$C_{PPM} = [m_A/(m_A + m_B)]10^6 \text{ (parts per million on a mass basis)}$$

If a material is pure, it can be described as 100% or 1 000 000 ppm. The relationship between percent and parts per million is demonstrated in Table 5-1.

It is critical to recognize that the same units must be used for the volume (mass) in the numerator and the denominator. An analogous situation exists in a dynamic system with gases diluted by mixing one gas stream with another gas stream or several other gas streams. This dilution can be expressed as:

$$C_{PPM, A} = [Q_A/(\Sigma_i Q_i)]10^6 \qquad i = a, b \ldots$$

where:

Q_A = flow rate of the A component in volume/unit time
Q_i = flow rate of the ith component in volume/unit time

Assume that material (A) flowing in the system is 100% pure A.

The concentration of impurity, volume V_A, in a solution with a solvent of volume V_B can be expressed as:

$$C_{PPM} = [V_A/(V_A + V_B)]10^6$$

Example 1

What is the length fraction of one inch in 16 miles?

Solution 1

To compute the length fraction requires a ratio of the lengths, both with the same units.

$$\text{Length fraction} = L(\text{in})/[L(\text{mi}) + L(\text{in})] =$$
$$\text{Length fraction} = 1 \text{ in}/(16 \text{ mi} + 1 \text{ in})$$
$$16 \text{ mi} = 16 \text{ mi}(5280 \text{ ft}/\text{mi})(12 \text{ in}/\text{ft}) = 1\,013\,760 \text{ in}$$
$$\text{Length fraction} = 1 \text{ in}/(1{,}013{,}760 \text{ in} + 1 \text{ in})$$
$$\text{Length fraction} \approx 1 \text{ in}/(1{,}013{,}760 \text{ in}) = 0.000\,000\,986$$

This is an awkward decimal fraction. Express the length fraction as a part per million as follows:

$$L_{\text{PPM}} = (\text{Length fraction})10^6 = (\text{Length inch}/\text{Length inch})10^6$$

$$L_{\text{PPM}} = (0.000\,000\,986)10^6 = 0.98 \text{ ppm} \approx 1 \text{ ppm}$$

Example 2

What is the length fraction of one inch in 16,000 miles?

Solution 2

To compute the length fraction requires a ratio of the lengths, both with the same units.

$$\text{Length fraction} = L(\text{in})/[L(\text{mi}) + L(\text{in})] =$$
$$\text{Length fraction} = 1 \text{ in}/(16\,000 \text{ mi} + 1 \text{ in})$$
$$16\,000 \text{ mi} = 16\,000 \text{ mi}(5280 \text{ ft}/\text{mi})(12 \text{ in}/\text{ft}) = 1\,013\,760\,000 \text{ in}$$
$$\text{Length fraction} = 1 \text{ in}/(1\,013\,760\,000 \text{ in} + 1 \text{ in})$$
$$\text{Length fraction} \approx 1 \text{ in}/(1\,013\,760\,000 \text{ in})$$
$$\text{Length fraction} = 0.000\,000\,000\,986$$

Express the length fraction as a part per billion as follows:

$$L_{\text{PPB}} = (\text{Length fraction})10^9 = (\text{Length inch}/\text{Length inch})10^9 =$$

$$L_{\text{PPB}} = (0.000\,000\,000\,986)10^9 = 0.986 \text{ ppb} \approx 1 \text{ ppb}$$

This technique will produce Table 5-2.

2. CONCENTRATION OF GASES AND VAPORS

The concentration of a gas in air can be expressed in many ways. The typical range is from parts per trillion by volume (from now on referred to as C_{PPT} or C_{PPTV}), up to and including concentration on a percent basis, also known

TABLE 5-2. Putting fractional units into perspective

Examples of 1 part per million	
Time	1 min in 2 years
Length	1 in in 16 miles
Weight	1 peanut M&M® out of 1 ton of chocolate M&Ms®
Area	1 sq ft in 23 acres, or 1 postage stamp compared to 4 copies of *The New York Times*, Sunday edition
Volume	1 drop in 185 cans of a soft drink
Quantity	1 bad byte in a 1 megabyte floppy disk
Events	1 swing in 10 seasons of professional baseball
Action	Tying the last knot in a 6 ft by 6 ft Kasha Persian rug

Examples of 1 part per billion	
Time	1 min in 32 years
Length	1 inch in 16,000 miles
Weight	1 peanut M&M® out of 1000 tons of chocolate M&Ms®
Area	1 sq ft in 36 sq miles or 1 period at the end of a sentence in *The New York Times*, Sunday edition
Volume	1 drop of liquid in 185,000 cans of a soft drink
Quantity	1 bad byte in a 1000 megabyte hard drive
Events	1 sour note in a lifetime of industrial rock and roll concerts
Action	burning 1 lb of household waste during 1 year of continuous operation of a 1500 ton per day municipal incinerator

Examples of 1 part per trillion	
Time	1 min in 320 centuries
Length	500 ft in the distance between the earth and the sun
Weight	1 M&M® out of 1 million tons of M&Ms®
Area	1 sq ft in 36,000 sq mi, or 1 period at the end of a sentence in 50 years of *The New York Times*, Sunday edition
Volume	1 drop of liquid in 185 million cans of a soft drink
Quantity	1 bad byte in 1000 1 gigabyte hard drives
Events	Adding 2 qt of oil to a car engine compared to the total crude oil production of the United States in 1994
Action	Spending 1 penny compared to the total copper production of the United States in 1994

as parts per hundred (referred to as $C_\%$). These concentrations can be calculated using the following expressions:

$$C_\% = \left[V_A/(V_A + V_B)\right]10^2 \qquad C_{\mathrm{PPM}} = \left[V_A/(V_A + V_B)\right]10^6$$

$$C_{\mathrm{PPB}} = \left[V_A/(V_A + V_B)\right]10^9 \qquad C_{\mathrm{PPT}} = \left[V_A/(V_A + V_B)\right]10^{12}$$

In the general case of i components in a mixture, the concentration of the ith component can be expressed as C_i:

$$C_i = \left[V_A/(V_A + V_B + \cdots + V_i)\right]10^j$$

where:

V_A = volume of the contaminant gas or vapor (solute)
V_B = volume of the container (bag, chamber, room, gas cell), the volume of air (diluent gas) added to a nonrigid container.
V_i = volume of the ith contaminant gas or vapor (solute)

The concentration of a gas in a mixture may be expressed as partial volume, partial pressure, flowrate, mass, number of molecules, or mole fraction (see Table 5-3).

The data in Table 5-3 may be summarized as shown in Table 5-4. The equations have various forms, depending on the values of j, which may vary from 0 to n. The typical range of values for j is 2, 3, 6, 9, 12, 15 (percent, %, to parts per quintillion, ppq). If $j = 2$, $k = \%$; if $j = 6$, $k =$ ppm; if $j = 9$, $k =$ ppb; if $j = 12$, $k =$ ppt.

Table 5-5 summarizes the expressions for various values of j.

The concentration of a gas or vapor in air, in a binary solution (two components A and B), may be determined by using the following equation:

$$C_k = [V_A/(V_A + V_B)]10^j$$

where:

V_A = volume of the contaminant, impurity gas or vapor, etc.
V_B = volume of air sampled, the dilution volume, room volume, chamber volume, etc.

Table 5-6 presents a summary of this calculation.

As noted earlier, in Examples 1 and 2, if the volume of a component, that is, component $A(V_A)$, is much smaller than that of component $B(V_B)$, the equation may be simplified. By applying this observation to the equation for C_k, it is possible to derive an expression that approximates the concentration. If V_A is small relative to V_B, the expressions for concentration may be rewritten as:

$$C_\% = (V_A/V_B)10^2 \qquad C_{PPB} = (V_A/V_B)10^9$$

$$C_{PPM} = (V_A/V_B)10^6 \qquad C_{PPT} = (V_A/V_B)10^{12}$$

In the general case:

$$C_k = (V_A/V_B)10^j$$

Table 5-7 demonstrates that the approximate method for calculating concentration is reasonable if the impurity (solute) is at a concentration less than 0.5% (5000 ppm).

TABLE 5-3. Concentration of gases, C_k, in a multicomponent mixture

Basis	Unit	Symbol, k	Formula
Volume	decimal	—	$V_j/\Sigma V_i$
Volume	percent	%	$(V_j/\Sigma V_i)10^2$
Volume	ppthousand	‰	$(V_j/\Sigma V_i)10^3$
Volume	ppm	ppm	$(V_j/\Sigma V_i)10^6$
Volume	ppb	ppb	$(V_j/\Sigma V_i)10^9$
Volume	ppt	ppt	$(V_j/\Sigma V_i)10^{12}$
Pressure	decimal	—	$P_j/\Sigma P_i$
Pressure	percent	%	$(P_j/\Sigma P_i)10^2$
Pressure	ppthousand	‰	$(P_j/\Sigma P_i)10^3$
Pressure	ppm	ppm	$(P_j/\Sigma P_i)10^6$
Pressure	ppb	ppb	$(P_j/\Sigma P_i)10^9$
Pressure	ppt	ppt	$(P_j/\Sigma P_i)10^{12}$
Flowrate	decimal	—	$Q_j/\Sigma Q_i$
Flowrate	percent	%	$(Q_j/\Sigma Q_i)10^2$
Flowrate	ppthousand	‰	$(Q_j/\Sigma Q_i)10^3$
Flowrate	ppm	ppm	$(Q_j/\Sigma Q_i)10^6$
Flowrate	ppb	ppb	$(Q_j/\Sigma Q_i)10^9$
Flowrate	ppt	ppt	$(Q_j/\Sigma Q_i)10^{12}$
Mass	decimal	—	$m_j/\Sigma m_i$
Mass	percent	%	$(m_j/\Sigma m_i)10^2$
Mass	ppthousand	‰	$(m_j/\Sigma m_i)10^3$
Mass	ppm	ppm	$(m_j/\Sigma m_i)10^6$
Mass	ppb	ppb	$(m_j/\Sigma m_i)10^9$
Mass	ppt	ppt	$(m_j/\Sigma m_i)10^{12}$
Molecules	decimal	—	$N_j/\Sigma N_i$
Molecules	percent	%	$(N_j/\Sigma N_i)10^2$
Molecules	ppthousand	‰	$(N_j/\Sigma N_i)10^3$
Molecules	ppm	ppm	$(N_j/\Sigma N_i)10^6$
Molecules	ppb	ppb	$(N_j/\Sigma N_i)10^9$
Molecules	ppt	ppt	$(N_j/\Sigma N_i)10^{12}$
Mole	decimal	—	$n_j/\Sigma n_i$
Mole	%	%	$(n_j/\Sigma n_i)10^2$
Mole	ppthousand	‰	$(n_j/\Sigma n_i)10^3$
Mole	ppm	ppm	$(n_j/\Sigma n_i)10^6$
Mole	pphm	pphm	$(n_j/\Sigma n_i)10^8$
Mole	ppb	ppb	$(n_j/\Sigma n_i)10^9$
Mole	ppt	ppt	$(n_j/\Sigma n_i)10^{12}$

Based on Butcher, S. S. and Carlson, R. J., *Introduction to Air Chemistry*, p. 212.

TABLE 5-4. Various fractional techniques for computing the concentration (C_k) of gases and vapors in a mixture

Basis of calculation	Symbol	Equation
Partial volume	V_k	$(V_j/\Sigma V_i)10^j$
Partial pressure	P_k	$(P_j/\Sigma P_i)10^j$
Quantity flowrate	Q_k	$(Q_j/\Sigma Q_i)10^j$
Mass	m_k	$(m_j/\Sigma m_i)10^j$
Molecules	N_k	$(N_j/\Sigma N_i)10^j$
Moles	X_k	$(n_j/\Sigma n_i)10^j$

$j = 2, 3, 6, 12, 15, 18 \ldots n$: k = %, ppm, ppb, ppt, ppq, etc.
i = number of components in the system

TABLE 5-5. Explanation of the values of j in Table 5-4

j value	Decimal fraction	Expressed in parts per...	Symbol (k)	Alternative expressions	Notes
0	1	—	—	—	
1	0.1	—	—	—	
2	0.01	hundred	%	1.0 pph	1
3	0.001	thousand	‰ ppht	1000 ppm	2
4	10^{-4}	ten thousand	—	100 ppm	
5	10^{-5}	hundred thousand	ppht	10 ppm	
6	10^{-6}	million	ppm	1000 ppb	
7	10^{-7}	—	—	0.1 ppm	
8	10^{-8}	hundred million	pphm	0.01 ppm	
9	10^{-9}	billion	ppb	0.001 ppm	
10	10^{-10}	—	—	0.1 ppb	
11	10^{-11}	hundred billion	pphb	0.01 ppb	2
12	10^{-12}	trillion	ppt	0.001 ppb	
13	10^{-13}	—	—	0.1 ppt	
14	10^{-14}	hundred trillion	—	0.01 ppt	
15	10^{-15}	quintillion	ppq	0.001 ppt	3
18	10^{-18}	attillion	ppa	0.001 ppq	3

1. The % symbol is used, not pph.
2. The ‰ (ppht) and pphb symbols are not commonly used.
3. Proposed abbreviation.

TABLE 5-6. Summary of concentration calculations: $C_k = [V_A/(V_A + V_B)]10^j$

$C_\%$	C_{PPM}	C_{PPB}	C_{PPT}
0.0001	1	1 000	1 000 000
0.001	10	10 000	10 000 000
0.01	100	100 000	100 000 000
0.1	1 000	1 000 000	1 000 000 000
0.5	5 000	5 000 000	5 000 000 000
1.0	10 000	10 000 000	10 000 000 000
10.0	100 000	100 000 000	100 000 000 000
100.0	1 000 000	1 000 000 000	1 000 000 000 000

Based on G. O. Nelson, *Controlled Test Atmospheres*.

TABLE 5-7. Summary of concentration calculations: $C_k = (V_A/V_B)10^j$

$C_\%$	C_{PPM}	C_{PPB}	C_{PPT}
0.0001000001	1.000001	1 000.001	1 000 001.
0.0010001	10.0001	10 000.100	10 000 100.
0.010001	100.01	100 010.	100 010 000.
0.1001	1 001.	1 001 000.	1 001 000 000.
0.5025	5 025.	5 025 000.	5 025 000 000.
1.010	10 101.	10 101 000.	101 010 000 000.
11.11	111 100.	111 100 000.	111 100 000 000.

Based on G. O. Nelson, *Controlled Test Atmospheres.*

3. GAS AND VAPOR CONCENTRATION AND IDEAL GASES

There is a basic assumption underlying gas and vapor calculations in industrial hygiene and air pollution: gases and vapors in air behave as ideal gases. At first this may appear to be an unreasonable statement. The concentration of contaminant is low, and the air can be described as an infinitely dilute solution of the contaminant gas or vapor. An infinitely dilute solution implies that the individual molecules of gases and vapors are separated by a sufficient distance that the interaction between the contaminant molecules is minimized.

The summary of concentration calculations given in Table 5-7 demonstrates that ignoring the volume of impurity in comparison to the dilution volume yields only a one percent error at 10,000 ppm (approximately calculated as 10 101 ppm).

4. CONCENTRATION IN PARTS PER MILLION AND MILLIGRAMS PER CUBIC METER

Industrial hygiene calculations often require conversion of concentration expressed as a volume per volume (ppm, ppb, ppt, etc.) and mass per volume (mg/m^3, μg/m^3, ng/m^3, etc.). A basic equation can be derived by combining the equation for C_{PPM}, C_{PPB}, and so on with the ideal gas law to calculate the concentration of an impurity in air on a mass per unit volume. Recall the ideal gas law, $PV_A = n_A RT$, where n_A is the number of moles of impurity, A:

$$n_A = (\text{mass of } A/\text{molecular weight of } A) = m_A/M_A$$

Solving the ideal gas equation for V_A gives:

$$V_A = n_A RT/P = m_A RT/M_A P$$

where V_A is the gas or vapor volume of component A. Substituting the ideal gas equation for V_A into the equation for gas concentration, on a volume per volume basis, where V_B is a *fixed volume* gives:

$$C_k = (V_A/V_B)10^j = (m_A RT/M_A PV_B)10^j$$

$$C_{PPM} = (V_A/V_B)10^6 = (m_A RT/M_A PV_B)10^6$$

The ratio of m_A/V_B is the mass of the impurity A in the dilution volume B. This is also the mass concentration per unit volume ($C_{M/V}$). Substituting ($m_A/V_B = C_{M/V}$) into the equation for concentration in parts per million (parts per billion, etc.):

$$C_{PPM} = (m_A RT/M_A PV_B)10^6 = (C_{M/V})(RT/M_A P)10^6$$

By specifying the normal temperature and pressure (NTP) or the standard temperature (STP) as given in Table 5-8, the conversion between volume per volume concentration and mass per volume concentration basis can be accomplished. Table 5-8 lists two sets of standard conditions: NTP, used in industrial hygiene and ambient air pollution, and STP, used in basic science, which is provided only for reference purposes.

The concentration conversion equations that results when NTP is specified are summarized in Table 5-9. Similar equations for the concentration in parts per billion (ppb) and parts per trillion (ppt) also are included.

Now that the mystery has been taken out of the relevant equations used to calculate the concentration of gases and vapors in air, the following examples will demonstrate how to apply these techniques in useful and productive ways.

TABLE 5-8. Normal conditions (NTP) for industrial hygiene and air pollution and standard conditions (STP) for basic science

Parameter	NTP	STP
Temperature	25°C = 298.15 K	0°C = 273.15 K
Pressure	1 atm, 101 325 Pa	1 atm 101 325 Pa
Dry air	28.96 g/mole	28.96 g/mole

TABLE 5-9. Summary of the conversion of concentration between volume per volume and mass per volume

	NTP	STP
C_{PPM}	24.45 l/mole $(C_{mg/m^3}/M_A)10^6$	22.4 l/mole $(C_{mg/m^3}/M_A)10^6$
C_{PPB}	24.45 l/mole $(C_{\mu g/m^3}/M_A)10^9$	22.4 l/mole $(C_{\mu g/m^3}/M_A)10^9$
C_{PPT}	24.45 l/mole $(C_{ng/m^3}/M_A)10^{12}$	22.4 l/mole $(C_{ng/m^3}/M_A)10^{12}$

The ACGIH (see Bibliography) recommends the conversion between TLVs in part per million by volume (ppm_V) and TLVs in milligram per cubic meter (mg/m^3) as:

$$TLV(ppm) = TLV(mg/m^3)(24.45)/Molec.\ wt.$$

$$TLV(mg/m^3) = TLV(ppm)(Molec.\ wt.)/24.45$$

The conversion equations, while appearing different from those listed in Table 5-9, are actually identical to them. The ACGIH has eliminated the "complication" of the units conversion and the need for 10^6 for converting units of grams to milligrams and liters to cubic meters. When converting from concentrations that are expressed in ppb, ppt, and so on, one must be careful when using the ACGIH equation. Using the methods outlined in this section (with all the units conversion factors) will assure the correct conversion.

Example 3

The ACGIH TLV for carbon dioxide is 5 000 ppm. Calculate the equivalent concentration in milligrams per cubic meter at NTP.

Solution 3

MW of carbon dioxide (CO_2) = 12.00(1) + 16.00(2) = 44.0 g/mole

$$C_{PPM} = 5\,000\ ppm$$

$$C_{M/V} = C_{PPM} M_A (P/RT) 10^{-6}$$

$$C_{M/V} = \frac{(5\,000\ ppm)(44.0\ g/mole)(1\ atm)}{(0.08205\ l\ atm/mole\ K)(298.15\ K)} 10^{-6}$$

$$C_{M/V} = 8\,998\ mg/m^3$$

$$TLV(mg/m^3) = TLV(ppm)(Molec.\ wt.)/24.45$$

$$TLV(mg/m^3) = 5\,000\ ppm(44.0)/24.45 = 8\,998\ mg/m^3$$

Example 4

The ACGIH TLV for toluene-2,4-diisocyanate (TDI) is 0.036 mg/m^3. Calculate the equivalent concentration in parts per billion at NTP.

Solution 4

Molecular weight of TDI $= CH_3C_6H_3(NCO)_2 = C_9H_6N_2O_2$
Molecular weight of TDI $= 12.00(9) + 1.008(6) + 14.00(2) + 16.00(2) = 174.1$
g/mole

$$C(\mu g/m^3) = C_{PPB}[M/(24.45 \text{ liter/mole})]10^{-9}$$
$$C(\mu g/m^3) = C_{PPB}[M/(24.45 \text{ liter/mole})]10^{-9}$$
$$C_{PPB} = (C_{\mu g/m^3} RT/M_A PV_B)10^9$$

$$C_{PPB} = \frac{(36 \ \mu g/m^3)(0.082 \ l \ atm/mole \ K)(298.15 \ K)}{(174.1 \ g/mole)(1.0 \ atm)} 10^9 = 5.0 \text{ ppb}$$

$$TLV(ppm) = TLV(mg/m^3)(24.45)/\text{Molec. wt.}$$

$$TLV(ppm) = (0.036)(24.45)/174.1 = 0.005 = 5.0 \text{ ppb}$$

Anyone using the equations listed by the ACGIH to convert between volume per volume and mass per volume concentration must remember that the conversion is valid only at NTP. If a conversion at other than NTP is needed, the molar volume (24.45) must be corrected to the prevailing temperature. Using the equations developed in this chapter, while requiring somewhat more effort, does not require remembering to convert the molar volume to NTP. The general form of the equation is self-correcting to any temperature and pressure owing to the term RT/P in the equation.

Example 5

Derive an equation to calculate the mass per volume equivalent concentration for 1 ppm, and convert a concentration of one part per million (1 ppm) toluene, formaldehyde, benzene, methyl cellosolve acetate, and acetone to milligrams per cubic meter (mg/m³). Compare the calculated values to the NIOSH *Pocket Guide to Chemical Hazards* (DHHS 90-117) and the ACGIH TLV list. (See Table 5-10.)

Solution 5

$$C_{PPM} = [(C_{M/V} RT)/MP]10^6$$

Solving this equation for $C_{M/V}$ yields:

$$C_{M/V} = C_{PPM}(MP)(10^6)/(RT)$$

TABLE 5-10. Example 5 comparison

Chemical name	Empirical formula	Molecular weight (g/mole)	Equivalent Concentration 1 ppm = ---mg/m³		
			Calculated	ACGIH (1992)	NOISH (1990)
Toluene	$C_6H_5CH_3$	92.13	3.77	3.76	3.83
Formaldehyde	CH_2O	30.04	1.23	1.23	NA
Benzene	C_6H_6	78.12	3.19	3.20	3.25
Methyl cellosolve acetate (EGMEA)	$C_5H_{10}O_5$	118.13	4.83	4.80	4.91
Acetone	C_3H_6O	58.05	2.38	2.37	2.42

Note: The mass concentration values (mg/m³) do not agree with the NIOSH *Pocket Guide to Chemical Hazards* (DHHS 90-117) or editions of the ACGIH TLV booklet published before 1990. Conditions other than normal temperature and pressure (25°C and 1 atmosphere) were used in developing the ACGIH values before 1990. In 1990 the ACGIH TLV committee recalculated all of the equivalent ppm vs. mg/m³ concentrations using the methods specified in this book. The NIOSH *Pocket Guide* specifies 68°F and one atmosphere; hence the difference.

Let $C_{PPM} = 1$ ppm

$$C_{M/V} = 1 \text{ ppm}(MP)(10^{-6})/(RT)$$

Specify a temperature and pressure, i.e., NTP:

$$C_{M/V} = 1 \text{ ppm}(M)(10^{-6})/(24.45 \text{ l/mole})$$

5. CALCULATING THE CONCENTRATION OF VAPORS IN AIR

A vapor is a liquid at room temperature; the vapor form is produced when a solvent (i.e., a liquid at room temperature) evaporates. Applying the ideal gas equation with a few assumptions, it is possible to calculate the concentration of a vapor in air. A solution of a vapor in air exists as an infinitely dilute solution. The vapor molecules are free of any interactions with themselves and the other molecules that constitute air. Working within this constraint, it is possible to calculate the concentration of the vapor in air using the ideal gas law.

Assume that A is a liquid at NTP with vapor pressure greater than about 10^{-3} mm Hg. It is possible to calculate the concentration that this liquid produces when it evaporates into a chamber of volume V_B. The chamber can be rigid, with a geometric volume V_B, or a bag filled to a volume V_B. Solve the ideal gas equation for the volume V_A as follows:

$$V_A = nRT/P = mRT/MP$$

The density of a liquid (expressed as ρ_L) that evaporates to become a vapor is given by:

$$\rho_L = \text{mass of the liquid/volume of the liquid}$$

$$\rho_L = m_L/V_L$$

The conservation of mass can be used to demonstrate that the mass of a vapor is equal to the mass of the liquid. In fact, $m_L = m_V = m_S$. The mass of material present does not change with the change in state of the material. Because of the conservation of mass, m in the ideal gas equation is the same mass as occurs in the density relationship ($\rho = m/v$). It is therefore possible to rewrite the ideal gas equation for V_A as:

$$V_A = mRT/PM = m_L RT/MP$$

This equation predicts the vapor volume (V_A) that will exist at a specified temperature and pressure when the mass of vapor present is equal to the mass of the liquid (m_L). Note: $m_L = m_G = m_V$ because of the conservation of mass during a phase change.

$$V_A = m_L RT/MP$$

The definition of density of a liquid (solid, vapor, or gas) is given by the mass of the material per unit volume of that material, all in the same physical state. The definition of the density of a liquid is given by:

$$\rho_L = m_L/V_L$$

This equation can be solved for m_L as:

$$m_L = \rho_L V_L$$

Substituting this expression for m_L into the equation for V_A gives:

$$V_A = m_L RT/MP$$

$$V_A = (\rho_L V_L RT/MP) = V_A$$

This equation permits the calculation of the concentration that a vapor will produce if it has a liquid density of ρ_L and a liquid volume of V_L and evaporates into a volume V_B. When the vapor volume is identified as V_A ($V_A = m_L RT/MP = \rho_L V_L RT/MP$) and substituted into the equation for concentration, it results in the following expression:

$$C_{PPM} = (V_A/V_B)10^6 = (\rho_L V_L RT/MPV_B)10^6$$

TABLE 5-11. Concentration of volatile liquids in air

	NTP	STP
C_{PPM}	24.45 l/mole ($\rho_L V_L/M_A V_B$)10^6	22.4 l/mole ($\rho_L V_L/M_A V_B$)10^6
C_{PPB}	24.45 l/mole ($\rho_L V_L/M_A V_B$)10^9	22.4 l/mole ($\rho_L V_L/M_A V_B$)10^9
C_{PPT}	24.45 l/mole ($\rho_L V_L/M_A V_B$)10^{12}	22.4 l/mole ($\rho_L V_L/M_A V_B$)10^{12}

This equation predicts the part per million concentration of vapor in air, given that the mass of liquid is m_L and the vapor follows the ideal gas equation. The liquid evaporates, producing a vapor volume V_A in an air volume V_B or a rigid chamber with a geometric volume V_B. The equation for concentration in ppm (C_{PPM}) can be solved for any of the variables (density, liquid volume, molecular weight, pressure, or dilution volume). Solutions to some of these variables will be demonstrated throughout this chapter. Table 5-11 is a summary of the calculation of concentration of a vapor in air, in ppm, ppb, and ppt at NTP and STP based on the density of the liquid, ρ_L.

Example 6

If one gallon of toluene, specific gravity of 0.86 and molecular weight of 92.1 g/mole, spills in a room 60 feet by 30 feet by 15 feet, what is the concentration in ppm of toluene present in this room?

Solution 6

As the temperature and pressure are not explicitly given in the problem, it is reasonable to assume a temperature and pressure, that is, 25°C and 1 atmosphere, NTP. It is also assumed that all of the liquid is evaporated, and there is no ventilation into or out from the space.

$$SG_L \equiv \rho_L/\rho_W$$

$\rho_L = SG_L(\rho_W)$, at 25°C, $\rho_W = 0.99707$ g/ml ≈ 1 g/ml. Toluene ($SG_L = 0.86$) has a liquid density of 0.86 g/ml at 25°C.

$$C_{PPM} = (V_A/V_B)10^6 = (\rho_L V_L RT/MPV_B)10^6$$

$C_{PPM} =$

$$\frac{(0.86 \text{ g/ml})(1 \text{ gal})(3.785 \text{ liter/gal})(10^3 \text{ ml/liter})(0.082 \text{ l atm/mole deg K})(298.15 \text{ K})10^6}{(92.1 \text{ g/mole})(1 \text{ atm})(27\,000 \text{ ft}^3)(28.32 \text{ l/ft}^3)}$$

$C_{PPM} = 1\,130$ ppm

6. PREPARATION OF KNOWN ATMOSPHERES

The preparation of known concentrations of a gas or a vapor in air is an essential technique in industrial hygiene and air pollution monitoring, using the equations developed in the previous section. A solution of a known concentration of a gas or a vapor in air may be used for:

- Multipoint calibration of continuous monitors.
- Respirator cartridge breakthrough testing.
- Permeability testing of personal protective clothing and glove materials.
- Toxicological exposure studies.
- Definitive testing of new or modified air sampling and analysis techniques.
- Single point calibration of detector tubes.

Multipoint instrument calibration also may be achieved by the techniques outlined below:

- Using a commercially prepared calibration gas mixture.
- Preparing a dynamic dilution of a test gas using flow dilution techniques.
- Drawing a sample of known concentration from a rigid chamber.

The calculation techniques needed to prepare known concentrations are based on an understanding of the ideal gas equation and the concentration calculation techniques discussed in this chapter. Recall the concentration equation:

$$C_{PPM} = (V_A/V_B)10^6$$

where V_A is the volume of the impurity gas or vapor present in the chamber or bag, and V_B is the volume of the chamber or the volume of gas added to the bag.

With a plastic bag, V_B is the volume of air or other diluent gas that is delivered to the bag. The volume, V_B, is determined by multiplying the flowrate of diluent gas and the time over which the bag was filled. If the container is rigid, then the volume, V_B, is the geometric volume (the geometric volume at one atmosphere pressure). If the mass of a liquid, m_L ($m_L = \rho_L V_L$), is injected into a bag and filled with a volume of air equal to V_B or injected into a rigid container of geometric volume V_B, the concentration of A (in ppm) is:

$$C_{PPM} = (\rho_L V_L RT/MPV_B)10^6$$

By solving the above equation for V_L, it is possible to calculate the volume of liquid (V_L) necessary to prepare a known concentration:

$$V_L = C_{PPM}(MPV_B)(10^{-6})/(\rho_L RT)$$

7. CALIBRATION OF A CONTINUOUS MONITOR

Assume that an air sampling instrument with large internal sample volume is going to be calibrated using a known concentration of a gas or a vapor, and the calibration gas or vapor is prepared in the laboratory. A few precautions are necessary to ensure that the concentrations being used to prepare a multipoint calibration curve are in fact the same concentrations that are calculated using the techniques discussed above. This is a consideration with continuous monitors using nondestructive flow through measuring techniques. When this occurs, the monitor's volume must be added to the volume of the chamber or bag used to prepare the calibration mixture. All the principles outlined in this section can be applied to this situation, as demonstrated in Figure 5-1.

A calibration gas is prepared in a chamber or bag according to the equation:

$$C_{\text{PPM}} = (V_A/V_B)10^6$$

where:

V_A = volume of the pollutant gas or vapor used to prepare the standard

V_B = volume of the calibration chamber or diluent air volume used to fill the bag

The concentration in parts per million, C_{PPM}, will be diluted when the flow system pump blends the sample cell volume, V_{CELL}, with the calibration chamber volume, V_B. The resulting concentration becomes:

$$C_{\text{PPM}} = [V_A/(V_{\text{CELL}} + V_B)]10^6$$

If V_{CELL} is much less than V_B, that is, $V_{\text{CELL}} \leq 0.01V_B$, this correction is not necessary. If there is a doubt about the effect of instrument sample cell dilution, this effect can be calculated, and if necessary a volume dilution correction can be applied.

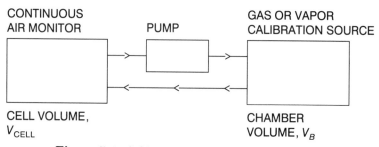

Figure 5-1. Calibration of a continuous monitor.

Example 7

An 85 liter indoor air sample is collected in a Tedlar bag in the crawl space of a building built on an old municipal dump. There is a suspicion that methylene chloride vapor may be seeping into the building. The temperature is 32°F and the pressure is 767.6 millimeters of mercury. The expanded bag is returned to the laboratory for analysis and allowed to equilibrate to 25°C and 760 millimeters of mercury. One milliliter of the sample is withdrawn from the bag with a gastight syringe. The mass of methylene chloride in the 1 ml aliquot is 28 μg. Calculate the concentration in parts per million by volume (ppm) methylene chloride in the air sample at the time of sampling.

Solution 7

Field conditions: 32°F (273.15 K) and 767.6 mm Hg.
Bag volume: 85 liters
Assume that the bag is filled to capacity in the field.
Laboratory conditions: 25°C (298.15 K) and 29.921 inches of mercury
Molecular weight of methylene chloride $(CH_2Cl_2) = M$

$$M = 12.011(1) + 1.0079(2) + 35.45(2) = 84.9 \text{ g/mole}$$

$$C_{M/V} = (28 \ \mu g/ml)(mg/1000 \ \mu g)(1000 \ ml/l)(1000 \ l/m^3)$$

$$C_{M/V} = 28\,000 \text{ mg/m}^3$$

$$C_{PPM} = (C_{M/V})(RT/MP)10^6$$

$$C_{PPM} = \frac{(28\,000 \text{ mg/m}^3)(0.08205 \text{ l atm/mole K})(298.15 \text{ K})}{(84.9 \text{ g/mole})(1 \text{ atm})}$$

$$C_{PPM} = 8064 \text{ ppm}$$

Alternate Solution 7

Recall:

$$P_1V_1/T_1 = P_2V_2/T_2$$

$$P_FV_F/T_F = P_LV_L/T_L$$

where F = field and L = laboratory.

$$V_L = V_F(P_F/P_L)(T_L/T_F)$$

$$V_L = (85 \text{ l})(767.6/760.0)(298.15/273.15)$$

$$V_L = 93.7 \text{ liters}$$

A 1 ml sample from the bag has 28 μg CH_2Cl_2, and the total mass of CH_2Cl_2 present in the 93.7 liter is:

$$\text{Total mass } CH_2Cl_2 = (93.7\ l)(28\ \mu g/ml)(10^3\ ml/l)(mg/10^3\ \mu g) = 2624\ mg$$

$$C_{M/V} = (2624\ mg/93.7\ l)(10^3\ l/m^3) = 28\,002\ mg/m^3$$

$$C_{M/V} = (28\ \mu g/ml)(1000\ ml/l)(1000\ l/m^3)(mg/1000\ \mu g)$$

$$C_{M/V} = 28\,000\ mg/m^3$$

$$C_{PPM} = (C_{M/V})(RT/MP)10^6$$

$$C_{PPM} = \frac{(28\,000\ mg/m^3)(0.08205\ l\ atm/mole\ K)(298.15\ K)}{(84.9\ g/mole)(1\ atm)}$$

$$C_{PPM} = 8064\ ppm$$

8. AIR SAMPLING CONTAINERS

Flexible and rigid containers of various nonreactive polymeric materials and glasses may be used to collect air samples for laboratory analysis or to contain gas and vapor solutions used to calibrate air sampling instruments. Nonreactive polymeric bags may be made of a single plastic layer or multiple layers of plastic and aluminum foil. The foil layer prevents the migration of gases and vapors through the polymeric materials, and improves the sample stability and longevity. It is important that the material used to contain an air sample (either bags or rigid chambers) not react with the sample in any way that will alter the concentration of the gas or vapor being collected, analyzed, or prepared. Reactions include adsorption on the walls of the chamber or chemical reactions with the surface material. It is equally important that the chamber not outgas materials that may contaminate the contents of the air sample. Outgassing can be controlled by aging the chamber and flushing dry nitrogen through it to enhance the outgassing before any test gases or vapors are added. If a pump is used to fill the bag or chamber or to flush the chamber, the active part of the pump that comes into contact with the gas or vapor stream *must also be nonreactive*. The active part of the pump *must not* add unwanted material to the container environment. Sampling pumps are always used to collect samples *upstream* from the pump inlet. Some air sampling pumps may use oil to lubricate moving pump parts. The oil is released and can become a contaminant on the chamber's walls. Smaller personal air sampling pumps contain moving parts that are elastomeric materials that can adsorb gases and vapors or emit previously sorbed material. To control these situations, background levels of potential contaminants must be determined.

9. AIR SAMPLING WITH BAGS

To determine the concentration of a pollutant in air integrated over time, a sample is drawn into an air sampling bag at a uniform rate for the desired sampling time. The concentration may be determined by measuring the pollutant mass, m_A, and dividing it by the volume of air sample collected in the bag, V_B. If the contents of the bag are well mixed, it often is adequate to withdraw only a small portion (an aliquot) of the bag contents with an uncontaminated, nonreactive, gastight syringe or a gas sampling loop, and then analyze the contents of the syringe using an appropriate analytical method. The calculated concentration in the syringe will be the same as that in the bag or in the air sampled if there has been no contamination or dilution of the sample between transfers, and if all operations have been conducted at the same temperature and pressure in a chamber or bag that is nonreactive.

Bag samples are collected at the temperature and pressure in the field (T_F and P_F) and brought to the laboratory, where they come to equilibrium at the prevailing laboratory temperature and pressure (T_L and P_L). During equilibration, the volume of the sample collected in the field, V_F, changes to V_L according to the ideal gas law:

$$P_F V_F / T_F = P_L V_L / T_L$$

$$V_L = V_F (P_F / P_L)(T_L / T_F)$$

(1)

The mass of the gas (or the masses of the components of a mixture of gases) is independent of temperature and pressure and does not change. Therefore, C_L, the mass concentration of the pollutant in the chamber or bag at laboratory conditions T_L, P_L, is C_L ($C_L = m/V_L$) and will not be the same as C_F ($C_F = m/V_F$), the mass concentration in the ambient atmosphere at the field conditions T_F, P_F. C_F may be determined from C_L in a simple manner. C_L ($C_L = m/V_L$) is determined by measuring the mass of the pollutant component in the sample by some instrumental or laboratory technique, and dividing the mass, m, by the volume of the bag sample at laboratory conditions (V_L). If a sample is drawn from this bag with a syringe and the syringe contents are analyzed, the contents of the syringe are used to calculate C_L. Thus, the mass concentration is given by:

$$C_L = m_B / V_B \equiv m_S / V_S$$

(2)

The subscripts B and S refer to bag and syringe, respectively. The term m_B is the mass of the pollutant component in the bag sample, and V_B is the volume of the bag or chamber, m_S is the mass of the sample in the syringe, and V_S is the volume of the syringe.

The field concentration C_F (C_F is the actual exposure concentration being determined) is obtained from C_L by correcting V_B in the denominator of equation (2) according to the temperature and pressure relationship given by the ideal gas equation. The numerator (mass) does not change with temperature or pressure. Recall that the temperature–pressure relationship for an ideal gas:

$$P_1 V_1 / T_1 = P_2 V_2 / T_2$$

can be rewritten to the field (F) and laboratory (L) conditions as:

$$P_L V_L / T_L = P_F V_F / T_F$$

Because m_F and m_B are independent of temperature and pressure, it is necessary only to correct the syringe concentration to the laboratory concentration and then calculate back to the field concentration, C_F.

Syringe concentration: $C_S = m_S / V_S \equiv C_L$
Bag concentration: $C_B = m_B / V_B \equiv C_L$

Temperature and pressure corrections to air sample volumes are discussed in Chapter 6.

10. STATIC DILUTION OF GASES AND VAPORS

Static dilution techniques are used to prepare solutions of gases and vapors in air. A volume of high-concentration gas or vapor is diluted with a volume of clean air. The concentration of gas or vapor in the final mixture can be calculated by using the conservation of mass principle. When a solution is diluted, the volume increases, and the concentration is decreased. The total amount (mass) of the contaminant present in the mixture remains constant. The two solutions of gas or vapor contaminants will be related because of the conservation of mass. The relationship is based on the product of the concentration and the volume:

$$C_I V_I = C_F V_F$$

where:

C_I = initial concentration of gas or vapor in the mixture
V_I = initial volume of gas or vapor delivered from the mixture
C_F = final concentration of gas or vapor
V_F = final volume of gas or vapor produced

Example 8

What dilution air volume is required to prepare 200 cm^3 of a 25 ppm solution from a standard mixture, that is, 1000 ppm, delivered from a cylinder?

Solution 8

The conservation of mass relationship is used, based on the product of the concentration and volume:

$$C_I V_I = C_F V_F$$

where:

C_I = initial concentration of gas or vapor in the 1000 ppm mixture.
V_I = initial volume of gas or vapor delivered from 1000 ppm mixture.
C_F = final concentration of gas or vapor, 25 ppm
V_F = final volume of gas or vapor produced, 200 cm^3

$$C_I V_I = C_F V_F$$

$$(1000 \text{ ppm})(V_I) = (25 \text{ ppm})(200 \text{ cm}^3)$$

$$V_I = (25 \text{ ppm})(200 \text{ cm}^3)/(1000 \text{ ppm})$$

$$V_I = 5 \text{ cm}^3$$

When 5 cubic centimeters of a 1000 ppm solution is diluted to 200 cubic centimeters, the resulting contaminant concentration is 25 ppm.

The following example is provided to demonstrate that working with gas and vapor solutions is the same as working with liquid solutions.

Example 9

Given a 5000 ppm nitrate ion (NO_3^-) standard liquid solution, prepare 200 cm^3 of a 125 ppm working liquid solution.

Solution 9

The conservation of mass relationship is used, based on the product of the concentration and volume:

$$C_I V_I = C_F V_F$$

where:

C_I = initial concentration of gas or vapor in the 5000 ppm mixture
V_I = initial volume of gas or vapor delivered from the 5000 ppm mixture

C_F = final concentration of gas or vapor, 125 ppm

V_F = final volume of gas or vapor solution produced, 200 cm^3

$$C_I V_I = C_F V_F$$

$$(5000 \text{ ppm})(V_I) = (125 \text{ ppm})(200 \text{ cm}^3)$$

$$V_I = (125 \text{ ppm})(200 \text{ cm}^3)/(5000 \text{ ppm})$$

$$V_I = 5 \text{ cm}^3$$

$$C_I V_I = C_F V_F$$

$$C_I = 1000 \text{ ppm}, V_I = ?$$

$$C_F = 25 \text{ ppm}, V_F = 100 \text{ cm}^3$$

$$V_I = C_F V_F C_I = (25 \text{ ppm})(100 \text{ cm}^3)/1000 \text{ ppm}$$

$$V_I = 2.5 \text{ cm}^3$$

When 2.5 cubic centimeters of a 1000 ppm liquid nitrate solution is diluted to 100 cubic centimeters, the final concentration is 25 ppm of nitrate in liquid solution.

11. DYNAMIC DILUTION OF GASES AND VAPORS

Dynamic dilution is used to prepare a continuously flowing solution of gas or vapor in air. A volume flowrate of a high-concentration gas or vapor mixture is diluted with a volume flowrate of clean air. The concentration of

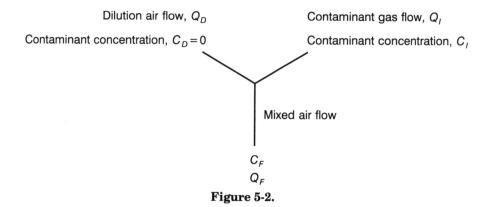

Figure 5-2.

gas or vapor flowing in the final mixture can be calculated by using the conservation of mass. When a solution is diluted, the volume increases, and the concentration is decreased; the total amount (mass) of the contaminant gas present in the mixture remains constant. The two solutions of a gas or a vapor contaminant in air will be related to each other; the relationship is based on the product of the concentration (C_I) and the volume flowrate (Q_I) (see Figure 5-2):

$$C_I Q_I = C_F Q_F$$

where:

C_I = concentration of gas or vapor in the initial mixture
Q_I = volume flowrate of gas or vapor flowing in the initial mixture
C_F = concentration of gas or vapor in the final mixture
Q_F = volume flowrate of gas or vapor flowing in the final mixture
C_D = concentration of gas or vapor in the dilution air flow
Q_D = volume flowrate of dilution air flowing in the system

Note: $Q_D + Q_I = Q_F$ (from the continuity equation).
   The continuity equation states that the total flow in a system is equal to the sum of the individual flows in the system.

Example 10

What diluent air flowrate is required to prepare a solution that is 25 ppm from a standard that is 1000 ppm delivered from a cylinder flowing at 5 cm^3/min (Figure 5-3)?

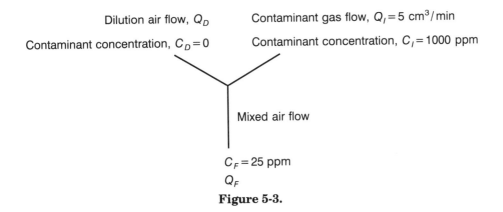

Dilution air flow, Q_D Contaminant gas flow, $Q_I = 5$ cm^3/min

Contaminant concentration, $C_D = 0$ Contaminant concentration, $C_I = 1000$ ppm

Mixed air flow

$C_F = 25$ ppm
Q_F

Figure 5-3.

Solution 10

$$Q_F C_F = Q_I C_I$$

$$Q_F = Q_I C_I / C_F$$

$$Q_F = (5 \text{ cm}^3)(1000 \text{ ppm})/(25 \text{ ppm}) = 200 \text{ cm}^3/\text{min}$$

$$Q_D + Q_I = Q_F \text{ (from the continuity equation)}$$

$$Q_D = Q_F - Q_I = (200 - 5)\text{cm}^3/\text{min} = 195 \text{ cm}^3/\text{min}$$

Using 195 cm^3/min diluent air to dilute 5 cm^3/min of a 1000 ppm solution will produce 200 cm^3/min of a 25 ppm solution. The assumption is that the diluent air has none of the contaminant present (i.e., so-called zero air).

Example 11

Given a cylinder of 500 ppm gaseous standard nitrogen dioxide (NO_2), prepare a 25 ppm solution flowing at 100 cm^3/min (see Figure 5-4).

Solution 11

$$Q_F C_F = Q_I C_I$$

$$Q_I = Q_F C_F / C_I$$

$$Q_F = (100 \text{ cm}^3)(10 \text{ ppm})/(500 \text{ ppm}) = 2 \text{ cm}^3/\text{min}$$

$$Q_D + Q_I = Q_F \text{ (from the continuity equation)}$$

$$Q_D = Q_F - Q_I$$

$$Q_D = Q_F - Q_I = (100 - 2)\text{cm}^3/\text{min} = 98 \text{ cm}^3/\text{min}$$

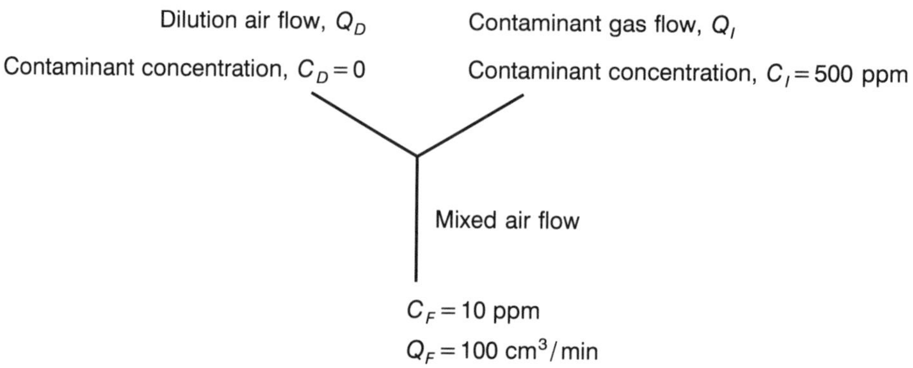

Dilution air flow, Q_D Contaminant gas flow, Q_I

Contaminant concentration, $C_D = 0$ Contaminant concentration, $C_I = 500$ ppm

Mixed air flow

$C_F = 10$ ppm
$Q_F = 100$ cm^3/min

Figure 5-4.

Using 98 cm^3/min of zero air to dilute 2 cm^3/min of a 500 ppm solution will produce 100 cm^3/min of a 10 ppm solution. The assumption is that the diluent air has no nitrogen dioxide contaminant present (i.e., so-called zero air).

BIBLIOGRAPHY

1. Butcher, S. S. and Carlson, R. J., *An Introduction to Air Chemistry*. Academic Press, New York (1972), p. 212.
2. Nelson, G. O., *Controlled Test Atmospheres*. Ann Arbor Science Publishers, Ann Arbor, MI (1971).
3. National Institute for Occupational Safety and Health, *Pocket Guide to Chemical Hazards* (DHHS/NIOSH Pub. No. 90-117). Government Printing Office, Washington, DC (1990).
4. American Conference of Governmental Industrial Hygienists, *Threshold Limit Values*. American Conference of Governmental Industrial Hygienists, Cincinnati, OH (editions prior to 1990).

PROBLEM SET

Problem 1

Calculate the equivalent concentration of 4.0 mg/m^3 of nitrogen dioxide in parts per million.

Solution 1

To solve this problem, derive an equation to convert ppm to mg/m^3. Recall:

$$C_{\text{PPM}} = (V_A/V_B)10^6$$

From the ideal gas law recall:

$$PV_A = (m_A RT/M_A)$$

This can be solved for V_A and substituted into C_{PPM} as:

$$C_{\text{PPM}} = (m_A RT/M_A PV_B)10^6$$

where:

m_A = the mass of contaminant A
V_B = the volume of air in which the mass m_A is contained.

The mass concentration of a contaminant in a volume of air can be identified as:

$$C_{M/V} = m_A/V_B$$

$$C_{PPM} = [(C_{M/V}RT)/MP]10^6$$

at NTP = 25°C, 298.15 K and one atmosphere.

$$C_{M/V} = 4 \text{ mg/m}^3$$

Molecular weight of nitrogen dioxide (NO_2)

$$= 14.0067(1) + 15.9994(2) = 46.0 \text{ g/mole}$$

$$C_{PPM} = \frac{(4.0 \text{ mg/m}^3)(0.082 \text{ l atm/mole K})(g/10^3 \text{ mg})(m^3/10^3 \text{ l})}{(46.0 \text{ g/mole})(1 \text{ atm})}$$

$$C_{PPM} = 2.1 \text{ ppm}$$

Problem 2

Calculate the equivalent length in inches of 1 ppm in the 8000-mile distance between Amherst, Massachusetts, and Maui.

Solution 2

$$8000 \text{ mi}(5280 \text{ ft/mi})(12 \text{ in/ft}) = 506.88 \times 10^6 \text{ in}$$

$$L_{PPM} = [(L_1)/(L_1 + L_2)]10^6 = (L_1/L_2)10^6 = L_{PPM}$$

$$L_2 = 506.88 \times 10^6 \text{ in} = 0.506688 \times 10^9 \text{ in}$$

$$L_1 = ? \qquad L_{PPM} = 1$$

$$(L_1/L_2)10^6 = L_{PPM}$$

$$L_1 = L_2 10^{-6} = (1)(506.88 \times 10^6 \text{ in}) \times 10^{-6} = 506.88 \text{ in}$$

$$L_1 = 42.24 \text{ ft is 1 ppm in the distance between Amherst and Maui.}$$

What is the distance in inches of 1 ppb between Amherst and Maui?

$$L_{PPB} = 1 \text{ ppb}$$

$$L_{PPB} = (L_1/L_2)10^9$$

$$L_2(10^{-9}) = L_1 = 1.0 \text{ ppm } (0.506688 \times 10^9 \text{ in})10^{-9} = L_1$$

$$L_1 = 0.507 \text{ in is 1 ppb in the distance between New York and Maui.}$$

Problem 3

What is the formula to convert from ppm to mg/m^3 at STP?

Solution 3

To solve this problem, derive an equation to convert ppm to mg/m^3. Recall:

$$C_{PPM} = (V_A/V_B)10^6$$

From the ideal gas law recall:

$$PV_A = (m_A RT/M_A)$$

This can be solved for V_A and substituted into C_{PPM} as:

$$C_{PPM} = (m_A RT/M_A PV_B)10^6$$

where:

m_A = mass of contaminant A
V_B = volume of air in which mass m_B is contained

Let $m_A/V_B = C_{M/V}$:

$$C_{PPM} = \left[(C_{M/V}RT)/MP\right]10^6$$

at STP = 0°C, 273.15 K, and one atmosphere.

$$C_{PPM} = \left[(C_{M/V})(22.4\,1/mole)/MW\right]10^6$$

$$C_{PPM} = \left[(C_{mg/m^3})(22.4\,1/mole)/MW\right]10^6$$

$$C_{mg/m^3} = C_{PPM}(MW)10^{-6}/(22.4\,1/mole)$$

Problem 4

What is the correct formula to convert from mg/m^3 to g/l?

Solution 4

$$mg/m^3 = (mg/m^3)(10^{-3}\,g/mg)(m^3/10^3\,1)$$

$$mg/m^3 = 10^{-6}\,g/l$$

Problem 5

A 10 liter sample of air collected at 25°C and one atmosphere contains 1 mg CCl_4. Calculate the concentration in ppm of CCl_4 in air.

Solution 5

MW of carbon tetrachloride $(CCl_4O) = 12.011(1) + 35.453(4) = 153.8$ g/mole
Given 10 liters of air at 25°C and 1 atmosphere, and 1 mg CCl_4:

$$C_{PPM} = (V_A/V_B)10^6$$

$$PV_A = m_A RT/M$$

$$V_A = m_A RT/MP$$

$$C_{PPM} = (V_A/V_B)10^6 = m_A RT/MPV_B$$

$$C_{PPM} = \frac{[(1 \times 10^{-3} \text{ g})(0.082 \text{ l atm/mole deg K})(298.15 \text{ K})10^6]}{[(1 \text{ atm})(153.8 \text{ g/mole})(10 \text{ l})]}$$

$$C_{PPM} = 15.8 \text{ ppm}$$

Problem 6

One gallon of perchloroethylene, specific gravity of 1.62, spills and completely evaporates in a room 60 feet by 30 feet by 15 feet. What is the concentration of perchloroethylene present in this room? Express the concentration in ppm.

Solution 6

Assume perfect mixing and no ventilation into or out of the space.
MW of perchloroethylene $(C_2Cl_4) = 12.011(2) + 35.453(4) = 165.8$ g/mole

$$C_{PPM} = (V_A/V_B)10^6 = (\rho_L V_L RT/MP)10^6$$

$$C_{PPM} = \frac{(1 \text{ gal})(1.62 \text{ g/ml})(3.785 \text{ l/gal})(10^3 \text{ ml/l})(0.082 \text{ l atm/mole deg K})(298.15 \text{ K})10^6}{(165.8 \text{ g/mole})(1 \text{ atm})(30 \text{ ft})(60 \text{ ft})(15 \text{ ft})(28.32 \text{ l/ft}^3)}$$

$$C_{PPM} = (1.18 \text{ l/ml})(10^6)(10^3 \text{ ml/l}) = 1\,183 \text{ ppm}$$

Problem 7

Given a vapor phase solution of a contaminant at its TLV concentration of 1000 ppm, what volume of the contaminant is required to prepare a 50 ppm calibration mixture in a 100 liter mylar bag?

Solution 7

Recall:

$$C_{PPM} = (V_A/V_B)10^6$$

This problem reduces to solving this equation for V_A, since V_B is fixed by the size of the 100 l mylar bag.

$$V_A = (C_{PPM})(V_B)10^{-6} = (50 \text{ ppm})(100 \text{ l})(10^{-6})/(1 \text{ l}/1000 \text{ ml})$$

$$V_A = 5 \text{ ml}$$

Problem 8

The vapor pressure of mercury at 77°F is 0.0018 mm Hg. The atomic weight of mercury is 200.6 g/mole. If the mercury vapor were allowed to reach equilibrium at this temperature in an enclosed space, what would be the mercury vapor concentration in the space?

Solution 8

Recall that the equilibrium vapor pressure equation is given by:

$$C_{PPM} = (P_{VP}/P_{ATM})10^6$$

$$C_{PPM} = (0.0018 \text{ mm Hg}/760 \text{ mm Hg})10^6 = 2.4 \text{ ppm}$$

$$C_{mg/m^3} = C_{PPM}(MW)10^{-6}/(24.45 \text{ l}/\text{mole})$$

$$C_{mg/m^3} = \frac{2.4 \text{ ppm}(200.6 \text{ g}/\text{mole})10^{-6}}{(24.45 \text{ l}/\text{mole})(10^3 \text{ mg}/\text{g})(m^3/10^3 \text{ l})}$$

$$C_{mg/m^3} = 19.4 \text{ mg}/m^3$$

Problem 9

A 1.0 μl aliquot of liquid ethyl alcohol is injected into a stream of metered clean air. A flow of 5 liters per minute (5 lpm) of clean air is maintained for 5 minutes. The alcohol is introduced early in the bag-filling procedure to ensure that it is all evaporated and carried into the bag. Calculate the concentration of alcohol in the bag.

Solution 9

MW of ethyl alcohol $(C_2H_5OH) = 12.011(2) + 1.0079(6) + 15.9994 = 46.07 \text{ g}/\text{mole}$

$$C_{PPM} = (V_A/V_B)10^6 = (\rho_L V_L RT/V_B MP)10^6$$

$$C_{PPM} = [\rho_L V_L(24.45 \text{ l}/\text{mole}/V_B M)]10^6$$

Given:

$$V_B = [5 \text{ lpm}][5 \text{ min}] = 25 \text{ l air in the bag}$$
$$V_L = 1.0 \ \mu\text{l} = 1 \times 10^{-6} \text{ l}$$
$$\rho_L = 0.785 \text{ g/ml}$$
$$RT/P = 24.45 \text{ l/mole at NTP}$$

$$C_{\text{PPM}} = \frac{(0.785 \text{ g/ml})(10^{-6} \text{ l})(10^3 \text{ ml/l})(24.45 \text{ l/mole})}{(46.07 \text{ g/mole})(25 \text{ l})} 10^6$$

$$C_{\text{PPM}} = 16.7 \text{ PPM}$$

$$C_{\text{mg/m}^3} = C_{\text{PPM}}(MW)10^{-6}/(24.45 \text{ l/mole})$$

$$C_{\text{mg/m}^3} = (16.7 \text{ ppm})(46.07 \text{ g/mole})10^{-6}/(24.45 \text{ l/mole})$$

$$C_{\text{mg/m}^3} = 31.5 \text{ mg/m}^3$$

Problem 10

A stream of gas containing 1000 ppm of carbon monoxide in nitrogen is metered at 50 ml/min and is mixed with a stream of clean air metered at 4950 ml/min until a total volume of 5 liters is reached. Calculate the concentration of carbon monoxide in the resulting mixture.

Solution 10

$$C_{\text{PPM}} = [(V_A)/(V_A + V_B)]10^6$$

$$V_A = \text{Volume of CO in nitrogen (CO = 1000 ppm)}$$

$$V_B = 50 \text{ ml}$$

$$C_{\text{PPM}} = [(V_A)/(V_A + V_B)]10^6 = [(0.05 \text{ l})/(0.05 + 4.950 \text{ l})](10^6)$$

$$C_{\text{PPM}} = 10 \text{ ppm carbon monoxide in nitrogen.}$$

Problem 11

A mixture is prepared by diluting 1.00 ml of sulfur dioxide gas with clean air to a final volume of one cubic meter. Calculate the concentration of sulfur dioxide in the mixture.

Solution 11

$$C_{\text{PPM}} = (V_A/V_B)10^6$$

$$C_{\text{PPM}} = (V_{\text{SO}_2}/V_{\text{FINAL}})10^6 = [(1 \text{ ml}_{\text{SO}_2})/(1 \text{ m}^3)]10^6$$

$$C_{\text{PPM}} = (1 \text{ ml}_{\text{SO}_2}/1 \text{ m}^3)(1 \text{ m}^3/1000 \text{ l})(1 \text{ l}/1000 \text{ ml})10^6 = 1 \text{ ppm SO}_2$$

Problem 12

The vapor pressure of benzene at 25°C is 97 mm Hg. What is the maximum concentration of benzene vapor in air that can be obtained at 25°C at a total pressure of 760 mm Hg?

Solution 12

$$C_{PPM} = (P_I/P_T)10^6 = [P_{VP}/P_T]10^6 = (97 \text{ mm Hg}/760 \text{ mm Hg})10^6$$

$$C_{PPM} = 1.28(10^5) \text{ ppm}$$

Problem 13

What is the concentration of toluene in air produced by vaporizing 1 ml of liquid toluene into clean air to produce a total volume of 100 liters? Toluene has a specific gravity of 0.86.

Solution 13

Molecular weight of toluene $(C_7H_8) = 12.011(7) + 1.0079(8) = 92.14$ g/mole

$$\rho_L = \rho_W(SG) = 0.86(1 \text{ g/ml}) = 0.86 \text{ g/ml}$$

$$C_{PPM} = (V_L \rho_L RT/V_B \ MW \ P)10^6$$

$$C_{PPM} = \frac{(1 \text{ ml})(0.86 \text{ g/ml})(24.45 \text{ l/mole})}{(92.14 \text{ g/mole})(100 \text{ l})}10^6$$

$$C_{PPM} = 2{,}282 \text{ ppm toluene}$$

Problem 14

What is the concentration in parts per million produced by the evaporation of 17 ml of CS_2 (specific gravity 1.26) in a room with that is 1700 cubic feet in volume?

Solution 14

Molecular weight of carbon disulfide $(CS_2) = 12.011(1) + 32.06(2) = 76.1$ g/mole

$$\rho_L = \rho_W(SG) = 1.26(1 \text{ g/ml}) = 1.26 \text{ g/ml}$$

The volume of CS_2 vapor present in the container that is 1700 ft^3 must be determined. Assumptions: NTP. No air is entering or leaving the room.

$$C_{PPM} = \left[(V_{CS_2})/(V_{CS_2} + V_{ROOM})\right]10^6 = \left[(V_{CS_2})/(V_{ROOM})\right]10^6$$

Assume that the vapor behaves as an ideal gas and calculate the vapor volume.

$$C_{\text{PPM}} = (V_L \, \rho_L RT)(V_R MP)10^6 = \frac{[V_L \, \rho_L(24.45 \text{ l/mole})]}{[V_R M_L]}10^6$$

$$V_R = \text{Room volume} = 1700 \text{ ft}^3$$

$$V_L = V_{\text{CS}_2} = 17 \text{ ml}$$

$$C_{\text{PPM}} = \frac{[(17 \text{ ml})(1.26 \text{ g/ml})(24.45 \text{ l/mole})]}{[(1700 \text{ ft}^3)(28.33 \text{ l/ft}^3)/(\text{mole}/76.1 \text{ g})]}10^6$$

$$C_{\text{PPM}} = 143.2 \text{ ppm}$$

$$C_{\text{mg/m}^3} = C_{\text{PPM}}(MW)10^{-6}/(24.45 \text{ l/mole})$$

$$C_{\text{mg/m}^3} = (143.2 \text{ ppm})(76.1 \text{ g/mole})10^{-6}/(24.45 \text{ l/mole})$$

$$C_{\text{mg/m}^3} = 445.7 \text{ mg/m}^3$$

Problem 15

The vapor pressure of a solvent in air is 7×10^{-3} mm Hg. What is the equilibrium concentration of this vapor in air in ppm? If the solvent is benzene, what would its concentration be in mg/m^3?

Solution 15

Molecular weight of benzene $(C_6H_6) = 12.011(6) + 1.0079(6) = 78.1$ g/mole
Vapor pressure $= P_{VP}$ in air $= 7 \times 10^{-3}$ mm Hg
What is the concentration in ppm?

$$C_{\text{PPM}} = (P_I/P_T)10^6 = (P_{VP}/P_{\text{TOTAL}})10^6$$

$$C_{\text{PPM}} = [(7 \times 10^{-3} \text{ mm Hg})/(760 \text{ mm Hg})]10^6$$

$$C_{\text{PPM}} = 9.2 \text{ ppm}$$

At NTP:

$$C_{\text{PPM}} = (V_A/V_B)10^6 = (m_A/MV_B)(RT/P)10^6$$

Notice $m_A/V_B = C_{m/V}$.

$$C_{PPM} = (C_{M/V})\left(\frac{RT}{MP}\right)10^6$$

$$C_{M/V} = (C_{PPM})\left(\frac{MP}{RT}\right)10^{-6}$$

$$C_{M/V} = \frac{(9.2)(78.1 \text{ g/mole})(1 \text{ atm})}{(0.08205 \text{ l atm/mole K})(298.15 \text{ K})}10^{-6}$$

$$C_{M/V} = 29.4 \text{ mg/m}^3$$

Problem 16

Given a concentration of 5 ppm ethylene oxide in air, calculate the corresponding concentration of ethylene oxide in mg/m^3, at NTP.

Solution 16

MW of ethylene oxide $(C_2H_4O) = 12.011(2) + 1.0079(4) + 15.9994(1) = 44.05$ g/mole

Temperature: $273.15 \text{ K} + 25°C = 298.15 \text{ K}$

$$C_{M/V} = (C_{PPM}M_A P/R_T)10^{-6}$$

$$C_{M/V} = \frac{5 \text{ ppm}(10^{-6})(44.05 \text{ g/mole})(1 \text{ atm})}{[0.082 \text{ l atm/mole K}(298.15 \text{ K})]}$$

$$C_{M/V} = (5)(10^{-6})(44.05)\text{g}/(0.082)(298.15)\text{l}$$

$$C_{M/V} = 9.009 \times 10^{-6}(\text{g/l})(10^3 \text{ mg/1 g})(10^{-3} \text{ l/m}^3)$$

$$C_{M/V} = [9.009 \times 10^{-6}(1000 \text{ mg})(1000)/\text{m}^3]$$

$$C_{M/V} = 9.0 \text{ mg/m}^3$$

Problem 17

The EPA 24-hour ambient air quality standard for sulfur dioxide (SO_2) is 0.14 ppm. Calculate the equivalent concentration in μg/m^3 at NTP.

Solution 17

MW of sulfur oxide $(SO_2) = 32.06(1) + 15.9994(2) = 64.06$ g/mole

$C_{PPM} = 0.14$ ppm

$$C_{M/V} = C_{PPM} M_A (P/RT) 10^{-6}$$

$$C_{M/V} = \frac{(0.14 \text{ ppm})(64.06 \text{ g/mole})(1 \text{ atm})}{[0.028 \text{ l atm/mole K}(298.15 \text{ K})]} 10^{-6} \text{ ppm}$$

$$C_{M/V} = \frac{0.14(64.06 \text{ g/mole})}{(0.082 \text{ l atm/mole K})(298.15 \text{ K})} [10^6 \ \mu g/1 \ g](10^{-6}) 10^3 \ 1/m^3$$

$$C_{M/V} = \frac{[(0.14)(64.06)(10^3) \ \mu g]}{[(0.082)(298.15) m^3]}$$

$$C_{M/V} = (8968.23 \ \mu g / 24.038 \ m^3) = 366.8 \ \mu g/m^3 = 367 \ \mu g/m^3$$

Problem 18

A one pound cylinder of chlorine gas (Cl_2) fell off a lab bench and broke. The contents leaked into a sealed room 60 feet by 30 feet by 15 feet. What is the concentration in ppm if the lab is at NTP?

Solution 18

Molecular weight of chlorine $(Cl_2) = 35.453(2) = 70.91$ g/mole
Room volume $= 27,000 \ ft^3 = V_B;$ $T = 298.15$ K; $P = 1$ atm;
$R = 0.082$ l atm/mole K; $V = nRT/P = (mRT/MP) = V_A$

$$C_{PPM} = [V_A/(V_A + V_B)](10^6) = (V_A/V_B)(10^6) = (mRT \times 10^6/MPV_B)$$

$$C_{PPM} = \frac{[1 \text{ lb}(0.082 \text{ l atm/mole K})(10^6 \ ft^3/28.36 \ l)298.15 \text{ K}(454 \text{ g/lb})]}{[(70.91 \text{ g/mole})(1 \text{ atm})27,000 \ ft^3]}$$

$$C_{PPM} = 204.4 \text{ ppm}$$

Problem 19

Calculate the concentration of sulfur hexafluoride (SF_6) gas after 1 cm³ is injected into a house and mixed into a volume of 35,000 ft³. Repeat the concentration in %, ppm, ppb, and ppt.

Solution 19

$$C = (V_A/V_B)10^n \quad n = 2 = \%; \; n = 9 = \text{ppb}; \; n = 12 = \text{ppt}$$

Assume the infiltration rate is initially zero, e.g., windows/doors sealed;

$$C_{PPM} = [V_A/(V_A + V_B)]10^n = (V_A/V_B)10^n$$

To solve this problem, V_A and V_B must be in the same units:

$$(35,000 \text{ ft}^3)(12 \text{ in/ft})^3(2.54 \text{ cm/in})^3 = 991.1 \times 10^6 \text{ cm}^3 = V_B$$

$$V_A = 1 \text{ cm}^3; \; V_B = 991.1 \times 10^6 \text{ cm}^3$$

$$C_{\%, SF_6} = (V_A/V_B)10^2 = (1/991.1 \times 10^6)10^2 = 1.008 \times 10^{-9} \times 10^2$$

$$C_{\%, SF_6} = 1.008 \times 10^{-7}\%$$

$$C_{PPM, SF_6} = (V_A/V_B)10^6 = (1/991.1 \times 10^6)10^6 = 1.008 \times 10^{-9} \times 10^6$$

$$C_{PPM, SF_6} = 1.008 \times 10^{-3} \text{ ppm}$$

$$C_{PPB, SF_6} = (V_A/V_B)10^9 = (1/991.1 \times 10^6)10^9 = (1.008 \times 10^{-9})10^9$$

$$C_{PPB, SF_6} = 1.008 \text{ ppb}$$

$$C_{PPT, SF_6} = (V_A/V_B)10^{12} = (1/991.1 \times 10^6)10^{12} = 1.008 \times 10^{-9} \times 10^{12}$$

$$C_{PPT, SF_6} = 1,008 \text{ ppt}$$

Problem 20

Fifty milliliters of ethylene oxide at 50°F and 30.9 inches Hg is added to a sterilizer 6 cubic meters in volume (6 m³). The sterilizer is subsequently heated to 180°F and 2 atm. What is the concentration of ethylene oxide inside the sterilizer, in parts per million (ppm) and in milligrams per cubic meter (mg/m³) at 25°C and one atmosphere?

Solution 20

MW of ethylene oxide $(C_2H_4O) = 12.011(2) + 1.0079(4) + 15.9994(1) = 44.05$ g/mole

Recall: $9(°C) = 5(°F) - 160$; $6 \text{ m}^3 \times 1000 \text{ l/m}^3 = 6000 \text{ l}$

Convert 50°F to °C: $°C = [(5)(°F) - 160]/9 = (5.50 - 160)/9 = 10°C$
Convert 180°F to °C: $°C = [(5)(°F) - 160]/9 = (5.180 - 160)/9 = 82°C$

At 10°C ethylene oxide is liquid (SG = 0.82, molecular weight = 44.1 g/mole). Calculate the volume change of the ETO when it goes from 10°C to 82°C and the pressure changes from 30.9 in Hg to 2 atm.

$$C_{PPM} = (V_A/V_B)10^6 = (m_A/MV_B)(RT/P)10^6 = (\rho_L V_L/MV_B)(RT/P)10^6$$

$$C_{PPM} = \frac{(0.82 \text{ g/ml})(50 \text{ ml})(0.082 \text{ l atm/mole K})(298.15 \text{ K})}{(44.1 \text{ g/mole})(1 \text{ atm})(6000 \text{ l})} 10^6$$

$$C_{PPM} = 3791 \text{ ppm}$$

$$C_{M/V} = 6838 \text{ mg/m}^3$$

Problem 21

How many cubic feet of SO_2 are necessary to produce a concentration of 100 ppm of the gas in a room 700 cubic feet in volume?

Solution 21

$$C_{PPM} = [(V_A)/(V_A + V_B)]10^6 = (V_A/V_B)10^6$$

$$V_A = [SO_2][V_B \times 10^{-6}]$$

$$V_A = (100)(700 \text{ ft}^3)10^{-6} = V_A = 0.07 \text{ ft}^3$$

Problem 22

What is the volume of liquid CCl_4 necessary to produce a concentration of 70 ppm in a room 1000 cubic feet in volume, if the liquid CCl_4 has a purity of 85% and a specific gravity of 1.6?

Solution 22

MW of carbon tetrachloride $(CCl_4) = 12.011(1) + 35.453(4) = 153.8$ g/mole $= M$

$$C_{PPM} = [(V_L \rho_L 24.45 \text{ l/mole} \times 10^6)/V_B M] \text{ at NTP}$$

Solve the equation for V_L:

$$V_L = (C_{PPM} V_B M)(24.45 \text{ l/mole})(1/\text{mole})(10^6)/\rho_L$$

$$V_L = \frac{(70 \text{ ppm})(100 \text{ ft}^3)(28.34 \text{ l/ft}^3)(154 \text{ g/mole})}{(1.6 \text{ g/ml})(24.45 \text{ l/mole})(10^6)}$$

$$V_L = (70 \times 1000 \times 28.24 \times 154 \text{ ml})/(1.6 \times 24.45 \times 10^6 \text{ ml})$$

$$V_L = 7.8 \text{ ml of 100\% pure } CCl_4$$

The CCl_4 is 85%; so increase the volume from 7.8 ml to 9.2 ml because 9.2 ml $\times$ 0.85 = 7.8 ml.

Problem 23

To prepare 15 liters of 5 ppm SO_2 in air, what volume of pure sulfur dioxide (SO_2) gas should be added to the 15 liters of clean air?

Solution 23

$$C_{PPM} = [(V_A)/(V_A + V_B)]10^6 = (V_A/V_B)10^6$$

V_A = volume of SO_2 needed, V_B = final volume required

$$C_{PPM} = (V_A/V_B)10^6$$

$$5 \text{ ppm} = (V_A \times 10^6/15 \text{ l})$$

Solving for V_A:

$$V_A = (5 \text{ ppm})(15 \text{ l})/(10^6 \text{ ppm})$$

$$V_A = 75 \times 10^{-6} \text{ l}(10^6 \text{ } \mu l/l) = 75 \text{ } \mu l$$

Problem 24

Given an analysis of X mg from a sample taken over a period of 24 hours at Y cfm, determine the concentration in mg/m^3.

Solution 24

For X mg of a sample collected over 24 hr at Y cfm: C = mass/volume

$$C = \frac{X \text{ mg}}{[(Y \text{ ft}^3/\text{min})(60 \text{ min/hr})(24 \text{ hr})(28.32 \text{ l/ft}^3)][m^3/10^3 \text{ l}]}$$

$$C = 0.0245 \text{ } X \text{ mg/}Y m^3$$

Problem 25

Calculate the volume of sulfur hexafluoride needed to prepare a gaseous solution of 250 ppb SF_6 in a house with a volume of 30,000 ft^3.

Solution 25

The first thing that we must do is determine the physical state of SF_6 (i.e., gas, liquid, or solid). SF_6 has a boiling point of $-63.8°C$, a molecular weight of 146.05 g/mole, and a gas density of 6.6 g/l.

$$C_{PPB} = \left[(V_{SF_6})/(V_{SF_6} + V_{HOUSE})\right]10^9 = (V_{SF_6}/V_{HOUSE})10^9$$

$$V_{SF_6} = C_{PPB} \times V_{HOUSE} \times 10^{-9} = 250 \times 30,000 \text{ ft}^3(28.32 \text{ l/ft}^3)10^{-9}$$

$$V_{SF_6} = 0.212 \text{ l}$$

$$V_{SF_6} = 212 \text{ ml}$$

Problem 26

Calculate the mass of formaldehyde that could potentially be present in a volume of 25,000 ft^3 when the formaldehyde concentration is 100 ppb.

Solution 26

At room temperature, formaldehyde exists as a polymer with a molecular formula $(-CH_2O)_n$; at 20°C it has a density of 0.815 g/ml. Any CH_2O that is present in this structure will be in a sufficiently dilute solution so that we can assume it exists as a monomer with a molecular weight of 30.03 g/mole.

$$C_{PPB} = \left[(V_A)/(V_A + V_B)\right]10^9 = (V_{CH_2O}/V_{HOUSE})10^9$$

where:

$$V_A = \text{volume of } CH_2O$$
$$V_B = \text{volume of the house} = V_{HOUSE}$$
$$V_{CH_2O} = C_{PPB}(V_{HOUSE})10^{-9}$$

$$C_{PPB} = (V_{CH_2O}/V_{HOUSE})10^9 = (m_A/MV_B)(RT/P)10^9$$

$$m_A = C_{PPB}(PMV_B/RT)10^{-9}$$

$$m_A = \frac{100(1 \text{ atm})(30.03 \text{ g/mole})(25,000 \text{ ft}^3)(28.32 \text{ l/ft}^3)}{(0.082 \text{ l atm/mole K})(298.15 \text{ K})}10^{-9}$$

$$m_A = 0.087 \text{ g } CH_2O$$

The house contains 0.087 gram of formaldehyde. This yields an indoor concentration of 100 ppb.

Problem 27

A cylinder loses 5 lb of ammonia (NH_3) into a 500 cubic meter chamber. What is the resulting concentration in (a) mg/l, (b) mg/m^3, and (c) ppm?

Solution 27

MW of ammonia $(NH_3) = 14.0067(1) + 1.0079(3) = 17.03$ g/mole

a. $[NH_3]$ in mg/liter (this is a straightforward conversion):

$$(5 \text{ lb } NH_3/500 \text{ m}^3)[(454 \text{ g/lb})(1000 \text{ mg/g})]/(1000 \text{ l/m}^3)$$

$$C_{mg/l} = (5 \text{ lb})(454 \text{ g/lb})(1000 \text{ mg/g})/(500 \text{ m}^3)(1000 \text{ l/m}^3)$$

$$C_{mg/l} = 2270 \text{ mg}/500 \text{ l} = 4.54 \text{ mg/l} = 4.54 \text{ mg/l}$$

b. $[NH_3]$ in mg/m^3 (this is a straightforward conversion):

$$(5 \text{ lb } NH_3/500 \text{ m}^3)[(454 \text{ g/lb})(1000 \text{ mg/g})]$$

$$C_{mg/m^3} = (5 \text{ lb})(454 \text{ g/lb})(1000 \text{ mg/g})/(500 \text{ m}^3)$$

$$C_{mg/m^3} = 4540 \text{ mg/m}^3$$

c. $[NH_3]$ in ppm; there are several routes to solve this problem:

$$C_{PPM} = [(V_A)/(V_A + V_B)]10^6 = (V_A/V_B)10^6 = (mRT/V_B MP)10^6$$

$$C_{PPM} = [24.45(1/\text{mole})/V_B M]10^6 \text{ (at NTP)}$$

$$C_{PPM} = \frac{[(24.45 \text{ l/mole})(5 \text{ lb})(454 \text{ g/lb})(10^6)]}{[(500 \text{ m}^3)(17.03 \text{ g/mole})(1000 \text{ l/m}^3)]}$$

$$C_{PPM} = 6518 \text{ ppm}$$

Problem 28

Calculate the volume of methane needed to prepare a gaseous solution of 2 ppm CH_4 in a chamber (a house) with a volume of 30,000 ft^3.

Solution 28

Determine the physical state of methane (i.e., gas, liquid, or solid). Methane's molecular weight is 16.03 g/mole, and its boiling point is $-161.49°C$. Clearly, this is a solution of a gas (methane) in a gas (air). The dilution of a gas in a gas is given by:

$$C_{PPM} = [V_A/(V_A + V_B)]10^6 = (V_A/V_B)10^6 \text{ (if } B \text{ is rigid)}$$

$$C_{PPM} = (V_{CH_4}/V_{AIR})10^6 \text{ or } (V_{CH_4}/V_{HOUSE})10^6$$

$$V_{CH_4} = C_{PPM} \times V_{AIR} \times 10^{-6}$$

$$V_{CH_4} = 2 \times 30,000 \text{ ft}^3[28.32 \text{ l/ft}^3]10^{-6} = 1.7 \text{ l}$$

Note: The CH_4 added should be at the same temperature as the house.
  Extra Credit. Why not use the following equation?

$$C_{PPM} = (22.4\rho_L V_L/V_B m_L)(T/273.15)(760/P)(10^6)$$

Because CH_4 is a gas and not a liquid with density ρ_L.

Problem 29

An industrial hygienist has several dozen detector tubes for measuring toluene between 50 ppm and 150 ppm (0.5 TLV to 1.5 TLV). These detector tubes are out of date, and the industrial hygienist cannot wait for an express shipment from the manufacturer. The only recourse is to calibrate the detector tubes versus a known concentration of toluene. An air sampling pump and a 10 liter Tedlar gas sampling bag in a test atmosphere are set up as indicated in Figure 5-5. The bag is filled until the water in the trap bubbles (1 inch of water column back pressure that keeps from overpressurizing the bag). How much toluene, which is a liquid at room temperature, must be injected into the bag to prepare a known atmosphere of toluene in air?

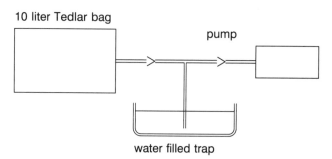

Figure 5-5. Schematic for a gas delivery system (Problem 29).

Solution 29

Recall:

$$C_{\text{PPM}} = (V_A/V_B)10^6 = (V_A/V_{\text{AIR}})10^6$$

where:

V_A = volume of the impurity (toluene vapor)
$V_B = V_{\text{AIR}}$ = in the volume in the 10 liter bag

Toluene is a liquid at room temperature, and this liquid is delivered to the bag. If the liquid is allowed to equilibrate, it will evaporate completely and form a vapor of volume V_A. It is possible to derive the expression below from the ideal gas equation:

$$C_{\text{PPM}} = (\rho_L V_L/MV_{\text{AIR}})(24.45)[(T_A/298.15 \text{ K})(760 \text{ mm Hg}/P_A)]10^6$$

Molecular weight of toluene $(C_7H_8) = 12.011(7) + 1.0079(8) = 92.14$ g/mole

ρ_L at $25°C = 0.86$ g/ml
$V_{\text{AIR}} = 10$ l (volume of the bag)
V_L = volume of liquid toluene added to the 10 l air to produce 50 ppm, 100 ppm, 150 ppm of toluene vapor in the bag

If $C_{\text{PPM}} = 50$ ppm, solve this equation for V_L:

$$V_L = (C_{\text{PPM}} MV_{\text{AIR}}/\rho_L 24.45)10^{-6}$$

$$V_L = \frac{[50(92.14 \text{ g/mole})10 \text{ l}]}{[(0.86 \text{ g/ml})(24.45 \text{ l/mole})]} 10^{-6} = 0.00219 \text{ ml}$$

$$V_L = (0.0022 \text{ ml})(10^3 \text{ } \mu\text{l/ml}) = 2.2 \text{ } \mu\text{l}$$

If 2.2 μl of liquid toluene evaporates into 10 l air, the concentration is 50 ppm.

Volume of liquid toluene (μl)	Resulting concentration in 10 l volume (ppm)
2.2	50
4.4	100
6.6	150
8.8	200
11.0	250

Problem 30

December 31, 1987, was a "slow" day for the news media; only three violent crimes were reported. More bad holiday news could easily send some people into depression. To lighten the tenor of the times, broadcast news anchors told the country of the addition of one leap second to be used to correct the time standard based on the earth's rotation. The one leap second was added to the beginning of the leap year (1988) to set all the clocks in the world to the same exact time. What is the magnitude of this time correction in parts per billion?

Solution 30

To solve this problem the fraction of one additional second in one standard year must be computed:

$$T_{PPB} = [(T_1)/(T_1 + T_2)]10^9 = (T_1/T_2)10^9$$

$$T_{PPB} = \frac{(1 \ sec)10^9}{(1 \ y)(365 \ d/y)(24 \ hr/d)(60 \ min/hr)(60 \ sec/min)}$$

$$T_{PPB} = 31.7 \ ppb$$

The organizers of the New Year's Eve celebration at New York's Times Square even provided a spectacular one second light show to welcome the additional leap second.

Problem 31

A laboratory ordered and received a mercury barometer. During shipment, mercury liquid spilled from a damaged reservoir. The cardboard and foam shipping container was contaminated. When the container was opened, the floor and air of the laboratory were contaminated. The laboratory's spill expert was called and performed a cleanup.

The health and safety coordinator for the trucking company is concerned with the potential mercury vapor exposure received by all the workers in the transportation system. You are asked to evaluate potential exposure to workers in the transportation system as a result of this spill. What would you find?

Solution 31

The health and safety coordinator's concern is to demonstrate whether by carelessly shipping the mercury barometer it is possible to potentially expose people in the transportation and handling network and risk contaminating other products being handled by the carrier. The occupational health standard recommended by American Conference of Governmental Industrial Hygienists for mercury vapor is 0.05 mg/m^3.

TABLE 5-12. The vapor pressure and concentration of mercury vapor in air as a function of temperature in a 27,568 liter truck.

Temperature		Mercury vapor pressure (mm Hg)	Mercury concentration (ppm)	(mg/m^3)	Multiple of the ACGIH standard
°F	°C				
32	0	0.000185	0.24	1.96	39
50	10	0.000490	0.65	5.29	106
68	20	0.001201	1.59	13.03	261
77	25	0.00185	2.43	19.92	398
86	30	0.002777	3.65	29.98	600
104	40	0.006079	8.0	65.62	1 312
122	50	0.01267	16.67	136.78	2 736

Mercury vapor concentration is a function of temperature and pressure. One way to estimate exposure is to calculate the possible mercury vapor concentration in air over a variety of temperatures that may be encountered in the handling and transportation of mercury liquid. On a winter day when the back of a delivery truck is at 32°F, the potential mercury vapor exposure could be nearly 39 times the occupational health (ACGIH) standard. On a summer day when the back of the delivery truck is 122°F, the potential mercury vapor exposure would be 2700 times the ACGIH standard. These values are for an unventilated truck, assuming that sufficient mercury is spilled to reach the equilibrium vapor pressure in the truck. The concentrations are calculated as indicated below:

$$C_{PPM} = (P_{VP, Hg}/P_{ATM})10^6$$

The vapor pressure of liquid mercury and the vapor concentration in the truck are given in Table 5-12. The dimensions of a "typical" truck are 16 feet long by 7.8 feet wide by 7.8 feet high.

$$V_{TRUCK} = (16 \text{ ft})(7.8 \text{ ft})(7.8 \text{ ft}) = 973.4 \text{ ft}^3 = 27,568 \text{ l}$$

$$C_{M/V} (mg/m^3) = C_{PPM}(MP/RT)10^{-6}$$

$$C_{M/V} (mg/m^3) = C_{PPM}[M/(24.45 \text{ l/mole})]10^{-6}$$

Problem 32

Recently a historian was talking about the death of King Tut. "The last breath he gasped occurred on..." During a class in Occupational Health, Professor I. M. Historical claimed to have measured a gasp of breath and it was 20 liters. Assume that the earth's atmosphere is uniformly thick and extends to a height of 2.5 miles above the surface and then it ends (a generous assumption!). Calculate the concentration of King Tut's last breath in the air surrounding the planet on a volume per volume basis (e.g., parts per million, etc.).

Solution 32

By inspection, this problem reduces to a calculation similar to that for C_{PPM}:

$$C_{PPM} = (V_A/V_B)10^6$$

where:

V_A = volume of the breath exhaled by King Tut
V_B = volume of the 2.5-mile-thick air layer uniformly surrounding the earth

Assume that there are no sinks for air in the environment. This is tough to defend in view of the massive amount of combustion that has occurred in the 4000 years since Tut's death, but assume that the number of air molecules present in the environment is so large relative to the amount combusted that one can safely say the number of molecules of air is a constant. The volume of air surrounding the earth may be calculated by the difference between a sphere with a diameter equal to the outside diameter (V_{OD}) of the earth including the air envelope minus the volume of the earth (V_E). Assume that the earth is a smooth, hard, round sphere of diameter equal to 8000 miles (D_E). Assume that the OD of the air envelope is 8005 miles (D_{OD}).

$$\text{Volume of air} = V_{OD} - V_E = \pi(D_{OD})^3/6 - \pi(D_E)^3/6$$

$$\text{Volume of air} = \pi/6\left[(D_{OD})^3 - (D_E)^3\right] = V_B$$

$$V_B = \pi/6(8005^3 - 8000^3) = 50.2(10^7)\text{mi}^3$$

$$V_B = 50.2(10^7 \text{ mi}^3)(5280^3 \text{ ft}^3/\text{mi}^3)(28.32\,1/\text{ft}^3) = 2.1 \times 10^{21}\,1$$

$$C_{PPM} = (V_A/V_B)10^6 = \left[20\,1/(2.1 \times 10^{21}\,1)\right]10^6 \text{ ppm} = 9.5 \times 10^{-15} \text{ ppm}$$

Problem 33

While you are driving a recreational vehicle (RV) through the Powder Pass (9 666 feet above sea level) on the road from Buffalo, Wyoming, to Cody, Wyoming, a 1.02 pound cylinder of propane gas falls out of a cabinet, hits the floor, and ruptures. The RV is 31 feet long by 10 feet wide by 7.2 feet high. Is this a fire or explosion problem?

Solution 33

Volume RV $= 2232$ ft^3, $63{,}210$ l; $P_{\text{ATM}} = P_S D_F = 0.71$ atm
Propane: 462.7 g C_3H_8, molecular weight 44.1 g/mole

$$C_{\text{PPM}} = (V_A/V_B)10^6 = (m_A/MV_B)(RT/P)10^6$$

$$C_{\text{PPM}} = \frac{(462.7 \text{ g})(0.082 \text{ l atm/mole K})(298.15 \text{ K})}{(44.1 \text{ g/mole})(0.71 \text{ atm})(63{,}210 \text{ l})}10^6$$

$$C_{\text{PPM}} = 5\,716 \text{ ppm}$$

Problem 34

A. While preparing to perform qualitative fit testing on a new group of workers, the industrial hygiene technician drops a one liter bottle of isoamyl acetate while traveling in the elevator. Is the technician at risk of overexposure to isoamyl acetate?
B. Assume that the elevator's dimensions are 6 feet by 6 feet by 8 feet.

Solution 34A

Isoamyl acetate is a liquid at room temperature, and this liquid is spilled into the elevator V_{ELEVATOR}. If the liquid has time to equilibrate (the elevator breaks down and the technician is stuck inside!), it will evaporate completely and form a vapor of volume V_A. It is possible to derive the expression from the ideal gas equation:

Molecular weight of isoamyl acetate $(CH_3COOCH_2\text{–}CH_2CH(CH_3)_2$

$$= 12.011(7) + 1.0079(14) + 15.9994(2) = 130.19 \text{ g/mole}$$

Recall:

$$C_{\text{PPM}} = (V_A/V_B)10^6 = (V_A/V_{\text{AIR}})10^6$$

where:

V_A = volume of the impurity (isoamyl acetate vapor)
$V_B = V_{\text{AIR}}$ = in the volume in the elevator

$$C_{\text{PPM}} = (\rho_L V_L/MV_{\text{ELEVATOR}})(24.45 \text{ l/mole})10^6$$

$T_A = 25°C$, $P_A = 1$ atm
ρ_L at $25°C = 0.87$ g/ml

$$C_{\text{PPM}} = \frac{(0.87 \text{ g/ml})}{(130.19 \text{ g/mole})(V_{\text{ELEVATOR}})}[24.45 \text{ l/mole}]10^6$$

Solution 34B

$$V_{\text{ELEVATOR}} = (6\ \text{ft})(6\ \text{ft})(8\ \text{ft})(28.32\ \text{l/ft}^3)(\text{m}^3/1000\ \text{l}) = 8.2\ \text{m}^3$$

$$C_{\text{PPM}} = \frac{(0.87\ \text{g/ml})(V_L)}{(130.19\ \text{g/mole})(V_{\text{ELEVATOR}})}(24.45\ \text{l/mole})10^6$$

$$C_{\text{PPM}} = \frac{(0.87\ \text{g/ml})(1\ \text{l})}{(130.19\ \text{g/mole})(8.2\ \text{m}^3)}(24.45\ \text{l/mole})10^6$$

$$C_{\text{PPM}} = 19{,}922\ \text{ppm}$$

When one is transporting hazardous materials through a building, secondary containment is critical!

Problem 35

What volume of benzene liquid must be vaporized to produce a concentration of 10 ppm in a test chamber that is 10 feet by 10 feet by 12 feet?

Solution 35

Molecular weight of benzene $(C_6H_6) = 12.011(6) + 1.0079(6) = 78.11\ \text{g/mole}$

ρ_L at $25°C = 0.879\ \text{g/ml}$

Chamber volume: $(10\ \text{ft})(10\ \text{ft})(12\ \text{ft}) = (1200\ \text{ft}^3)(28.32\ \text{l/ft}^3) = 33{,}984\ \text{l} = 33.9(10^6)\ \text{ml}$

$$C_{\text{PPM}} = \left[V_A/(V_A + V_B)\right]10^6 = (V_A/V_B)10^6$$

$$PV_A = nRT = (mRT/M) = (\rho_L V_L RT/M)$$

$$V_A = (\rho_L V_L RT/MP)$$

$$C_{\text{PPM}} = (V_A/V_B)10^6 = (\rho_L V_L RT/MPV_B)10^6$$

Solve for V_L:

$$V_L = (C_{\text{PPM}} MPV_B/\rho_L RT)10^{-6} \quad V_B = \text{chamber volume in cm}^3$$

$$V_L = \frac{\left[(10\ \text{ppm})(78.1\ \text{g/mole})(1\ \text{atm})(33.9 \times 10^6\ \text{cm}^3)(10^{-6})\right]}{\left[(0.082\ \text{l atm/mole K})(298.15\ \text{K})(0.879\ \text{g/cm}^3)(1000\ \text{cm}^3/\text{l})\right]}$$

$$V_L = 1.23\ \text{cm}^3$$

Alternate Solution 35

$$C_{PPM} = [V_{Benzene}/(V_{Benzene} + V_{Room})]10^6$$

$$C_{PPM} = (V_{Benzene}/V_{Room})10^6$$

$$V_B = (C_{PPM}V_R)(10^{-6}) = (10)(33.9)(10^6 \text{ ml})/10^{-6}$$

$$V_B = 339 \text{ ml of benzene vapor in a } 1200 \text{ ft}^3 \text{ room to give}$$

$$a \ 10 \text{ ppm concentration}$$

Assume that the room is at NTP, and then calculate the volume of benzene liquid that, when evaporated, will give 339 ml of vapor:

$$PV_V = nRT = (mRTV_L/MV_L) = (\rho RTV_L/M)$$

$$PV_V = (\rho RTV_L/M); V_L = (PV_VM/\rho RT) = 0.879 \text{ g/cm}^3$$

$$V_L = \frac{[(1 \text{ atm})(339 \text{ ml})(78.1 \text{ g/mole})(10^{-3} \text{ l/ml})]}{[(0.879 \text{ g/cm}^3)(0.082 \text{ l atm/mole K})(298.15 \text{ K})]}$$

$$V_L = 1.23 \text{ cm}^3$$

Problem 36

Preparing to clean and sterilize a kidney dialysis apparatus, a technician drops a one liter bottle of formalin (37% formaldehyde plus 12% methanol) while washing out the apparatus in the laboratory. Is there a potential for an adverse exposure to formaldehyde or methanol if the room is 10 feet by 12 feet by 8 feet?

Solution 36

Recall:

$$C_{PPM} = (V_A/V_B)10^6 = (V_A/V_{LAB})10^6$$

where:

$$V_A = \text{volume of the impurity (formaldehyde and methanol vapor)}$$
$$V_{LAB} = \text{volume of the laboratory} = 960 \text{ ft}^3 = 27.2 \text{ m}^3$$

$$C_{PPM} = [(\rho_L V_L/MV_{LAB})(24.45 \text{ l/mole})][(T_A/298.15 \text{ K})(760 \text{ mm Hg}/P_A)]10^6$$

Formaldehyde: molecular weight $M = 30.02$ g/mole; $T_A = 25°C$; $P_A = 1$ atm; ρ_L at $25°C = N/A$; ρ_L at $20°C = 0.81$ g/ml

$$C_{PPM} = \frac{0.81 \text{ g/ml}}{(30.02 \text{ g/mole})(27.2 \text{ m}^3)}(24.45 \text{ l/mole})\left[(T_A/298.15 \text{ K})(760 \text{ mm Hg}/P_A)\right]10^6$$

$$C_{PPM} = 8\,975 \text{ ppm}$$

Methanol: molecular weight $M = 32.04$ g/mole; $T_A = 25°C$; $P_A = 1$ atm; ρ_L at $25°C = 0.79$ g/ml

$$C_{PPM} = \frac{0.79 \text{ g/ml}}{(32.04 \text{ g/mole})(27.2 \text{ m}^3)}(24.45 \text{ l/mole})\left[(T_A/298.15 \text{ K})(760 \text{ mm Hg}/P_A)\right]10^6$$

$$C_{PPM} = 2\,660 \text{ ppm}$$

Problem 37

A permeation tube containing vinyl chloride monomer is 5 cm long, and it permeates vinyl chloride at a rate of 128 ng/cm/min into a dry air stream (at 22°C and 638.2 mm Hg) flowing at 2.5 liters per minute. What is the concentration of vinyl chloride in this air stream?

Solution 37

Molecular weight of vinyl chloride $(CH_2 = CHCl) = 12.011(2) + 1.0079(3) + 35.453(1) = 62.5$ g/mole
Mass permeated in one minute $= (128 \text{ ng/cm/min})(1 \text{ min})(5 \text{ cm}) = 640$ ng

$$C_{M/V} = 640 \text{ ng}/2.5 \text{ l}$$

$$C_{M/V} = (640 \text{ ng}/2.5 \text{ l})(1000 \text{ l/m}^3)(\mu g/1000 \text{ ng})[1 \text{ mg}/1000 \text{ } \mu g]$$

$$C_{M/V} = 0.256 \text{ mg/m}^3$$

$$C_{PPM} = (C_{M/V}RT/MP)10^6$$

$$C_{PPM} = \frac{(0.265 \text{ mg/m}^3)(0.08205 \text{ l atm/mole K})(295.15 \text{ K})}{(62.5 \text{ g/mole})(638.2 \text{ atm}/760)}10^6$$

$$C_{PPM} = 0.10 \text{ ppm}$$

Problem 38

In the process of preparing an indoor air quality survey, an industrial hygienist decided to collect continuous air samples for carbon dioxide. The carbon dioxide analyzer samples air at 100 cm³/min. To maintain a reliable quality assurance program, a multipoint calibration is necessary. The calibration gas is 2500 ppm carbon dioxide in zero air (carbon dioxide–free air), and the diluent air is zero (carbon dioxide–free) air. Specify the rotameter necessary for this calibration, and give examples of the calibration and zero air flow rates.

Solution 38

The zero air is prepared by blending 79.0% nitrogen and 21.0% oxygen. Because the analyzer samples at 100 cm³/min, the final calibration gas mixture will be prepared at 110 cm³/min. The extra airflow volume will vent into the laboratory. The calibration gas mixture is 2500 ppm carbon dioxide in zero air. (See the sketch in Figure 5-6.)

   A reasonable multipoint calibration should include 0, 500, 1000, 1500, 2000, 2500 ppm CO_2; that is, C_{FINAL} varies over the range 0, 500, 1000, 1500, 2000, 2500 ppm CO_2.

   $Q_{\text{FINAL}} = 110$ cm³/min
Using the relationship for mass flow balance:

$$Q_{CO_2} C_{CO_2} = Q_{\text{FINAL}} C_{\text{FINAL}} = Q_F C_F$$

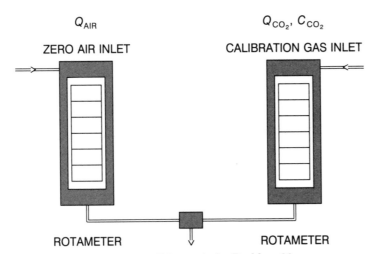

Figure 5-6. Schematic for Problem 38.

Solve for Q_{CO_2}:

$$Q_{CO_2} = Q_{FINAL}C_{FINAL} = Q_F C_F / C_{CO_2}$$

$$Q_{CO_2} = (110 \text{ cm}^3/\text{min})C_F/2500 \text{ ppm}$$

$$Q_{CO_2} = (0.0440 \text{ cm}^3/\text{min ppm})C_F$$

Substitute the various values for C_F:
  $C_F = 500$ ppm:

$$Q_{CO_2} = (0.0440 \text{ cm}^3/\text{min ppm})500 \text{ ppm} = 22 \text{ cm}^3/\text{min}$$

$C_F = 1000$ ppm:

$$Q_{CO_2} = (0.0440 \text{ cm}^3/\text{min ppm})1000 \text{ ppm} = 44 \text{ cm}^3/\text{min}$$

$C_F = 1500$ ppm:

$$Q_{CO_2} = (0.0440 \text{ cm}^3/\text{min ppm})1500 \text{ ppm} = 66 \text{ cm}^3/\text{min}$$

$C_F = 2000$ ppm:

$$Q_{CO_2} = (0.0440 \text{ cm}^3/\text{min ppm})2000 \text{ ppm} = 88 \text{ cm}^3/\text{min}$$

$C_F = 2500$ ppm:

$$Q_{CO_2} = (0.0440 \text{ cm}^3/\text{min ppm})2500 \text{ ppm} = 110 \text{ cm}^3/\text{min}$$

Recall:

$$Q_F = Q_{AIR} + Q_{CO_2}$$

$$Q_{AIR} = Q_F - Q_{CO_2}$$

$$Q_{AIR} = \frac{110 \text{ cm}^3}{\text{min}} - Q_{CO_2}$$

Q_{CO_2} CO$_2$ Flowrate (cm^3/min)	Q_{AIR} Diluent air flowrate (cm^3/min)	C_{FINAL} [CO$_2$] Concentration (ppm)
0	110	0
22	88	500
44	66	1000
66	44	1500
88	22	2000
110	0	2500

The flow meters that are selected must be capable of delivering diluent air and carbon dioxide calibration gas between 0 cm^3/min and 200 cm^3/min.

Problem 39

Silane gas is exhausted into a chamber exhaust duct (a branch duct that is a part of a larger system) at 3.0 liters per minute.

> **A.** How many cubic feet per hour of nitrogen are needed to dilute the silane to 0.50% before it reaches the main duct?
> **B.** The silane/nitrogen mixture then enters a main exhaust duct. The total flow rate in the main exhaust duct is 2500 cubic feet per minute (ft^3/min). What is the concentration of silane (in parts per million) in the main duct?

Solution 39

Silane (silicon tetrahydride) is SiH_4. Assume that the silane is 100.0% pure SiH_4. Assume that pure nitrogen is used as the diluent gas flow (see Figure 5-7).

$$Q_F C_F = Q_I C_I$$
$$(Q_I + Q_D) C_F = Q_I C_I$$
$$Q_I C_F + Q_D C_F = Q_I C_I$$
$$Q_D C_F = Q_I C_I - Q_I C_F$$
$$Q_D = (Q_I C_I - Q_I C_F)/C_F$$
$$Q_D = (300 \text{ lpm\%} - 1.5 \text{ lpm\%})/0.5\%$$
$$Q_D = (298.5 \text{ lpm\%})/0.5\% = 597 \text{ lpm nitrogen}$$

Therefore, 597 lpm of N_2 is needed to dilute the 100% SiH_4 flowing at 3 lpm to 0.5% SiH_4. The total volume flow entering the main duct is Q_T (Q_{TOTAL}).

$$Q_F = Q_I + Q_D = (3 + 597)\text{lpm} = 600 \text{ lpm.}$$
$$Q_{TOTAL} = Q_{SiH_4} + Q_{N_2} = (3 + 597)\text{lpm} = 600 \text{ lpm}$$
$$(600 \text{ lpm})(60 \text{ m/h})(ft^3/28.32 \text{ l}) = 1271 \text{ cfh of nitrogen}$$

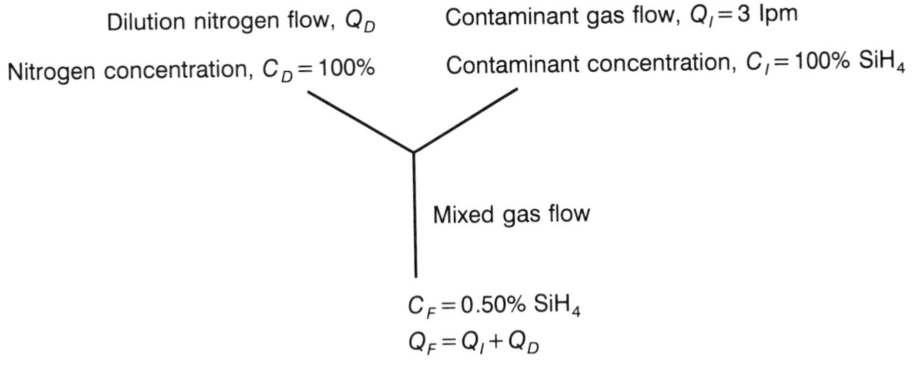

Dilution nitrogen flow, Q_D Contaminant gas flow, $Q_I = 3$ lpm

Nitrogen concentration, $C_D = 100\%$ Contaminant concentration, $C_I = 100\%$ SiH_4

Mixed gas flow

$$C_F = 0.50\% \text{ } SiH_4$$
$$Q_F = Q_I + Q_D$$

Figure 5-7.

6

Temperature and Pressure Effects

Outcome Competencies   *After studying this chapter you will be able to:*

- *Explain volume and volume flowrate.*
- *Derive temperature effects.*
- *Derive pressure effects.*
- *Develop combined temperature and pressure effects.*
- *Correct field and laboratory volume for temperature and pressure effects.*
- *Develop temperature and pressure corrections to calculate mass per volume concentration.*

1. INTRODUCTION

The review of the laws of Boyle, Charles, Gay-Lussac, and Dalton presented in Chapter 3 is the basis for understanding temperature and pressure effects on air sample volume. The volume of a collected air sample changes if the temperature and the pressure at the sampling location differ from the laboratory calibration temperature and pressure. To compare an individual's exposure to occupational exposure limits (i.e., TLVs, PELs, RELs, WEELs, etc.) conditions are established at normal temperature and pressure. To calculate exposures, air sample volumes measured in the field must be corrected to NTP conditions if the field conditions vary substantially from NTP. Examples of substantial variations from standard conditions will be given later in this chapter. Every time an instrument, sampling method, or monitor is used to measure contaminant concentration in air, there must be assurance that the device is correctly calibrated for sample volume, flowrate, and concentration. The determination of sample mass is an analytical laboratory concern and will be discussed in a later chapter. This chapter describes how to incorporate temperature, pressure, and humidity differences between standard conditions, laboratory calibration conditions, and field conditions into a monitoring program to assess worker exposure to air contaminants.

Chapter 3 demonstrated that air is a dynamic mixture of gases and must be given a "standardized definition" to describe its composition. For industrial hygiene and air pollution, standard air is defined as air at 25°C, one atmosphere pressure; dry air has an apparent molecular weight of 28.96 grams per mole. Without an environmental chamber with extensive temperature, humidity, and barometric pressure controls, the standard temperature and pressure condition is almost impossible to achieve. Attempting to reproduce standard conditions is not an inexpensive engineering design problem; neither is it a very practical one. After the definition of standard air is established, it is possible to calculate back to the standard condition from either the calibration conditions or field conditions, using the ideal gas equation.

2. VOLUME AND VOLUME FLOWRATE

The volume of a gas or vapor collected during air sampling is the product of volume flowrate delivered by the air sampling pump (Q) and time (t):

$$V = Qt$$

Volume flowrate (Q) is the volume of a gas or vapor delivered per unit of time. As in all the other chapters in this book, there are typical units to consider. The volume unit (V) may be in liters (l), cubic meters (m^3), or cubic centimeters (cm^3). Volume flowrate (Q in volume per unit time) may be in units of liters per minute (lpm or l/min), cubic meters per second (m^3/s), cubic meters per minute (m^3/min), or cubic centimeters per minute (cc/min). This list covers the usual allowed exceptions in the SI system. Typical SI values for volume flowrates are cubic meters per second (m^3/s), liters per minute (lpm), and cubic centimeters per minute (cc/min). The minute is usually the most convenient time interval to use. Flowrates in the English system of units include cubic feet per minute (cfm or ft^3/min). Fortunately, the time dimension (minutes, second, hours, etc.) is independent of temperature and pressure.

Later in this chapter, air sampling pumps that deliver a wide range of volume flowrates from 0.20 lpm to 4.0 lpm will be employed in exposure assessments. Pumps deliver their rated volume flowrate whether they are operating at the calibration location or in the field location as long as their batteries are sufficiently charged or the line voltage is constant. The volume flowrates that air sampling pumps deliver are not normally affected by the conditions at which they operate. To compare exposure to an occupational health standard, it is necessary to determine the *volume* of air sampled corrected to standard conditions. This requires the procedures outlined in this chapter.

3. DERIVATION OF TEMPERATURE EFFECT FACTOR

Recall what happens when a gas or a vapor changes from a lower temperature, T_1, to a higher temperature, T_2. This temperature increase causes the gas to expand, from V_1 to V_2 (Charles' law). Reasoning through the effect of this temperature change on the gas volume may be done intuitively. Solving the ideal gas equation at two conditions yields a ratio of temperatures. For example, the ideal gas equation can be written at two different environmental conditions, standard condition (S) and field condition (F):

$$P_F V_F = nRT_F \qquad P_S V_S = nRT_S$$

$$P_F V_F / T_F = nR \qquad P_S V_S / T_S = nR$$

Since both equations equal nR, this yields:

$$P_F V_F / T_F = P_S V_S / T_S$$

At a constant pressure (isobaric) condition, $P_F = P_S$, solving for V_S gives:

$$V_S = V_F (T_S / T_F)$$

It is critical to remember that V_S is the air sample volume corrected from the field condition (V_F) to the volume that would exist if the field volume were returned to standard condition (V_S at 25°C and one atmosphere). The volume corrected to standard conditions is the volume that is used in calculating the mass concentration of the contaminant (mg/m³, μg/m³, etc.).

If T_S is larger than T_F, the ratio T_S / T_F will be a number greater than one ($T_S / T_F > 1.0$). Any ratio greater than one will cause a calculated increase in the volume V_F to a new and larger volume V_S:

$$V_S = V_F (T_S / T_F)$$

If T_S is less than T_F, the ratio T_S / T_F will be a number less than one ($T_S / T_F < 1.0$). Any ratio less than one will cause a calculated decrease in the volume V_F to a new and smaller volume, V_S:

$$V_S = V_F (T_S / T_F)$$

The temperature effect factor, T_S / T_F, can be expressed as F_T.

4. DERIVATION OF PRESSURE EFFECT FACTOR

A change in the pressure exerted on a gas of volume V_F from a higher pressure P_F to a lower pressure P_S is predicted by the ratio P_F/P_S. This ratio will be a number greater than one ($P_F/P_S > 1.0$; Boyle's law). Solving the ideal gas equation at two conditions yields a ratio of temperatures and pressure. For example, the ideal gas equation can be written at two different environmental conditions, F and S:

$$P_F V_F = nRT_F \qquad P_S V_S = nRT_S$$

$$P_F V_F/T_F = nR \qquad P_S V_S/T_S = nR$$

Since both equations equal nR, this yields:

$$P_F V_F/T_F = P_S V_S/T_S$$

At a constant temperature (isothermal) condition, $T_F = T_S$, solving for V_S gives:

$$V_S = V_F(P_F/P_S)$$

A ratio of pressures greater than one will cause an increase in the volume V_F to a new and larger volume V_S:

$$V_S = V_F(P_F/P_S)$$

A ratio of pressures less than one will cause a decrease in the volume V_F to a new and smaller volume V_S:

$$V_S = V_F(P_F/P_S)$$

The pressure effect factor, P_F/P_S can be expressed as F_P.

A change in pressure is readily observed when one is flying in a commercial airliner. The increase in volume of air in the headspace of a cream container that was filled at sea level expands to a new and larger volume (V_F). This occurs because of the decrease in cabin pressure ($P_F < P_S$ or $P_S/P_F > 1.0$). The cabin pressure in commercial airliners is maintained at a nominal value of about 0.76 atmosphere ($P_F = 0.76$). This is an atmospheric pressure equivalent to an altitude of 8000 feet. The field pressure is less than standard sea level pressure ($P_S/P_F = 1.0$ atm$/0.76$ atm $= 1.3$), and the foil closure on a container of cream, sealed at sea level, appears to have expanded and feels like a drum head. The decrease in pressure from P_S to P_F ($P_S/P_F = 1.3$) results in an increase in volume from V_S to V_F:

$$V_F = V_S(P_S/P_F) \text{ or } V_F = 1.3V_S$$

If the traveler is not careful opening the container, it is likely to erupt and spray cream everywhere. Image what would happen if the ink bladder of an expensive fountain pen ruptured under the same conditions!

5. DERIVATION OF PRESSURE EFFECT FACTOR FOR ALTITUDE

Tables that list factors for temperature (F_T) and factors for pressure (F_P) are available in the literature (1, 2). They can be derived as indicated in this section. The American Society of Heating, Refrigeration and Air-Conditioning Engineers (ASHRAE)(2) lists two empirically derived equations to predict barometric pressure:

- For altitudes less than 4000 feet:

$$P_{ATM} = 29.921 \text{ inches of mercury} - 0.001025\ H$$

- For altitudes greater than 4000 feet and less than 10,000 feet:

$$P_{ATM} = 29.42 \text{ inches of mercury} - 0.00090\ H$$

where:

P = local atmospheric pressure in inches of mercury
H = local elevation, feet above sea level

Pressure correction factors (F_P) can be calculated using the ASHRAE values for pressure:

- At 4000 feet ($H = 4000$):

$$F_P = (29.921 - 0.001025H)/(29.921)$$

$$F_P = [29.921 - 0.001025(4000)]/(29.921)$$

$$F_P = (25.821)/(29.921) = 0.863$$

- At 10,000 feet ($H = 10,000$):

$$F_P = (29.420 - 0.00090H)/(29.921)$$

$$F_P = [29.420 - 0.00090(10,000)]/(29.921)$$

$$F_P = (20.420)/(29.921) = 0.682$$

A reasonable approximation to the pressure correction factor can be derived based on a few simple assumptions (see Figure 6-1). The relation-

In meters above sea level:

$$F_P = e^{-0.000109A}$$

(A is in meters)

$$P_{ACTUAL} = F_P(P_{STD})$$

Pressure one meter above sea level:

$$P_1 = 101\,289\ \text{Pa}$$

Force one meter above sea level:

$$F_1 = 101\,289\ \text{N}$$

Pressure at sea level:

$$P_0 = 101\,300\ \text{Pa}$$

Force at sea level:

$$F_0 = 101\,300\ \text{N}$$

In feet above sea level:

$$F_P = e^{-0.00003493A}$$

(A is in feet)

$$P_{ACTUAL} = F_P(P_{STD})$$

Pressure one foot above sea level:

$$P_1 = 2116.14\ \text{PSF}$$

Force one foot above sea level:

$$F_1 = 14.621\ \text{lb}_F$$

Pressure at sea level:

$$P_0 = 2116.22\ \text{PSF}$$

Force at sea level:

$$F_0 = 14.695\ \text{lb}_F$$

Figure 6.1. The variation of atmospheric pressure with altitude.

ship will predict the change in barometric pressure within 5% for altitudes less than 10,000 feet.

- At the earth's surface, the pressure exerted by the atmosphere is:

$$P_0 = 101\,300\ \text{Pa} = 101\,300\ \text{N/m}^2 = 101\,300\ \text{kg m/s}^2\text{m}^2$$

- The force (F_0) exerted on one square meter at the earth's surface can be calculated:

$$F_0 = (101\,300\ \text{kg m/s}^2\text{m}^2)(1\ \text{m}^2) = 101\,300\ \text{kg m/s}^2 = 101\,300\ \text{N}$$

Moving up one meter from the earth's surface is identical to moving up through the column of air that has a volume ($V = \text{area} \times \text{height}$) of one cubic meter ($m^3$). A decrease in the force results by moving above the surface one meter. This can be calculated from the standard density ($\rho_{STD} = 1.1184\ \text{kg/m}^3$). Recall density equals mass per volume:

$$\rho_{STD} = m/v; \quad v\rho_{STD} = m$$

$$F = ma = \rho_{STD}va = (1.1184\ \text{kg/m}^3)(1\ \text{m}^3)(9.808\ \text{m/s}^2)$$

$$F = 10.969267\ \text{kg m/s}^2$$

By moving up one meter, the force will decrease by $10.969267 \text{ kg m/s}^2$. This is the force exerted by a column of air one meter above the surface. The new force at one meter (F_1) is:

$$F_1 = F_0 - \rho_{STD} v a = 101300 \text{ kg m/s}^2 - 10.969267 \text{ kg m/s}^2 = 101289 \text{ kg m/s}^2$$

The ratio of the force at one meter (F_1) to the force at the surface (F_0) is F_1/F_0:

$$F_1/F_0 = \frac{(101289 \text{ kg m/s}^2)}{(101300 \text{ kg m/s}^2)} = 0.999891$$

$$F_1/F_0 = 0.999891$$

Ignore the temperature effect with changes in altitude and assume that the barometric pressure decreases similarly to the first order decay of radiation, some chemical reactions, and bacterial growth. This may sound like an unreasonable assumption, but it will predict the correction factor for atmospheric pressure (F_P) rather well for altitudes below 3048 meters or 10000 feet! Recall the radioactive decay equation, which is a first order decay equation:

$$R = e^{-kt}$$

where $-k$ is the rate constant, or the rate at which the radiation decreases with time (t). A similar equation can be used to calculate the correction factor for atmospheric pressure (F_P) with respect to altitude. The atmospheric pressure correction factor F_P is given by:

$$F_P = e^{-kA}$$

where $-k$ is the rate constant for the decrease in barometric pressure with respect to altitude (A) in meters; thus:

$$k = F_1/F_0 = 0.999891$$

$$F_P = e^{-kA} = 0.999891$$

When $A = 1$ meter, this equation can be solved for k by taking the logarithm of both sides:

$$0.999891 = e^{-k(1)}$$

$$\ln 0.999891 = -k = -0.000109$$

In the general case, the barometric pressure correction factor (F_P) for altitude in meters (Figure 6-1) is:

$$F_P = e^{-0.000109A} \quad (\text{A is in meters})$$

Given a sea level pressure of 14.695 lb/in^2 and a density of 0.07391 lb/ft^3, a similar derivation can be developed. In the general case, the barometric pressure correction factor (F_P) for altitude in feet (Figure 6-1) is:

$$F_P = e^{-0.00003493A} \ (A \text{ is in feet})$$

The pressure effect factor (F_P) relates variation in barometric pressure to altitude. Once F_P is calculated, the approximate barometric pressure (P_F, which excludes the variation caused by local weather patterns) can be calculated from:

$$P_F = F_P(P_S)$$

Example 1

Calculate the pressure effect factor F_P and normal barometric pressure for Denver, Colorado, using the ASHRAE equation as well as the exponential equation derived in this section. The elevation for Denver is $A = 1524$ meters = 5000 feet.

- ASHRAE method:

$$F_P = P_{ATM}/P_{STD} = (29.42 - 0.00090H)/(29.921)$$

$$F_P = P_{ATM}/P_{STD} = [29.42 - 0.00090(5000)]/(29.921) = 0.83$$

- Exponential equation method:

$$F_P = e^{-0.000109A} \ (A \text{ is in meters})$$

$$F_P = e^{-0.000109A} = e^{-0.000109(1\,524)} = 0.85$$

$$F_P = e^{-0.00003493A} \ (A \text{ is in feet})$$

$$F_P = e^{-0.00003493A} = e^{-0.00003493(5\,000)} = 0.84$$

$$F_P = 0.83 \text{ (literature value) (1)}$$

$$P_F = F_P(P_S) = 0.84(760 \text{ mm Hg}) = 630.4 \text{ mm Hg}$$

The barometric pressure in Denver is 630.4 mm Hg and is equivalent to 760 mm Hg at sea level.

The calculated values for F_P differ by less than 2.5% from the literature value. The calculation resulting from the use of the exponential equation and ASHRAE correction is summarized in Table 6-1 (1, 2).

TABLE 6-1. Calculated pressure correction factors for altitudes to 10 000 meters (32 808 feet)

Altitude		Exponential Calculated				ASHRAE Calculated			
(Meters)	(Feet)	F_P	P_{ATM} (mm Hg)	P_{ATM} (in Hg)	Pa (Pascals)	F_P	P_{ATM} (mm Hg)	P_{ATM} (in Hg)	Pa (Pascals)
−500	−1640	1.06	805.6	31.72	107 405	1.056	802.6	31.60	106 999
	−1000	1.04	790.4	31.12	105 378	1.034	785.8	30.94	104 770
0	0	1.00	760.0	29.92	101 325	1.00	760.0	29.92	101 325
	1000	0.97	737.2	29.02	98 285	0.966	734.2	28.90	97 880
500	1640	0.95	722.0	28.42					
	2000	0.93	706.8	27.83	94 232	0.94	714.4	28.13	95 246
	3000	0.90	684.0	26.93	91 193	0.897	681.7	26.84	90 889
1000	3281	0.89	676.4	26.63	90 179	0.90	684.0	26.93	91 193
	4000	0.87	661.2	26.03	88 153	0.863	655.9	25.82	87 443
	5000	0.84	638.4	25.13	85 113	0.83	630.8	24.83	84 100
	6000	0.81	615.6	24.24	82 073	0.79	600.4	23.64	80 047
2000	6562					0.80	608.0	23.94	81 060
	7000	0.78	592.8	23.34	79 034	0.772	586.7	23.10	78 223
	8000	0.76	577.6	22.74	77 007	0.73	554.8	21.84	73 967
	9000	0.73	554.8	21.84	73 976				
3000	9843					0.72	547.2	21.54	72 954
	10000	0.71	539.6	21.24	71 941	0.682	518.3	20.41	69 104
4000	13 123	0.65	494.0	19.45	65 861	—	—	—	—
5000	16 404	0.58	440.8	17.35	58 769	—	—	—	—
6000	19 685	0.52	395.2	15.56	52 689	—	—	—	—
7000	22 966	0.47	357.2	14.06	47 623	—	—	—	—
8000	26 247	0.42	319.2	12.57	42 557	—	—	—	—
9000	29 528	0.37	281.2	11.07	37 490	—	—	—	—
10000	32 808	0.34	258.4	10.17	34 451	—	—	—	—

Source: ASHRAE, *Handbook of Fundamentals* (1981), p. 5.1.
ACGIH, *Industrial Ventilation: A Manual of Recommended Practice*, 21st Edition (1992), p. 5-44.

6. COMBINED TEMPERATURE AND PRESSURE EFFECTS

The individual temperature and pressure effects can be combined to predict changes in volume. To adjust a volume to the standard condition (V_S, 298.15 K and 1 atmosphere) from the volume during calibration (V_C) or field sampling volume (V_F), the ideal gas equation must be written for each condition [i.e., the calibration condition (C), the field condition (F), and the standard condition (S)]:

$$P_C V_C = nRT_C \qquad P_S V_S = nRT_S \qquad P_F V_F = nRT_F$$

These equations may be solved for nR and set equal to each other:

$$nR = P_C V_C / T_C = P_S V_S / T_S = P_F V_F / T_F$$

To correct the volume from the calibration condition to standard condition, solve the equation for V_S:

$$V_S = V_F (P_F / P_S)(T_S / T_F) = V_F (F_{TP})$$

$$V_S = V_C (P_C / P_S)(T_S / T_C) = V_C (F_{TP})$$

This equation demonstrates the change in pressure and temperature on the volume, V_C, the volume handled under calibration conditions, to produce volume V_S, the volume that would exist at standard conditions. The magnitude of this change in volume is given by F_{TP}, the temperature and pressure correction factor.

7. COMBINED TEMPERATURE AND PRESSURE EFFECTS ON VOLUME FLOWRATE

Field (F) and calibration (C) conditions vary with time, location, and climate. By defining a standard (S) condition, that is, normal temperature and pressure (NTP = 25°C, 1 atmosphere, and dry air), it is possible to correct the calibration condition and/or the field condition to the standard condition. The standard condition is independent of where and when the samples are collected (the joy of the standard condition!).

What do the combined temperature and pressure effects have to do with air sampling and analysis? The purpose of an air sampling program is to determine an individual's exposure by measuring the concentration of a pollutant. An air sample is collected and sent to an analytical laboratory, which determines the mass of contaminant or the number of fibers of material collected. Mass concentration then is determined by dividing the mass by the volume of air sampled *corrected to the normal temperature and pressure (NTP) condition*. The mass concentration exposure is compared to occupational exposure limits, which are expressed at NTP. Concentration may be expressed as the mass of pollutant per volume of air (at NTP), for example, mg/m^3, $\mu g/m^3$, ng/m^3, and pg/m^3, or the number of fibers per cubic centimeters (f/cc). Mass concentration for gases and vapors can be converted to concentration in parts per million, as described in Chapter 5. Worker exposure is compared to the occupational exposure limit in parts per million or milligram per cubic meter *if and only if* the conversion between parts per million and milligram per cubic meter is performed correctly, as outlined in Chapter 5 and later in this chapter.

The volume or volume flowrate multiplied by time ($V = Qt$) of air sampled at the field (F) condition will be adjusted to the equivalent volume at NTP. This correction also must be applied if the pump was calibrated in a laboratory at another set of temperature and pressure conditions. This will be called the calibration condition (e.g., P_C and T_C). To avoid the complication introduced by calibrating the volume flow off-site (away from the location where sampling is performed), it is recommended that the pump be calibrated at the location under conditions similar to those to be encountered during the actual field sampling (T_F and P_F conditions must be correctly recorded for volume correction). The volume sampled in the field will be corrected to the volume at NTP before the exposure concentration is calculated. If this procedure is not followed, the exposure concentration will be incorrect.

In summary, changes in temperature and pressure affect the volume occupied by all gases and vapors. As it is assumed that the gases and vapors behave as ideal gases, the pressure, volume, and temperature relationship follows the ideal gas equation.

8. APPLYING TEMPERATURE AND PRESSURE CORRECTION TO VOLUME

An important step in using an air sampling device or air monitor is to correct the volume delivered during the field procedure (or calibration procedure) to the standard condition. It is necessary to correct the sample volume to normal temperature and pressure condition so that the correct exposure concentration can be calculated. The concentration that results from an exposure measurement is compared to an occupational exposure limit (TLVs, PELs, RELs, WEELs, etc.), which is specified in part per million by volume (which is independent of temperature and pressure) or milligrams per cubic meter at NTP. Applying a temperature and pressure correction to the air volume returns it to the volume at normal temperature and pressure. The standard volume during the calibration procedure is:

$$V_S = V_C(T_S/T_C)(P_C/P_S)$$

The standard volume during the field procedure is:

$$V_S = V_F(T_S/T_F)(P_F/P_S)$$

It is also necessary to determine if the volume collected is sufficient to meet the conditions imposed by the air sampling protocol (5, 6) to collect the limit of detection (LOD) mass. The limit of detection mass will be discussed in Chapter 7.

To correct the volume of air delivered by a pump, to the normal temperature and pressure condition, calculate the volume ($V_F = Qt$). This volume (V_F) is corrected to the volume (V_S) that would exist at NTP. Each of these effects for pressure and temperature will be demonstrated separately, and then they will be combined.

Temperature Correction

Temperature correction is the adjustment to the volume (the volume flowrate multiplied by time) required by the difference between the calibration temperature (T_C) or field sampling temperature (T_F) and the desired standard temperature (T_S) of 25°C (298.15 K). The volume delivered at the standard condition (V_S) either increases or decreases by the ratio of the absolute temperatures (the temperature effect factor, T_S/T_F).

Example 2

Determine the NTP volume of air collected at 0.2 lpm for 20 minutes when an air sampling pump is operating at a sampling location at 15°C. The pump was calibrated at the field location.

$$Q_F = \text{the volume flowrate, at the calibration and field condition}$$
$$t_F = \text{time interval, at the field condition}$$
$$V_F = \text{volume delivered, at the field condition}$$
$$T_F = \text{temperature at the field condition}$$
$$Q_F = 0.20 \text{ lpm}$$
$$t_F = 20.0 \text{ min}$$
$$V_F = (Q_F)(t_F)$$
$$T_F = 15°C \ (288.15 \text{ K})$$
$$V_S = V_F(T_S/T_F)$$
$$V_F = (Q_F)(t_F) = (0.20 \text{ lpm})(20 \text{ min}) = 4.0 \text{ l}$$
$$T_S/T_F = 298.15K/288.15K = 1.035$$
$$V_S = V_F(T_S/T_F) = 4.0 \text{ l } (1.035) = 4.14 \text{ l}$$

Percent difference from NTP $= [(V_S - V_F)/V_F] 100$

Percent difference from NTP $= [(4.14 \text{ l} - 4.0 \text{ l})/4.0 \text{ l}] 100 = 3.5\%$

This volume change between field and standard conditions is less than 5% and may be considered too small to correct, but this is not always the situation. In this example the volume flowrate measured is 0.20 lpm. The volume delivered is (0.2 lpm)(20 min) = 4.0 l. When corrected, the field volume becomes the temperature corrected standard volume (V_S) of 4.14 l. This volume (4.14 l) would exist if the air moving through the system were at the standard condition (298.15 K).

Example 3

Determine the NTP volume of air collected at 0.2 lpm for 20 minutes when a firefighter is working close to an oil well fire in Kuwait. The sampling temperature is 140°F behind a reflective aluminum shield.

$$Q_F = \text{the volume flowrate, at the field condition} = 0.2 \text{ lpm}$$
$$t_F = \text{time interval, at the field condition} = 20.0 \text{ min}$$
$$V_F = \text{volume delivered, at the field condition} = (Q_F)(t_F)$$
$$= (0.20 \text{ lpm})(20 \text{ min}) = 4.0 \text{ l}$$
$$T_F = \text{temperature at the field condition} = 140°F = 60.0°C$$
$$= 333.15 \text{ K}$$
$$F_T = 298.15 \text{ K}/333.15 \text{ K} = 0.895$$
$$V_S = V_F(F_T) = V_F(T_S/T_F) = 4.0(0.895) = 3.58 \text{ l}$$

$$\text{Percent difference from NTP} = \left[(V_S - V_F)/V_F\right]100$$

$$\text{Percent difference from NTP} = \left[(3.58 \text{ l} - 4.0 \text{ l})/4.0 \text{ l}\right]100$$

$$= -10.5\%$$

This extreme temperature produces a -10.5% change in the volume and must be considered in subsequent calculations to assess worker exposure. In this example the volume flowrate measured is 0.20 lpm. The volume delivered (the volume flowrate multiplied by time is 4.0 l) is corrected to standard temperature and results in a temperature-corrected standard volume (V_S) of 3.58 l. This volume (3.58 l) would exist if the air moving through the system were at the standard condition (298.15 K).

A temperature change ranging from 15°C (283.15 K) to 40°C (313.15 K) results in a temperature effect on volume of $\pm 5\%$ (Table 6-2). If a change in

TABLE 6-2. The temperature range with a minimum effect on volume

T_I (°C/K)	T_S (°C/K)	T_S/T_I	Change from normal temperature (%)
15/283.15	25/298.15	1.05	+5
40/313.15	25/298.15	0.95	-5

Note: T_I is either T_F or T_C, depending on whether the correction is from field or calibration conditions.

volume of $\pm 5\%$ can be tolerated in an exposure assessment, then a change in temperature between 15°C and 40°C will not change the volume by more than 5%. This effect should be evaluated to determine the effect of temperature on volume before the decision is made to ignore the effect of temperature on the volume sampled.

Pressure Correction

Pressure correction is the adjustment to the volume (the volume flowrate multiplied by time) required by the difference between the calibration pressure (P_C) or field sampling pressure (P_F) and the desired standard pressure (P_S) of one atmosphere (760 mm Hg). The volume delivered at the standard condition (V_S) either increases or decreases by the ratio of the field and standard pressure (the pressure effect factor, P_F/P_S).

Example 4

Determine the NTP volume of air collected at 0.2 lpm for 20 minutes when an air sampling pump is operating at a sampling location that is at an elevation of $+1000$ feet. The pump was calibrated at the field location.

$$Q_F = \text{volume flowrate, at the calibration and field condition}$$
$$t_F = \text{time interval, at the field condition}$$
$$V_F = \text{volume delivered, at the field condition} = (Q_F)(t_F)$$
$$= (0.20 \text{ lpm})(20 \text{ min}) = 4.0 \text{ l}$$
$$P_F = \text{pressure at the field condition} = 733.9 \text{ mm Hg}$$
$$V_S = V_F(P_F/P_S)$$
$$P_F/P_S = 733.9 \text{ mm Hg}/760 \text{ mm Hg} = 0.966$$
$$V_S = V_F(P_F/P_S) = 4.0 \text{ l}(0.966) = 3.86 \text{ l}$$

Percent difference from NTP $= [(V_S - V_F)/V_F]100$

Percent difference from NTP $= [(3.86 \text{ l} - 4.0 \text{ l})/4.0 \text{ l}]100 = -3.5\%$

This volume change between field and standard conditions is less than 5% and may be considered too small to correct, but this is not always the situation. In this example the volume flowrate measured is 0.20 lpm. The volume delivered is $(0.2 \text{ lpm})(20 \text{ mins}) = 4.0 \text{ l}$. When corrected, the field volume becomes the pressure-corrected standard volume (V_S) of 3.86 l. This volume (3.86 l) would exist if the air moving through the system were at the standard condition (one atmosphere).

Example 5

Determine the NTP volume of air collected at 0.2 lpm for 20 minutes when an air sampling pump is operating at a sampling location that is at an elevation of +5000 feet. The pump was calibrated at the field location.

$$Q_F = \text{volume flowrate, at the calibration and field condition}$$
$$t_F = \text{time interval, at the field condition}$$
$$V_F = \text{volume delivered, at the field condition} = (Q_F)(t_F)$$
$$= (0.20 \text{ lpm})(20 \text{ min}) = 4.0 \text{ l}$$
$$P_F = \text{pressure at the field condition} = 638.2 \text{ mm Hg}$$
$$V_S = V_F(P_F/P_S)$$
$$P_F/P_S = 638.2 \text{ mm Hg}/760 \text{ mm Hg} = 0.84$$
$$V_S = V_F(P_F/P_S) = 4.0 \text{ l}(0.84) = 3.36 \text{ l}$$

$$\text{Percent difference from NTP} = \left[(V_S - V_F)/V_F\right]100$$

$$\text{Percent difference from NTP} = \left[(3.36 \text{ l} - 4.0 \text{ l})/4.0 \text{ l}\right]100 = -16\%$$

This extreme temperature produces a −16% change in the volume and must be considered in subsequent calculations to assess worker exposure. In this example the volume flowrate measured is 0.20 lpm. The volume delivered (the volume flowrate multiplied by time is 4.0 l) is corrected to standard pressure and results in a pressure corrected standard volume (V_S) of 3.36 l. This volume (3.36 l) would exist if the air moving through the system were at the standard condition (one atmosphere).

A pressure change ranging from 722 mm Hg (+1500 feet in elevation) to 798 mm Hg (−1400 feet in elevation) results in a pressure effect on volume of ±5% (Table 6-3). If a change in volume of ±5% can be tolerated in an exposure assessment, then a change in pressure between 722 mm Hg and 798 mm Hg will not change the volume by more than 5%. This effect should be evaluated to determine the effect of pressure (elevation) on volume before a decision is made to ignore the effect of pressure on the volume sampled.

TABLE 6-3. The barometric pressure range (altitude) with a minimum effect on volume

Elevation (Feet)	F_P	P_I (mm Hg)	P_S (mm Hg)	P_S/P_I	Change from normal pressure (%)
−1400	1.05	798	760	0.95	−5
+1500	0.95	722	760	1.05	+5

Note: P_I is either P_F or P_C, depending on whether the correction is from field or calibration conditions.

Apparatus Flow Diagram

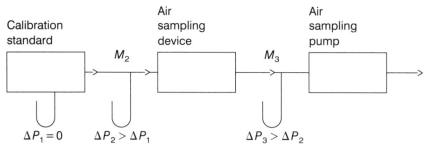

Figure 6-2. Apparatus flow diagram used to calibrate air sampling devices.

The need for pressure corrections to air volumes are not limited to changes in altitude. Some calibration of air sampling systems will introduce changes in pressure caused by the vapor pressure of water from some calibration devices and static pressure changes due to the air sampling devices. Figure 6-2 is the schematic diagram for calibrating an air sampling train. Note the locations of the manometers in Figure 6-2. Pressure correction is the adjustment to the volume (the volume flowrate multiplied by time) caused by the difference between the atmospheric pressure at the calibration location (P_C) and the desired standard pressure (P_S) of one atmosphere and dry air (1 atm). The volume delivered at the standard condition (V_S) either increases or decreases by the ratio of the pressures (the pressure effect factor, $F_P = P_C/P_S$).

The static pressure on the suction side of an air sampling system is always less than the atmospheric pressure. The sign for static pressure is *negative* on the suction or inlet side of an air sampling pump ($\Delta P_{SP} < 0$). As air moves through a calibration system, the static pressure drop (ΔP_{SP}) increases and becomes more negative through the system. The manometers indicate larger and more negative static pressures throughout the system. Static pressure is *positive* ($\Delta P_{SP} > 0$) on the pressure or outlet side of the air sampling pump or compressed gas supply.

Volume and flowrate calibration devices essentially are water-sealed systems (spirometer, manual and electronic soap bubble flowmeter, wet test meter) and operate at 100% relative humidity (% R.H.) with an inlet static $\Delta P_{SP} \approx 0$ inches of water column (inches H_2O or inches w.c.). The static pressure at the inlet to and within the calibration standard (spirometer, manual and electronic soap bubble flowmeter, wet test meter) is approximately zero inches of water. Therefore, the calibration device is delivering moist air, essentially at atmospheric pressure, when the calibration device is in thermal equilibrium with the surrounding environment.

It is imperative to recall that water vapor will always exert its own partial pressure or vapor pressure at the prevailing temperature according to Dalton's law of partial pressure ($P_T = \Sigma_i P_i$) in the calibration system. (The vapor pressure of water as a function of temperature is given in the Appendix.) The vapor pressure of water affects the volume of dry air passing through the calibration system. The volume of standard (dry) air passing through the system is the quantity of interest. To find the dry air volume, one must remove the effect of the partial pressure that water exerts at the calibration condition. Because the calibration system is not at the standard condition, a temperature and pressure correction must be applied to the volume delivered by that system to return it to the standard condition.

The air in the water-sealed calibration system is saturated with water vapor from the volume standard measuring device at local atmospheric pressure while it is at the prevailing static pressure of the system. The static pressure in the system also is treated as a component of the Dalton equation. It is important to remember that the sign of the static pressure is negative in a system that is under suction (i.e., it is less than the atmospheric pressure surrounding the system). Recall Dalton's law of partial pressure:

$$P_T = \Sigma_i P_i$$

Perhaps this is somewhat clearer:

$$P_T = P_{\text{ATM}} - P_{\text{VP}} + P_{\text{SP}}$$

where:

P_T = corrected dry air pressure
P_{ATM} = atmospheric pressure measured at the location of interest
P_{VP} = vapor pressure of water exerted on the air flowing through the water-sealed calibration device
P_{SP} = static pressure at which the calibration system operates, indicated by manometer M_3 in Figure 6-2

When calculating a pressure correction on the moist air volume delivered at the calibration condition, consider the system static pressure and the vapor pressure of water. The result of this correction is the total pressure of the dry air—the pressure exerted on that system without the influence of the static pressure ($P_{\text{SP}} = 0$) or vapor pressure ($P_{\text{VP}} = 0$). The volume is corrected to the standard pressure (dry air) because it is the actual pressure that influences the air volume as if the system were dry air operating without static pressure.

Combined Temperature and Pressure Correction

The next several examples demonstrate the combination of temperature and pressure effects on sample volumes.

Table 6-4 gives generic definitions applied to the examples that follow, to describe the measurements made in an air sampling system. These exam-

TABLE 6-4. Definition of terms used to correct the volume and volume flowrate through an air sampling train

Symbol	Generic definition	Value for this example only
C	Calibration condition	—
Q_C	Volume flowrate delivered during calibration	0.20 lpm
t_C	Duration (in minutes) at the calibration process	20 min
V_C	Volume delivered during calibration	4.0 l ($V_C = Q_C t_C$)
T_C	Temperature during calibration	27°C = 300.15 K
P_{ATM}	Atmospheric pressure as measured by a mercury in glass barometer	763.2 mm Hg
P_{VP}	Vapor pressure of liquid used in the liquid-sealed calibration device	26.7 mm Hg (vapor pressure of water at 27°C) (Note 1)
P_{SP}	Static pressure difference between room environment and calibration device ($P_{SP} < 0$ under suction)	-3.8 mm Hg (M_3, Figure 6-2); may also be in inches of water (Note 2)
P_C	The calculated pressure in the calibration (C) train: $P_C = P_{ATM} - P_{VP} + P_{SP} = P_{DRY}$ (Note 3)	$763.2 - 26.7 - 3.8 = 732.7$ mm Hg

Note 1: Vapor pressure of water is given in the Appendix.

Note 2: This P_{SP} is inserted here to demonstrate a principle and is not a value normally encountered, especially with a solid sorbent tube. This is common with a cassette mounted membrane filter used for sampling asbestos, metal fumes, or particles not otherwise classified (PNOC).

Note 3: P_{DRY} will be used later in this chapter.

ples will demonstrate the combined temperature and pressure correction calculations.

In the calibration laboratory at $Q_C = 0.2$ lpm, the volume delivered at the laboratory is:

$$V_C = (Q_C)(t_C) = (0.20 \text{ lpm})(20 \text{ min}) = 4.0 \text{ l}$$

Example 6

In this example a pump is being calibrated at conditions C, and is operating at the conditions given in Table 6-4. Calculate the volume of air at standard condition delivered by the pump.

Q_C = volume flowrate, at the calibration condition = 0.20 lpm
t_C = time interval, at the calibration condition 20.0 min
V_C = volume delivered, at the calibration condition
$V_C = (Q_C)(t_C) = (0.20 \text{ lpm})(20 \text{ min}) = 4.0 \text{ l}$

P_C = pressure at the calibration condition:

$$P_C = P_{ATM} - P_{VP} + P_{SP}$$

P_{ATM} = Atmospheric pressure measured at the calibration location at the time of calibration = 763.2 mm Hg in this example

P_{VP} = Vapor pressure of water over the air flowing through the water-sealed calibration device = 26.7 mm Hg in this example at $T_C = 27.0°C$ (Appendix)

P_{SP} = Static pressure at which the calibration system operates, as indicated by manometer M_3 in Figure 6-2 = −3.8 mm Hg in this example (usually read in inches of water and converted to millimeters of mercury)

$$P_C = P_{ATM} - P_{VP} + P_{SP} = 763.2 - 26.7 - 3.8 = 732.7 \text{ mm Hg}$$

$$V_S = V_C F_{TP} = V_C(P_C/P_S)(T_S/T_C)$$

$$(P_C/P_S)(T_S/T_C) = (732.7/760)(298.15/300.15) = (0.964)(0.993) = 0.957$$

$$V_S = (0.957)(4.0 \text{ l}) = 3.83 \text{ l}$$

In the calibration system described above the volume flowrate measured is 0.20 lpm, and the uncorrected (moist air) volume delivered is 4.0 liters. When the volume is corrected to a dry air volume, at NTP, without a static pressure effect, it results in a volume of 3.83 liters at NTP. This is the volume that would exist if the air moving through the system were at standard conditions (25°C, one atmosphere and *dry*).

Percent difference from NTP = $[(V_S - V_C)/V_C]100$

Percent difference from NTP = $[(3.83 \text{ l} - 4.0 \text{ l})/3.83 \text{ l}]100 = -4.4 \text{ l}$

Example 7: Cold Climate Corrections, Part A

Table 6-5 gives an example of standard, calibration, and field conditions that might be experienced in a cold region (e.g., inside the Arctic Circle).

Example 7: Cold Climate Corrections, Part B

See Table 6-5 for cold climate air sampling conditions. A pump operating in the calibration laboratory at $Q_C = 0.20$ lpm, and the volume delivered at the calibration condition is V_C:

$$V_C = (Q_C)(t_C) = (0.20 \text{ lpm})(20 \text{ min}) = 4.0 \text{ l}$$

TABLE 6-5. Conditions for cold climate air sampling

Parameter	Calibration condition (C)	Standard condition (S)	Field condition (F)
Relative humidity (%)	100	0	10 (-0.01 mm Hg)
Elevation (feet)	257	0	500
Temperature, °C (K)	27 (300.15)	25 (298.15)	-40 (233.15)
P_{ATM} (mm Hg) (Note 1)	763.2	760.0	746.8 (Note 2)
P_{VP} (mm Hg) (Note 1)	26.7	0.0	0.01
P_{SP} (mm Hg)	-3.8	0.0	-3.8
Local station pressure	(Note 3)		(Note 4)
Pressure (mm Hg)	$732.7 = P_C$	$760.0 = P_S$	$743.0 = P_F$
Flowrate (lpm)	$Q_C = 0.20$	$Q_S = 0.20$	$Q_F = 0.2$
Time (minutes)	$t_C = 20.0$	N/A	$t_F = 35$
Volume (liters, l)	$V_C = 4.0$	$V_S = —$	$V_F = 7.0$

Correction from the field condition to the standard condition:

$$V_S = V_F(P_F/P_S)(T_S/T_F)$$

$$V_S = 7.0(743.0/760.0)(298.15/233.15)$$

$$V_S = 7.0(1.25) = 8.8 \text{ l (at NTP)}$$

Note 1: The relative humidity in the field is 10%, and it may be ignored. One may wish to calculate 0.1 (10%) times the partial pressure of water at -40°C (0.0966 mm Hg) and then subtract 0.1(0.0966) = 0.0096 mm Hg from the atmospheric pressure.

Note 2: This is the local station pressure recorded on site. Beware: many airport weather stations and United States Weather Bureau stations report atmospheric pressures corrected to sea level and 0°C (8).

Note 3: $P_C = P_{ATM} - P_{VP} + P_{SP} = 763.2 - 26.7 - 3.8 = 732.7$ mm Hg.

Note 4: $P_F = P_{ATM} - P_{VP} + P_{SP} = 746.8 - 0.01 - 3.8 = 743.0$ mm Hg.

If the volume is corrected to standard conditions, then V_S is:

$$V_S = V_C(P_C/P_S)(T_S/T_C)$$

$$(P_C/P_S)(T_S/T_C) = (732.7/760)(298.15/300.15) = (0.96)(0.99) = 0.95$$

$$V_S = (0.95)(4.0 \text{ l}) = 3.8 \text{ l}$$

Example 7: Cold Climate Corrections, Part C

See Table 6-5 for cold climate air sampling conditions. When the pump operates in the field, in a cold location, (-40°C and 0.2 liter per minute, $Q_F = 0.2$ lpm), calculate the field volume (V_F) that must be collected to produce a volume at NTP (V_S) equal to 14.0 liters. Recall:

$$V_S = V_F(P_F/P_S)(T_S/T_F)$$

Solve for V_F as follows:

$$V_F = V_S/(P_C/P_S)(T_S/T_C) = V_S/F_{TP}$$

$$(P_C/P_S)(T_S/T_C) = (743.0/760)(298.15/233.15) = (0.98)(1.28) = 1.25$$

$$V_F = (14.0 \text{ l})/(1.25) = 11.2 \text{ l}$$

Calculate the time (t_F) that the pump must operate in the field to deliver 11.2 liters:

$$V_F = (Q_F)(t_F)$$

$$t_F = (V_F)/(Q_F) = (11.2 \text{ l}/0.2 \text{ lpm})$$

$$t_F = 56.0 \text{ min}$$

If a pump is operating at a flowrate of 0.2 lpm and a 14.0 liter air sample is needed at NTP, then the air sampling pump must be operated for 56.0 minutes at the field conditions to deliver the required volume. The air volume collected in the field, 11.2 liters, is less than the volume required at the standard condition because cold air is denser, and a smaller volume of denser air will become the required 14.0 liters at NTP. A simple ideal gas calculation can verify this.

In Chapter 7 the analytical laboratory protocol is used to determine if the air volume sampled is sufficient to enable the laboratory to exceed the limit of detection.

Example 8: Hot Climate Corrections, Part A

Table 6-6 gives an example of standard, calibration, and field conditions that might be experienced in a hot region, i.e., a mechanical room located on the 50th floor of a high rise in Denver, Colorado, 5500 feet above sea level.

Example 8: Hot Climate Corrections, Part B

See Table 6-6 for hot climate air sampling conditions. A pump operates in the calibration laboratory at $Q_C = 4.0$ lpm, and the volume delivered at the calibration condition is:

$$V_C = (Q_C)(t_C) = (4.0 \text{ lpm})(20 \text{ min}) = 80.0 \text{ l}$$

If the volume is corrected to standard condition, then V_S is:

$$V_S = V_C(P_C/P_S)(T_S/T_C)$$

$$(P_C/P_S)(T_S/T_C) = (732.7/760)(298.15/300.15) = (0.964)(0.993) = 0.97$$

$$V_S = (80.0 \text{ l})(0.97) = 76.6 \text{ l}$$

TABLE 6-6. Conditions for hot climate air sampling

Parameter	Calibration condition (C)	Standard condition (S)	Field condition (F)
Relative humidity (%)	100	0	100 (92.6 mm Hg)
Elevation (feet)	257	0	5500
Temperature, °C (K)	27 (300.15)	25 (298.15)	+50 (323.15)
P_{ATM} (mm Hg)	763.2	760.0	626.9 (Note 2)
P_{VP} (mm Hg) (Note 1)	26.7	0.0	92.6
P_{SP} (mm Hg)	−3.8	0.0	−3.8
Local station pressure	(Note 3)		(Note 4)
Pressure (mm Hg)	$732.7 = P_C$	$760.0 = P_S$	$530.5 = P_F$
Flowrate (lpm)	$Q_C = 4.0$	$Q_S = 4.0$	$Q_F = 4.0$
Time (minutes)	$t_C = 20.0$	N/A	$t_F = 23.2$
Volume (liters, l)	$V_C = 80.0$	$V_S = -$	$V_F = 126.6$

Correction from the field condition to the standard condition:

$$V_S = V_F(P_F/P_S)(T_S/T_F)$$

$$V_S = 126.6(530.5/760.0)(298.15/323.15)$$

$$V_S = 126.6(0.64) = 81.5 \text{ l sampled (at NTP)}$$

Note 1: The relative humidity is 100% and must be considered. Calculate the vapor pressure of water at +50°C (92.6 mm Hg), and then subtract 92.6 mm Hg and the system static pressure from the atmospheric pressure.

Note 2: This is the local station pressure recorded on-site. Beware: many airport weather stations and United States Weather Bureau stations report atmospheric pressures corrected to sea level at 0°C (8).

Note 3: $P_C = P_{ATM} - P_{VP} + P_{SP} = 763.2 - 26.7 - 3.8 = 732.7$ mm Hg.

Note 4: $P_F = P_{ATM} - P_{VP} + P_{SP} = 626.9 - 92.6 - 3.8 = 530.5$ mm Hg.

Example 8: Hot Climate Corrections, Part C

When the same pump operates in the field in a hot location (50°C and 4.0 liters per minute, $Q_F = 4.0$ lpm) calculate the field volume (V_F) that must be collected to produce a volume at NTP (V_S) equal to 400.0 liters. Recall:

$$V_S = V_F(P_F/P_S)(T_S/T_F)$$

Solve for V_F as follows:

$$V_F = V_S/[P_C/P_S][T_S/T_C] = V_S/F_{TP}$$

$$(P_C/P_S)(T_S/T_C) = (530.5/760)(298.15/323.15) = (0.70)(0.92) = 0.644$$

$$V_F = (400.0 \text{ l})/(0.644) = 621.1 \text{ l}$$

Calculate the time (t_F) that the pump must operate in the field to deliver 615.4 liters:

$$V_F = (Q_F)(t_F)$$

$$t_F = (V_F)/(Q_F)$$

$$t_F = (621.1\ l/4.0\ \text{lpm})$$

$$t_F = 155.3\ \text{min}$$

If a pump is operating at a flowrate of 4.0 lpm and a 400.0 liter air sample is needed at NTP, then the air sampling pump must be operated for 155.3 minutes at the field conditions to deliver the required volume. The actual volume delivered is 621.1 liters, which is more than the volume required at the standard condition because hot air is less dense and a larger volume of less dense air will become the required 400.0 liters at NTP. An ideal gas calculation will verify this.

In Chapter 7 the analytical laboratory protocol is used to determine if the air volume sampled is sufficient to enable the laboratory to exceed the limit of detection.

9. EFFECT OF VOLUME CORRECTION ON MASS CONCENTRATION

To assess what happens to the mass concentration if the uncorrected volume flowrate is used, consider Examples 9 through 12.

Example 9

During a worker exposure assessment for acetone vapor the sorbent tube(s) and the requisite number of field blanks are analyzed. The pump was calibrated at 0.19 lpm. The outdoor operation was sampled for 27 minutes. The worker wore the pump in her armpit to keep it from freezing in the $-40°C$ ambient temperature. Two possible mass concentration (expressed in mg/m^3) can be calculated, depending on the air sample volume selected. In one sample the laboratory reports that the acetone mass was 5.20 mg. Assume that the air sampling pump ran for 27 minutes at 0.19 lpm in the field at $-40°C$ and 743.0 mm Hg.

Summary: NIOSH Method 1300, Ketones I (3, 6, 7)

1993–94 ACGIH TLV-TWA 1780 mg/m^3	Molecular weight = 58.2 g/mole
Range studied: 1200–4500 mg/m^3; or	Estimated LOD: 20 μg/sample
2.4–14.2 mg/sample	Sample flow rate: 0.01–0.2 lpm
Air sampling media: 100 mg/50 mg	1 ppm = 2.38 mg/m^3
coconut shell charcoal	

Solution 9

Concentration Using the Field (Sampling) Condition (−40°C, 743.0 mm Hg) In this example, using the volume as sampled in the field will overestimate the exposure.

$$Q_F = 0.19 \text{ lpm}; V_F = Q_F(t_F) = 0.19 \text{ lpm}(27 \text{ min}) = 5.13 \text{ l sampled}$$

$$V_F = 5.13 \text{ l sampled}$$

$$C_{M/V} = (\text{mass, mg}/V_F, \text{liters})(1000 \text{ l/m}^3)$$

$$C_{M/V} = (5.20 \text{ mg}/5.13 \text{ l})(1000 \text{ l/m}^3) = 1014 \text{ mg/m}^3$$

$$C_{M/V} = 1014 \text{ mg/m}^3 = 426 \text{ ppm} \qquad (incorrect\ exposure)$$

Note: Calculating concentration based on this field condition yields a mass concentration that is high because the volume of air collected (V_P) is less than the volume at NTP.

Concentration Calculated at NTP (25°C, 760 mm Hg)

$$Q_F = 0.19 \text{ lpm}; V_F = Q_F(t_F) = 0.19 \text{ lpm}(27 \text{ min}) = 5.13 \text{ liters sampled}$$

$$V_S = V_F(P_F/P_S)(T_S/T_F)$$

$$V_S = 5.13(743.0/760.0)(298.15/233.15) = 5.13(1.25)$$

$$V_S = 6.4 \text{ liters sampled at NTP}$$

$$C_{M/V} = (\text{mass, mg}/V_S, \text{liters})(1000 \text{ l/m}^3)$$

$$C_{M/V} = (5.20 \text{ mg}/6.4 \text{ l})(1000 \text{ l/m}^3) = 813 \text{ mg/m}^3$$

$$C_{M/V} = 813 \text{ mg/m}^3 = 342 \text{ ppm} \qquad (correct\ exposure\ at\ NTP)$$

Note: Correcting the field volume (V_F) to the normal temperature and pressure (NTP) yields the correct exposure. Not correcting the volume to NTP may make a difference in the final recommendation.

Example 10

During a worker exposure assessment for acetonitrile vapor, the sorbent tube(s) and the requisite number of field blanks are analyzed. In one sample the laboratory reports an acetonitrile mass of 0.22 mg. Two mass concentrations can be calculated, depending on the selection of the air sample volume selected. Assume that the air sampling pump ran for 30 minutes at 0.2 lpm in the field at 50°C and 462.3 mm Hg.

Summary: NIOSH 1606 (3, 6, 7)

1993–94 ACGIH TLV-TWA 67 mg/m^3
Range studied: 31–140 mg/m^3; or
  0.2–2.0 mg/sample
Air sampling media: 400 mg/200 mg
  coconut shell charcoal

Molecular weight = 41.1 g/mole
Estimated LOD: 10 μg/sample
Sample flow rate: 0.01–0.2 lpm
1 ppm = 1.68 mg/m^3

Solution 10

Calculating Concentration Using Field (Sampling) Condition (50°C, 462.3 mm Hg) In this example, using the volume as sampled in the field will underestimate the exposure.

$$Q_F = 0.2 \text{ lpm}; V_F = Q_F(t_F) = 0.2 \text{ lpm}(30 \text{ min}) = 6.0 \text{ l sampled}$$

$$C_{M/V} = (\text{mass, mg}/V_F, \text{liters})(1000 \text{ l/m}^3)$$

$$C_{M/V} = (0.22 \text{ mg}/6.0 \text{ l})(1000 \text{ l/m}^3) = 36.7 \text{ mg/m}^3$$

$$C_{M/V} = 36.7 \text{ mg/m}^3 = 22 \text{ ppm} \qquad (incorrect\ exposure)$$

Note: Calculating the concentration based on this field condition yields a mass concentration that is low because the volume of air collected at the field condition is higher than the volume at NTP.

Calculating the Volume Using NTP (25°C, 760 mm Hg)

$$Q_F = 0.2 \text{ lpm}; V_F = Q_F(t_F) = 0.2 \text{ lpm}(30 \text{ min}) = 6.0 \text{ l sampled}$$

$$V_S = V_F(P_F/P_S)(T_S/T_F)$$

$$V_S = 6.0(462.3/760.0)(298.15/323.15) = 6.0(0.56)$$

$$V_S = 3.37 \text{ l sampled at NTP}$$

$$C_{M/V} = (\text{mass, mg}/V_S, \text{liters})(1000 \text{ l/m}^3)$$

$$C_{M/V} = (0.22 \text{ mg}/3.37 \text{ l})(1000 \text{ l/m}^3) = 65.3 \text{ mg/m}^3$$

$$C_{M/V} = 65.3 \text{ mg/m}^3 = 38.8 \text{ ppm} \qquad (correct\ exposure\ at\ NTP)$$

Note: Correcting the field volume to the normal temperature and pressure (NTP) yields the correct exposure. Not correcting the volume to NTP may make a difference in the final recommendation.

Example 11

During a worker exposure assessment for ethylene glycol vapor and mist, the sorbent tube(s) and filter(s) and the requisite number of field blanks are analyzed. In one sample the laboratory reports an ethylene glycol mass of 1.0 mg. Two possible mass concentrations (mg/m^3) can be calculated, depending on the selection of the air sample volume selected. The air sampling pump ran for 15 minutes at 0.2 lpm in the field at 50°C and 462.3 mm Hg.

Summary: NIOSH 5500 (3, 6, 7)

1993–94 ACGIH TLV-TWA 127 mg/m^3	Molecular weight = 62.1 g/mole
Range studied: 45–98 mg/m^3; or	Estimated LOD: 4 μg/sample
0.02–1.0 mg/sample	Sample flow rate: 0.2 lpm
Air sampling media: 520 mg/260 mg	1 ppm = 2.54 mg/m^3
silica gel + fiberglass filter	

Solution 11

Calculating Concentration Using Field (Sampling) Condition (50°C, 462.3 mm Hg)

$$Q_F = 0.2 \text{ lpm}; V_F = Q_F(t_F) = 0.2 \text{ lpm}(15 \text{ min}) = 3.0 \text{ l sampled}$$

$$V_F = V_C(P_C/P_F)(T_F/T_C)$$

$$C_{M/V} = (\text{mass, mg}/V_F, \text{ liters})(1000 \text{ l/m}^3)$$

$$C_{M/V} = (1.0 \text{ mg}/3.0 \text{ l})(1000 \text{ l/m}^3) = 333 \text{ mg/m}^3$$

$$C_{M/V} = 333 \text{ mg/m}^3 = 131 \text{ ppm} \qquad (incorrect\ exposure)$$

Note: Calculating the concentration based on this field condition yields a mass concentration that is low because the volume of air collected at the field condition is higher than the volume at NTP.

Calculating the Concentration Using NTP (25°C, 760 mm Hg)

$Q_F = 0.2$ lpm; $V_F = Q_F(t_F) = 0.2$ lpm$(30$ min$) = 3.0$ l sampled

$V_S = V_F(P_F/P_S)(T_S/T_F)$

$V_S = 3.0(462.3/760.0)(298.15/323.15) = 3.0(0.56)$

$V_S = 1.68$ l sampled (at NTP)

$C_{M/V} = ($mass, mg$/V_S$, liters$)(1000$ l/m$^3)$

$C_{M/V} = (1.0$ mg$/1.68$ l$)(1000$ l/m$^3) = 595.2$ mg/m^3

$C_{M/V} = 595.2$ mg/m$^3 = 234.4$ ppm   (*correct exposure at NTP*)

Note: Correcting the field volume to the normal temperature and pressure (NTP) yields the correct exposure. Not correcting the volume to NTP may make a difference in the final recommendation.

Example 12

As a result of a clearance sample taken for asbestos fibers inside containment located at Powder Pass in the Rocky Mountains (elevation 9 222 feet) at 57°C, in one sample the laboratory reports that the filter contains 3.2×10^6 fibers. Two possible concentrations (fibers/cm^3) can be calculated, depending on the selection of the air sample volume selected. The air sampling pump ran for 480 minutes at 3.5 lpm in the field at 57°C and 550.7 mm Hg.

Solution 12

Calculating Concentration Using Field (Sampling) Condition (57°C, 550.7 mm Hg)

$Q_F = 3.5$ lpm; $V_F = Q_F(t_F) = 3.5$ lpm$(480$ min$) = 1680.0$ l sampled

$V_F = V_C(P_C/P_F)(T_F/T_C)$

$C($f/cm$^3) = ($fibers$/V_F$, liters$)($liter$/1000$ cm$^3)$

$C($f/cm$^3) = (3.2 \times 10^6$ fibers$/1680$ l$)(1/1000$ cm$^3) = 1.9$ fibers/cm^3

$C($f/cm$^3) = 1.9$ fibers/cm^3 (*incorrect exposure*)

Note: Calculating the concentration based on this field condition yields a fiber concentration that is low because the volume of air collected at the field condition is higher than the volume at NTP.

Calculating the Concentration Using NTP (25°C, 760 mm Hg)

$$Q_F = 3.5 \text{ lpm}; \; V_F = Q_F(t_F) = 3.5 \text{ lpm}(480 \text{ min}) = 1\,680.0 \text{ l sampled}$$

$$V_S = V_F(P_F/P_S)(T_S/T_F)$$

$$V_S = 1\,680(550.7/760.0)(298.15/330.15) = 1\,680(0.654)$$

$$V_S = 1\,066.6 \text{ l sampled (at NTP)}$$

$$C(\text{f/cm}^3) = (\text{fibers}/V_F, \text{ liters})(\text{liter}/1000 \text{ cm}^3)$$

$$C(\text{f/cm}^3) = (3.2 \times 10^6 \text{ fibers}/1\,066.6 \text{ l})(1/1000 \text{ cm}^3) = 3.0 \text{ fibers/cm}^3$$

$$C(\text{f/cm}^3) = 1.9 \text{ fibers/cm}^3 \qquad \qquad (\textit{correct exposure at NTP})$$

Note: Correcting the field volume to the normal temperature and pressure (NTP) yields the correct exposure. Not correcting the volume to NTP may make a difference in the final recommendation.

10. TEMPERATURE AND PRESSURE CORRECTION TO MASS CONCENTRATION

Recall from Chapter 5 and the ideal gas equation:

$$C_{\text{PPM}} = (V_A/V_B)10^6$$

$$PV_A = (m_A RT/M_A)$$

The ideal gas equation can be solved for V_A and substituted into C_{PPM} as:

$$C_{\text{PPM}} = (m_A RT/M_A PV_B)10^6$$

where:

m_A = the mass of contaminant A
V_B = the volume of air in which the mass of contaminant, m_A, is
      contained

The mass concentration of a contaminant (m_A) in a volume of air (V_B) can be identified as:

$$C_{M/V} = m_A/V_B$$

$$C_{\text{PPM}} = \left[(C_{M/V} RT)/MP\right]10^6$$

At NTP = 25°C, 298.15 K and one atmosphere:

$$C_{PPM} = \left[(C_{M/V} RT)/MP \right] 10^6$$

$$= C_{M/V} \left\{ \left[(0.08205 \text{ l atm/mole K})(298.15 \text{ K}) \right] / \left[M(1 \text{ atm}) \right] \right\} 10^6$$

$$C_{PPM} = C_{M/V} \left[(24.45 \text{ l/mole})/M \right] 10^6$$

This can be rewritten as:

$$C_{PPM} = (\text{mass of impurity/volume of air}) \left[(24.45 \text{ l/mole})/M \right] 10^6$$

$$C_{PPM} = (\text{mass of impurity}/V_S) \left[(24.45 \text{ l/mole})/M \right] 10^6$$

The volume of air sampled (V_F) must be adjusted from the field condition (V_F) to the standard condition (NTP) by applying the temperature and pressure adjustment factor, F_{TP}, as indicated below:

$$V_S = V_F (P_F/P_S)(T_S/T_F)$$

$$C_{PPM} = \left[\text{mass of impurity}/V_F \right] \left[(P_F/P_S)(T_S/T_F) \right] \left[(24.45 \text{ l/mole})/M \right] 10^6$$

$$C_{PPM} = \frac{(\text{mass of impurity})(24.45 \text{ l/mole}) 10^6}{\left[V_F \left[(P_F/P_S)(T_S/T_F) \right] \right] (\text{molecular weight})}$$

The units of volume may have to be reduced to a standard volume (e.g., cubic meters) from liters or cubic centimeters; hence the units conversion factor (unit factor = 1000 l/m³, etc.). The units of mass may have to be reduced to milligrams (mg) from whatever value the laboratory reported. Apply conversions to give the final concentration in mg/m³, μg/m³, etc.:

$$C_{PPM} = \frac{(\text{mass of impurity})}{(V_F)(\text{unit factor})} \frac{P_S T_F}{P_F T_S} \frac{[24.45 \text{ liter/mole}] 10^6}{[\text{molecular weight}]}$$

$$C_{PPM} = \frac{(\text{mass of impurity})}{(V_F)(\text{unit factor})} \frac{(760)(T + 273.15)}{(P_F)(298.15)} \frac{(24.45 \text{ liter/mole}) 10^6}{(\text{molecular weight})}$$

$$C_{PPM} = \frac{(\text{mass of impurity})}{(V_F)(\text{unit factor})} \frac{(24.45 \text{ liter/mole})}{(\text{molecular weight})} \frac{(760)}{(P_F)} \frac{(t + 273.15) 10^6}{(298.15)}$$

Notice the relationship between the equation above and the equation recommended by NIOSH (6) to calculate the concentration in parts per million:

$$\text{ppm} = \frac{\text{mg}}{\text{cu m}} \times \frac{24.45}{M.W.} \times \frac{760}{P} \times \frac{t + 273}{298}$$

where:

P = barometric pressure (mm Hg) of air at the sampling location

t = temperature (°C) of air sampled

24.45 = molar volume (liter/mole) at NTP (25°C and 760 mm Hg)

$M.W.$ = molecular weight (g/mole) of analyte

760 = normal pressure (mm Hg)

298 = normal temperature (K)

A lowercase t denotes Celsius temperature (°C); an uppercase T denotes Kelvin temperature (K).

It is essential to recognize that the temperature effect factor (T_S/T_F) and the pressure effect factor (P_F/P_S) are *applied to the air sample volume in cubic meters and not the molar gas volume*. However, if the molar gas volume is corrected to the same temperature and pressure condition that the air sample volume was corrected to, the resulting concentration in parts per million is identical. Because concentration in parts per million is independent of temperature and pressure (i.e., it is calculated on a volume per volume basis) and both volumes *are expressed at the same condition*, the concentrations are identical.

It is an individual choice to decide whether to write the conversion equation at 25°C and one atmosphere and to temperature and pressure correct the air sample volume:

$$\text{ppm} = \frac{\text{mg}}{\text{cu m}} \times \frac{24.45}{M.W.} \times \frac{760}{P} \times \frac{t + 273}{298}$$

or to use the general equation and substitute the temperature and pressure into the general equation *if and only if* the concentration is expressed at the same temperature and pressure:

$$C_{\text{PPM}} = (C_{\text{mg/m}^3}) \frac{(24.45\ 1/\text{mole})}{M} \frac{(760\ \text{mm Hg})}{P} \frac{(t + 273.15)\ \text{K}}{298.15\ \text{K}}$$

Example 9 Alternate

Field (Sampling) Condition (−40°C, 743.0 mm Hg)

Q_F = 0.2 lpm; 4.0 l sampled at the field condition

$V_S = V_F(P_F/P_S)(T_S/T_F)$

$V_S = 4.0(743.0/760.0)(298.15/233.15) = 4.0(1.25)$

$V_S = 5.0$ l sampled (at NTP, Table 6-4)

Acetone molecular weight = 58.2 g/mole

Acetone mass reported by the laboratory is 5.20 mg.

$C_{M/V} = (5.20 \text{ mg}/4.0 \text{ l})(1000 \text{ l}/\text{m}^3) = 1300 \text{ mg}/\text{m}^3$ (*incorrect exposure*)

$C_{M/V} = (5.20 \text{ mg}/5.0 \text{ l})(1000 \text{ l}/\text{m}^3)$

$C_{M/V} = 1040 \text{ mg}/\text{m}^3$ (*correct exposure at NTP*)

Using the general equation and substituting the temperature and pressure:

$$C_{\text{PPM}} = (C_{\text{mg/m}^3}) \frac{(24.45 \text{ l/mole})}{M} \frac{(760 \text{ mm Hg})}{P} \frac{(t + 273.15)\text{K}}{298.15 \text{ K}} = 436.8 \text{ ppm}$$

Using the equation recommended by NIOSH (6) to calculate the concentration in ppm:

$$\text{ppm} = \frac{\text{mg}}{\text{cu m}} \times \frac{24.45}{M.W.} \times \frac{760}{P} \times \frac{t + 273}{298}$$

$$\text{ppm} = \frac{5.20 \text{ mg}}{0.004 \text{ cu m}} \times \frac{24.45}{58.2} \times \frac{760}{743} \times \frac{-40 + 273}{298}$$

$$= 436.8 \text{ ppm} = 1040 \text{ mg}/\text{m}^3$$

Note: Correcting the air sample volume to the normal temperature and pressure (NTP) yields the correct exposure. An error in correcting the volume to NTP will not make a difference in the recommendation because the exposure to acetone is 58% of the TLV (at NTP) or if calculated incorrectly (1300 mg/m^3) or 73% of the TLV.

Example 10 Alternate

Field (Sampling) Condition (50°C, 462.3 mm Hg)

$Q_F = 0.2$ lpm; 6.0 l sampled at the field condition

$V_S = V_F(P_F/P_S)(T_S/T_F)$

$V_S = 6.0(462.3/760.0)(298.15/323.15) = 6.0(0.56)$
$\quad = 3.37$ l sampled (at NTP, Table 6-4)

Acetonitrile molecular weight $= 41.1$ g/mole

Acetonitrile mass reported by the laboratory is 0.22 mg.

$C_{M/V} = (0.22 \text{ mg}/6.0 \text{ l})(1000 \text{ l}/\text{m}^3) = 36.7 \text{ mg}/\text{m}^3$

           (*Incorrect exposure*)

$C_{M/V} = (0.22 \text{ mg}/3.37 \text{ l})(1000 \text{ l}/\text{m}^3)$

$C_{M/V} = 65.3 \text{ mg}/\text{m}^3$ (*Correct exposure at NTP*)

Use the general equation and substituting the temperature and pressure:

$$C_{\text{PPM}} = (C_{\text{mg/m}^3})\frac{(24.45 \text{ l/mole})}{M} \frac{(760 \text{ mm Hg})}{P} \frac{(t + 273.15) \text{ K}}{298.15 \text{ K}} = 38.8 \text{ ppm}$$

Using the equation recommended by NIOSH (6) to calculate the concentration in ppm:

$$\text{ppm} = \frac{\text{mg}}{\text{cu m}} \times \frac{24.45}{M.W.} \times \frac{760}{P} \times \frac{t + 273}{298}$$

$$\text{ppm} = \frac{0.22 \text{ mg}}{0.006 \text{ cu m}} \times \frac{24.45}{41.1} \times \frac{760.0}{462.3} \times \frac{+50 + 273}{298} = 38.8 \text{ ppm}$$

Note: Correcting to the normal temperature and pressure (NTP) yields the correct exposure. An error in correcting the volume to NTP may make a difference in the recommendation because the exposure to acetonitrile is 97% of the TLV. If the incorrect concentration is used, the exposure to acetonitrile is only 55% of the TLV.

Example 11 Alternate

Field (Sampling) Condition (50°C, 462.3 mm Hg)

$Q_F = 0.2$ lpm; 6.0 l sampled at the field condition

$V_S = V_F(P_F/P_S)(T_S/T_F)$

$V_S = 6.0(462.3/760.0)(298.15/323.15) = 6.0(0.56)$
$V_S = 3.37$ l sampled (at NTP, Table 6-4)

Ethylene glycol molecular weight = 62.1 g/mole

Ethylene glycol mass reported by the laboratory is 1.0 mg.

$C_{M/V} = (1.0 \text{ mg}/6.0 \text{ l})(1000 \text{ l/m}^3) = 166.7 \text{ mg/m}^3$ (*incorrect exposure*)

$C_{M/V} = (1.0 \text{ mg}/3.37 \text{ l})(1000 \text{ l/m}^3)$

$C_{M/V} = 296.7 \text{ mg/m}^3$ (*correct exposure at NTP*)

Using the general equation and substituting the temperature and pressure:

$$C_{\text{PPM}} = (C_{\text{mg/m}^3})\frac{(24.45 \text{ l/mole})}{M} \frac{(760 \text{ mm Hg})}{P} \frac{(t + 273.15) \text{ K}}{298.15 \text{ K}} = 116.8 \text{ ppm}$$

Using the equation recommended by NIOSH (6) to calculate the concentration in ppm:

$$\text{ppm} = \frac{\text{mg}}{\text{cu m}} \times \frac{24.45}{M.W.} \times \frac{760.0}{P} \times \frac{t + 273}{298}$$

$$\text{ppm} = \frac{1.00 \text{ mg}}{0.006 \text{ cu m}} \times \frac{24.45}{62.1} \times \frac{760.0}{462.3} \times \frac{+50 + 273}{298} = 116.9 \text{ ppm}$$

Note: Correcting to the normal temperature and pressure (NTP) yields the correct exposure. An error in correcting the volume to NTP will not make a difference in the recommendation because the exposure to ethylene glycol is 233% of the TLV. If the incorrect concentration is used, the exposure to ethylene glycol is 131% of the TLV.

Conclusion

Apply the temperature and pressure effect $[(P_F/P_S)(T_S/T_F)]$ *to the field air sample volume and not the molar gas volume.* Applying the temperature and pressure effect $[(P_F/P_S)(T_S/T_F)]F_{TP}$ to the air sample volume returns it to the volume at NTP. The mass per volume concentration (mg/m^3) is then converted to parts per million. The equation to calculate the concentration in parts per million is:

$$C_{\text{PPM}} = \frac{\text{mass of contaminant}}{V_F[(P_F/P_S)(T_S/T_F)]M} \times \frac{24.45 \text{ liters/mole}}{(\text{units conversion})} \times 10^6$$

Example 13

Develop and plot a family of curves that relate air sample volumes collected over a range of field temperature conditions $(+50°C \text{ to } -50°C)$ to the

TABLE 6-7. Data for Example 13

Std. temp. (K)	Field temp. (°C)	Field temp. (K)	Temp. ratio, F_T	$V_F = 1.0\,l$ $V_S =$ $V_F(F_T)$ (liters)	$V_F = 10\,l$ $V_S =$ $V_F(F_T)$ (liters)	$V_F = 100\,l$ $V_S =$ $V_F(F_T)$ (liters)	$V_F = 1000\,l$ $V_S =$ $V_F(F_T)$ (liters)
298.15	50	323.15	0.923	0.923	9.23	92.3	923.
298.15	35	308.15	0.968	0.968	9.68	96.8	968.
298.15	25	298.15	1.000	1.000	10.00	100.0	1000.
298.15	15	288.15	1.035	1.035	10.35	103.5	1035.
298.15	0	273.15	1.092	1.092	10.92	109.2	1092.
298.15	−15	258.15	1.155	1.155	11.55	115.5	1155.
298.15	−25	248.15	1.201	1.201	12.01	120.1	1201.
298.15	−40	233.15	1.279	1.279	12.79	127.9	1279.
298.15	−50	223.15	1.336	1.336	13.36	133.6	1336.

Note: $F_T = (T_S/T_F)$.

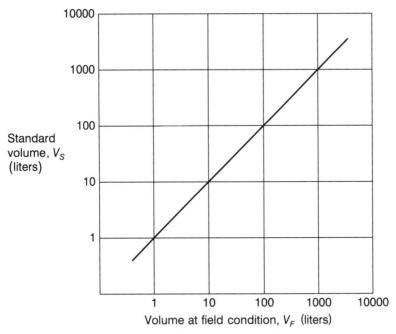

Figure 6-3. Plot for Example 13.

volumes at the standard condition. Assume that $V_F = 1.0$ liter, 10 liters, 100 liters, and 1000 liters, and calculate the temperature correction for each volume (see Table 6-7 and Figure 6-3). Recall:

$$V_S = V_F(T_S/T_F)$$

The temperature effect ratio (T_S/T_F) is the slope of the plot of V_S versus V_F:

$$(T_S/T_F) = (V_S/V_F)$$

11. TEMPERATURE AND PRESSURE EFFECTS ON GAS DENSITY

Applying the ideal gas equation with a few assumptions, it is possible to calculate the variation of density with temperature and pressure using the ideal gas law.

Assume that S represents the standard condition and F represents the field condition. It is possible to calculate the change in density represented by the change in the condition from field condition (F) to the standard condition (S):

$$P_S V_S = nRT_S = m_S RT_S/M_S$$
$$P_F V_F = nRT_F = m_F RT_F/M_F$$

These equations can be rearranged and used to produce an expression for density:

$$P_S = m_S RT_S / M_S V_S$$

$$P_F = m_F RT_F / M_F V_F$$

Recall that density equals mass of a material per volume of the same material and the units are typically g/cm^3, kg/cm^3, lb_M/ft^3, etc. An expression for density at the standard condition and field condition is:

$$\rho_S = m_S / V_S$$

$$\rho_F = m_F / V_F$$

Substituting the density relationship into the ideal gas equation yields:

$$P_S = \rho_S RT_S / M_S$$

$$P_F = \rho_F RT_F / M_F$$

Solving both of these equations for R/M_i yields:

$$P_S / \rho_S T_S = P_F / \rho_F T_F = R/M_i$$

This equation can be established for either the standard condition or the field condition:

$$\rho_S = \rho_F (P_S / P_F)(T_F / T_S)$$

This equation predicts the actual density, ρ_F, when the standard density, ρ_S, that exists at normal temperature and pressure is specified:

$$\rho_F = \rho_S (P_F / P_S)(T_S / T_F)$$

Recall that $F_P = (P_F / P_S)$ and $F_T = (T_S / T_F)$. Recall that $F_{TP} = (F_T)(F_P) = (P_F / P_S)(T_S / T_F)$ is the combined pressure and temperature correction factor. Hence:

$$\rho_F = \rho_S (F_P)(F_T)$$

Table 6-1 lists the coefficients F_P used to calculate the density change with altitude.

BIBLIOGRAPHY

1. American Conference of Governmental Industrial Hygienists, *Industrial Ventilation; A Manual of Recommended Practice*, 21st Edition (1992), p. 5-44, Table 5-7.
2. American Society of Heating, Refrigeration and Air-Conditioning Engineers, *ASHRAE Handbook of Fundamentals* (1993), p. 6.1.
3. National Institute for Occupational Safety and Health, *Pocket Guide to Chemical Hazards* (DHHS/NIOSH Pub. No. 90-117). U.S. Government Printing Office, Washington, DC (1990).
4. Powell, Charles, Evaluation of exposure to chemical agents. In *Patty's Industrial Hygiene and Toxicology*, Vol. III, *Theory and Rationale of Industrial Hygiene Practice*, ed. Cralley, J. V. and Cralley, L. J., Second Edition. John Wiley & Sons New York (1985), pp. 319–358.
5. Occupational Safety and Health Administration, *OSHA Analytical Methods* (DOL/OSHA Pub. No. 825), OSHA Analytical Laboratories, Salt Lake City, UT. U.S. Government Printing Office, Washington, DC.
6. National Institute for Occupational Safety and Health, *Manual of Analytical Methods*, ed. Eller, P. E., Third Edition (DHHS/NIOSH Pub. No. 84-100). U.S. Government Printing Office, Washington, DC (1984, revised 1987).
7. American Conference of Governmental Industrial Hygienists, *Threshold Limit Values and Biological Indices 1993–1994*. American Conference of Governmental Industrial Hygienists, Cincinnati, OH (1993).
8. *Handbook of Chemistry and Physics*, ed. Weast, R. C., 70th Edition. CRC Press, Boca Raton, FL (1989), p. E-37.

PROBLEM SET

Problem 1

Given a concentration of 5 ppm ethylene oxide in air, calculate the corresponding concentration of ethylene oxide in mg/m^3, at NTP and STP and at 150°F and 2 atmospheres.

Solution 1

The solution begins with the familiar equation: $C_{\text{PPM}} = (C_{M/V}(RT/PM)10^6$
Ethylene oxide (C_2H_4O), $M = 44.1$ g/mole
At NTP = 25°C, 298.15 K, $R = 0.082$ latm/mole K, and $P = 1$ atm:

$$C_{\text{PPM}} = \left[(C_{M/V})(24.45 \text{ l/mole})/M\right]10^6$$

$$C_{\text{PPM}} = \left[(C_{\text{mg/m}^3})(24.45 \text{ l/mole})/M\right]10^6$$

$$C_{\text{mg/m}^3} = C_{\text{PPM}}(44.1 \text{ g/mole}/24.45 \text{ l/mole})10^{-6} = 9.0 \text{ mg/m}^3$$

At STP = 0°C, 273.15 K, $R = 0.082$ l atm/mole K, and $P = 1$ atm:

$$C_{PPM} = \left[(C_{M/V})(22.4\ \text{l/mole})/M \right]10^6$$

$$C_{PPM} = \left[(C_{mg/m^3})(22.4\ \text{l/mole})/M \right]10^6$$

$$C_{mg/m^3} = C_{PPM}(44.1\ \text{g/mole}/22.4\ \text{l/mole})10^{-6} = 9.8\ \text{mg/m}^3$$

At 150°F, 65.6°C = 338.7 K, $R = 0.082$ l atm/mole K, and $P = 2$ atm:

$$C_{mg/m^3} = C_{PPM}(PM/RT)10^{-6}$$

$$C_{mg/m^3} = C_{PPM}\left[(2\ \text{atm})(44.1\ \text{g/mole})/(0.082\ \text{l atm/mole K})(338.7\ \text{K}) \right]10^{-6}$$

$$C_{mg/m^3} = 15.9\ \text{mg/m}^3$$

Problem 2

For the EPA 24-hour ambient sulfur dioxide (SO_2) standard in ppm, calculate the equivalent concentration in $\mu g/m^3$ at NTP and STP. EPA Ambient Air Quality Standard (AAQS) for sulfur dioxide is 0.14 ppm.

Solution 2

The solution begins with the familiar equation: $C_{PPM} = (C_{M/V})(RT/PM)10^6$
Sulfur dioxide (SO_2), $M = 64.1$ g/mole
At NTP = 25°C, 298.15 K, $R = 0.082$ l atm/mole K, and $P = 1$ atm:

$$C_{PPM} = \left[(C_{M/V})(24.45\ \text{l/mole})/M \right]10^6$$

$$C_{PPM} = \left[(C_{mg/m^3})(24.45\ \text{l/mole})/M \right]10^6$$

$$C_{mg/m^3} = C_{PPM}\left[64.1\ \text{g/mole}/24.45\ \text{l/mole} \right]10^{-6} = 0.3670\ \text{mg/m}^3$$

$$C_{\mu g/m^3} = 367.0\ \mu g/m^3$$

At STP = 0°C, 273.15 K and 1 atm:

$$C_{PPM} = \left[(C_{M/V})(22.4\ \text{l/mole})/M \right]10^6$$

$$C_{PPM} = \left[(C_{mg/m^3})(22.4\ \text{l/mole})/M \right]10^6$$

$$C_{mg/m^3} = C_{PPM}(M)10^{-6}/(22.4\ \text{l/mole}) = 0.4006\ \text{mg/m}^3$$

$$C_{\mu g/m^3} = 400.6\ \mu g/m^3$$

Problem 3

During a worker exposure assessment for toluene-2,4-diisocyanate (TDI) vapor, coated glass wool tubes are used as a collecting device, and the laboratory uses NIOSH Method 2535 for analysis. The tube(s) and the requisite number of field blanks are analyzed. In one sample the laboratory reports the TDI mass to be 9.0 μg for the sample. Two possible mass concentrations (mg/m^3) can be calculated, depending on the selection of the air sample volume. The air sampling pump ran for 380 minutes at 0.5 lpm.

Summary: NIOSH Method 2535, Toluene-2,4-diisocyanate

1993–94 ACGIH TLV-TWA 0.036mg/m^3
Range studied: 0.039–0.53 mg/m^3; or
  0.3–25 μg/sample
Air sampling media: Sampling tube,
  glass wool coated with
  N-[(4-nitrophenyl)methyl]propylamine
Sample flow rate: 0.2–1.0 lpm

Molecular weight = 174.2 g/mole
Estimated LOD: 0.1 μg/sample
1 ppm = 7.12 mg/m^3

Solution 3

Concentration Using the Field (Sampling) Condition ($-40°C$, 743.0 mm Hg)
In this example, using the volume as sampled in the field will overestimate the exposure.

$$Q_F = 0.5 \text{ lpm}; \ V_F = Q_F(t_F) = 0.5 \text{ lpm}(380 \text{ min})$$

$$= 190.0 \text{ l sampled}$$

$$V_F = 190.0 \text{ l sampled}$$

$$C_{M/V} = (\text{mass, mg}/V_F, \text{ liters})(1000 \text{ l/m}^3)$$

$$C_{M/V} = (0.009 \text{ mg}/190.0 \text{ l})(1000 \text{ l/m}^3) = 0.047 \text{ mg/m}^3$$

$$C_{M/V} = 0.047 \text{ mg/m}^3 = 0.0066 \text{ ppm} = 6.6 \text{ ppb} \quad (\textit{incorrect exposure})$$

Note: Calculating concentration based on this field condition yields a mass concentration that is high because the volume of air collected (V_F) is less than the volume at NTP.

Concentration Calculated at NTP (25°C, 760 mm Hg)

$Q_F = 0.5$ lpm; $V_F = Q_F(t_F) = 0.5$ lpm$(380$ min$) = 190.0$ l sampled

$V_S = V_F(P_F/P_S)(T_S/T_F)$

$V_S = 190.0(743.0/760.0)(298.15/233.15)$

$\quad = 190.0(1.25) = 237.5$ l sampled at NTP

$C_{M/V} = ($mass, mg$/V_S,$ liters$)(1000$ l/m$^3)$

$C_{M/V} = (0.009$ mg$/237.5$ l$)(1000$ l/m$^3) = 0.038$ mg/m^3

$C_{M/V} = 0.038$ mg/m$^3 = 0.0053$ ppm $= 5.3$ ppb (*correct exposure at NTP*)

Note: Correcting the field volume (V_F) to the normal temperature and pressure (NTP) yields the correct exposure. Not correcting the volume to NTP will not make a difference in the final recommendation.

Problem 4

Repeat the calculation in Example 5 for Leadville, Colorado, elevation 12,000 feet above sea level. Determine the NTP volume of air collected at 0.2 lpm for 20 minutes when an air sampling pump is operating at a sampling location that is at an elevation of $+12\,000$ feet. The pump was calibrated at the field location.

Solution 4

$Q_F =$ volume flowrate, at the calibration and field condition
$t_F =$ time interval, at the field condition
$V_F =$ volume delivered, at the field condition
$P_F =$ pressure at the field condition
$Q_F = 0.20$ lpm
$t_F = 20.0$ min
$V_F = (Q_F)(t_F)$
$P_F = 499.8$ mm Hg
$V_S = V_F(P_F/P_S)$
$V_F = (Q_F)(t_F) = (0.20$ lpm$)(20$ min$) = 4.0$ l
$P_F/P_S = 499.8$ mm Hg$/760$ mm Hg $= 0.66$
$V_S = V_F(P_F/P_S) = 4.0$ l$(0.66) = 2.63$ l

Percent difference from NTP $= [(V_S - V_F)/V_F]100$

Percent difference from NTP $= [(2.63$l$ - 4.0$ l$)/4.0$ l$]100 = -34.3\%$

This extreme pressure effect produces a -34.3% change in the volume and must be considered in subsequent calculations to assess worker exposure. In this example the volume flowrate measured is 0.20 lpm. The volume delivered (the volume flowrate multiplied by time, 4.0 liters) is corrected to standard pressure and results in a pressure-corrected standard volume (V_S) of 2.63 liters. This volume (2.63 l) would exist if the air moving through the system were at the standard condition (1 atmosphere).

Problem 5

It is a cold and dreary winter day, about two weeks before the Christmas holiday. You are extremely busy with holiday chores, shopping, and year-end reports for your consulting clients. The telephone rings; a former classmate whom you have not heard from since graduation calls you long distance from Prudhoe Bay, Alaska. She has been working as an industrial hygienist for a major oil company for three years, the last one on-site in Alaska. After reviewing the weather in the lower forty-eight, and the fact that your former industrial hygiene professor has gone off the deep end and is now wearing beads on a beach in Baja, presumably still writing the definitive book on antique car restoration, she got to the heart of the phone call.

The Northern Oil Waste Away Yahoo Company (NOWAY-C) has been sued by the Chemical, Oil and Particle Makers Association (COPMA) in Fairbanks, Alaska. The suit alleges that NOWAY-C was negligent in its air sampling and analysis program of the roughnecks on the North Slope. At best the North Slope is a mean and vicious place to be. Typical winter temperatures are $-30°F$, and with the wind chill it can seem as cold as $-100°F$. Obviously most of the work is performed in weatherproof shelters. The workers do spend about 45 minutes each day outdoors performing some critical activities with extremely toxic diethylacetyldecane (DEAD).

Your former classmate has modified the NIOSH standard method normally used for sampling and analysis of DEAD to enable its use in this climatic extreme. NOWAY-C's defense attorney, the famous Herschel Bailey, wants you to prepare some temperature and pressure correction factors to compare the NOWAY-C modified sampling method to the NIOSH standard sampling method. Bailey wants to know the correct response to the critical questions on air sampling that the plaintiffs' attorney will present to the corporate industrial hygienist while she is on the witness stand.

In addition, the correction factors that you develop will be used by a team of external auditors under the direction of your former industrial hygiene professor (finally getting bored playing volleyball on the Baja beach all day) to critically evaluate the alleged overexposure of the COPMA members. COPMA is suing the Company for 500 million dollars. Moreover, COPMA's experts include the editors of the NIOSH *Manual of Analytical Methods*, which is at the heart of this suit. Attorney Bailey would like for you to: develop temperature and pressure criteria for comparison of the modified

NIOSH method with the official NIOSH method including the relevant equations; and to explain the correct application of the temperature and pressure criteria that you developed for use on the North Slope site.

Solution 5

There is no single solution to this problem. It is, however, an excellent group discussion project.

Problem 6

Dr. Ivan Ivanowich, the Minister of the Russian Institute for Occupational Safety and Health (RIOSH), has invited you to visit the Siberian Center for Occupational Research and Education (SCORE) to recommend workplace health standards for this region of his country. Upon your review of the situation you recommend that RIOSH adopt the ACGIH TLV's for workplace standards. Dr. Ivanowich agrees, but is concerned that the ACGIH standards are based upon 25°C and 760 mm Hg. You suggest that the TLV's be adopted and corrected for the prevailing Siberian environment, 15°C and 710 mm Hg. Dr. Ivanowich agrees and asks you to produce the conversion factor for these standards as you are waiting to board your flight to Helsinki and home.

Solution 6

Use the ACGIH TLV's for gases and vapors expressed in parts per million. The remainder of the problem will take some discussion.

Problem 7

A high pressure gas cylinder contains nitrogen at 2200 psi. The inside diameter of the gas cylinder is 8 inches, and the cylinder is 54 inches high. What is the volume of nitrogen at NTP?

Solution 7

Volume of the cylinder with a radius r and height H: $V = \pi r^2 h = \pi d^2 h / 4$

$$V = \pi d^2 h / 4 = \pi (8/12 \text{ ft})^2 (54/12 \text{ ft}) / 4 = 1.57 \text{ ft}^3 \text{ at } 2200 \text{ psi}$$

$$V_S = V_F (P_F / P_S) / (T_S / T_F)$$

$$= 1.57 \text{ ft}^3 (2200 \text{ psi} / 14.7 \text{ psi}) / (298.15 \text{ K} / 298.15 \text{ K})$$

$$V_S = 234.97 \text{ ft}^3 \text{ at NTP}$$

7

Fundamentals of Air Sampling

Outcome Competencies   *After studying this chapter you will be able to:*

- *Apply limit of detection to air sampling study design.*
- *Apply limit of quantification to air sampling study design.*
- *Compute appropriate air sample volumes.*
- *Employ the coefficient of variation to interpret air sampling results.*

1. INTRODUCTION

This chapter emphasizes calculation techniques used in designing air sampling protocols. It is not a complete guide to the process of air sampling to characterize workplace air. The objectives of this characterization are to determine if the worker is exposed to chemicals, determine if the exposure is adverse, and then design controls to protect the worker from adverse exposure. Air sampling also is used to evaluate the efficacy of engineering controls. This may be done by using area sampling (environmental sampling).

Federal and state occupational health compliance officials, insurance companies, and corporate industrial hygienists survey workplace air quality. It is in the interest of the worker, industry, and regulatory agencies to use standard sampling and analytical methods. Standard methods are those that have been critically evaluated by collaborative test methods for reliability, accuracy, precision, bias, limits of detection (LOD), limits of quantification (LOQ), range, and other characteristics.

Standard methods to assess exposure to chemical agents in the workplace are developed and published by NIOSH and OSHA. The NIOSH *Manual of Analytical Methods* contains these methods (9). Similarly, OSHA has developed and validated its own set of analytical methods (8). There are other sources of air sampling methods, including the United States Environmental Protection Agency (10), ASTM (formerly the American Society for Testing and Materials) (11), the World Health Organization (12), the American Public Health Association (13), and the published industrial hygiene and air pollution literature. Recognized standard air sampling and analytical methods exist to provide a comparable database for these surveys. However, if it is believed that a method adopted by NIOSH or OSHA is not appropriate, it need not be used. The rationale for method substitution for the NIOSH or OSHA adopted method must be documented. This documentation must be sufficient to withstand a critical review.

Eight-hour Threshold Limit Values–Time Weighted Averages (TLV-TWA) exist for some four hundred plus chemical agents commonly found in the workplace (14). NIOSH (9) lists sampling and analytical methods for most of these agents. This chapter will elaborate on calculation techniques for air sampling using existing air sampling protocols and procedures (8, 9, 17) for developing reliable exposure assessment.

2. AIR SAMPLE VOLUME

The *OSHA Analytical Methods* (8) and the NIOSH *Manual of Analytical Methods* (9) list a range of air sample volumes, minimum volume (VOL-MIN) to maximum volume (VOL-MAX), that should be collected for an exposure assessment. The volume is based on the sampler's sorptive capacity and assumes that the measured exposure is at the OSHA PEL. The range of volumes listed may not collect a sufficient mass for accurate laboratory analysis if the actual contaminant concentration is less than the PEL or the Time Weighted Average–Threshold Limit Value (TWA-TLV). If a collection method recommends sampling 10 liters of air, the hygienist may not be sure if an 8.5 liter air sample will collect sufficient mass for the laboratory to quantify. Finding that an insufficient air volume (i.e., too little mass) was sampled after the laboratory results are returned can turn out to be an enormous waste of resources and a professional embarrassment! To avoid this situation, it is essential to understand the restrictions faced by analytical laboratories: Limit of Detection (LOD) and Limit of Quantification (LOQ). To compute a minimum air sample volume to provide useful information for evaluating airborne contaminant concentration in the workplace, the hygienist must understand how to manipulate the LOD and the LOQ. Knowledge of these limits will provide increased flexibility in sampling. This chapter describes the techniques needed to select appropriate air sampling parameters (sample flowrate and duration).

3. LIMIT OF DETECTION

The limit of detection (LOD) has many definitions in the literature (5, 6). In this book the limit of detection (LOD) is the lowest concentration that can be determined to be statistically different from a blank. The analytical instrument output signal produced by the sample must be three to five times the instrument's background noise level to be at the limit of detection; that is, the signal-to-noise ratio (S/N) is three-to-one $(3/1)$ to five-to-one $(5/1)$. The chemical mass that produces a $3/1$ S/N ratio is the analytical method's lower limit of detection. In reality, a $3/1$ signal-to-noise ratio is a "wiggle" in the baseline and not a value to be cited with much confidence. Attempts to report definitive results when the minimum mass is present are fraught with potential difficulty. A sufficient air volume must be sampled to collect a mass that will exceed the limit of detection and reach the limit of quantification. The LOD should be used only when the recommended sample volume cannot be collected (e.g., the pump fails). Unless the pump has an elapsed time meter, pump failure results in an invalid sample. If the exposure is the result of a very short operation performed once a day, a mass less than the LOD may be collected. The discussion later in this chapter and in Chapter 8 will resolve this sampling problem.

The laboratory may elect to report a datum as below the LOD, or a less than value (L.T.). A less than value is reported as a numerical value preceded by a "$<$" symbol. For example, if the LOD is 20 ng and a contaminant is not detected, the laboratory will report the result as < 20 ng or U20 ng (under 20 ng). The mass represented by the LOD is useful and may be used to *estimate* the airborne contaminant concentration. If the LOD is not exceeded, for example, if an insufficient mass is collected in/on the sampling media, the sample mass will be reported as a "less than" value. This *must not* be considered the same as zero mass [0 milligrams (mg)] or zero concentration [0 parts per million (ppm) or 0 milligrams per cubic meter (mg/m^3)]. If the laboratory reports zero, beware! Instead, a datum reported as "$< $LOD" means that the actual mass collected [in milligrams (mg), micrograms (μg), nanograms (ng), etc.] lies somewhere between zero and the LOD. When "none detected" is reported, the actual mass of the contaminant is unknown, and the actual contaminant concentration in the workplace cannot be computed. It is possible to use the LOD mass and the sample volume to compute an *estimated* concentration. Sometimes called a limit of detection concentration, this may be useful in estimating the airborne contaminant concentration (as described in Example 1 below).

4. LIMIT OF QUANTIFICATION

The limit of quantification (LOQ) is the minimum mass of the analyte above which the precision of the reported result is better than a specified level.

Precision is the reproducibility of replicate analyses of the same sample (mass or concentration). For example, how close to each other is a target shooter able to place a set of shots anywhere on the target? Accuracy is the degree of agreement between measured values and an accepted reference value. For example, how close does a target shooter come to the bull's-eye? Bias is the difference between the average measured mass or concentration and a reference mass or concentration, expressed as a fraction of the reference mass or concentration. For example, how far from the bull's-eye is the target shooter able to place a cluster of shots?

5. COEFFICIENT OF VARIATION AND RELATIVE STANDARD DEVIATION

This section only reviews terms commonly encountered in the air sampling literature. It is not intended as a primer for air sampling statistics. The reader not familiar with these terms can consult the references cited in the Bibliography or any basic statics textbook (6, 19, 21).

The specified level referred to above is reported by NIOSH (9) and can be achieved by skilled analysts. It does not represent the absolute lower mass of detection (i.e., the limit of detection). The LOQ is between the lower end and the higher end of the range of concentration values that can be measured with a minimum coefficient of variation. The coefficient of variation (C_V) is the sample standard deviation divided by the sample mean:

$$\text{Standard deviation, } s_r = \frac{\left[\Sigma(x_i - M)^2\right]^{1/2}}{n-1}$$

$$\text{Arithmetic mean, } M = \frac{[\Sigma(x_i)]}{n}$$

$$\text{Coefficient of variation} = C_V = s_r/M$$

$$\text{Coefficient of variation, } C_V = \frac{\left\{\left[\Sigma(x_i - M)^2\right]^{1/2}/n - 1\right\}}{\left\{[\Sigma(x_i)]/n\right\}}$$

The coefficient of variation is about ten times the noise level and is sometimes expressed as a percent. NIOSH (9) renamed the coefficient of variation, changing from C_V to relative standard deviation (s_r). The relative standard (s_r) is computed exactly as the coefficient of variation (C_V) is, by dividing the estimated standard deviation (s) by the mean of a series of measurements. This gives a measure of precision or the reproducibility of individual measurements of mass or concentration. Because the standard deviation is less than the mean in a normal distribution, the ratio of the standard deviation to the mean is a decimal, and when multiplied by 100 can be reported as a percent precision.

Chapter 8 describes using the relative standard deviation (s_r) to evaluate air sampling data.

Example 1

What is the toluene concentration in a workplace if the analytical result from the laboratory is "None detected" (ND), and the volume of air collected is 0.159 liter?

Solution 1

NIOSH method number 1500 (9) describes the evaluation of hydrocarbons and gives the following information on toluene:

Range studied: 548–2190 mg/m^3; or 1.13–4.51 mg/sample
Estimated LOD: 53 μg/sample;   1 ppm = 3.77 mg/m^3
Air sample flow rate: ≤ 0.2 lpm   1993–94 ACGIH TLV-TWA 188 mg/m^3
Air sampling media: 100 mg/50 mg coconut shell charcoal

Mass concentration is the actual mass reported by the analytical laboratory divided by the sample volume, corrected to normal temperature and pressure (F_{TP}) and with the units converted so that concentration is reported in mg/m^3, μg/m^3, ng/m^3, etc. For example:

$$[\text{Actual mass}/\text{Volume sample } (F_{TP})](\text{Unit conversion factor})$$

$$= \text{Actual mass concentration}$$

where actual mass is the mass reported by the laboratory or the LOD (mg, μg, ng, etc.), and volume sampled (liters) is the product of the air flowrate (lpm) and time, corrected to NTP. F_{TP} is the temperature and pressure correction factor (see Chapter 6). Units conversion is needed to convert liters to cubic meters and mass to mg or ng, etc.

Because the analytical result is "none detected," the actual mass is not known. Although a specific number for the actual mass cannot be used, it is known that the value lies between zero and the LOD (0.053 mg in this example). Assuming the most conservative case, substitute the LOD for the actual mass:

$$[\text{LOD}/\text{Volume sampled } (F_{TP})](\text{Unit conversion factor})$$

$$= \text{LOD concentration}$$

The LOD is 0.053 mg and the sample volume is 0.159 l (NTP, F_{TP} = 1). The LOD concentration is:

$$[0.053 \text{ mg}/0.159 \text{ l}(1)](1000 \text{ l/m}^3) = 333 \text{ mg/m}^3$$

This means that the actual concentration is somewhere between "zero" and 333 mg/m^3 and should be reported as " < 333 mg/m^3." Because the TLV for toluene is 188 mg/m^3, knowing that the actual concentration is less than 333 mg/m^3 is of concern in evaluating the workplace. One does not know if the actual concentration is 5 mg/m^3 or 333 mg/m^3. If the volume of air sampled is increased by a factor of ten, the concentration that is reported will be lowered by a factor of ten. For example, if 1.59 liters of air is sampled rather than 0.159 liter and the laboratory reports "none detected" at 0.053 mg, then the LOD concentration (NTP, $F_{TP} = 1$) becomes:

$$[53 \ \mu g/1.59 \ l(1)](mg/10^3 \ \mu g)(1000 \ l/m^3) = 33.3 \ mg/m^3$$

The actual concentration is between zero and 33.3 mg/m^3, and is reported as " < 33.3 mg/m^3." This 33.3 mg/m^3 is approximately 18% of the TLV-TWA for toluene (33.3 mg/m^3 divided by 188 mg/m^3 = 18%). In this situation the LOD and the volume sampled can be very useful in evaluating a workplace. Determining the range of concentration requires application of the relative standard deviation to the concentration that results from the laboratory analysis. This will be described in a later section.

If an analytical result is "none detected" (at a specified mass), what percent of the TLV would be an "acceptable" sample result? Some chemicals listed in the OSHA PELs have an action limit, which usually is one-half the PEL. Exceeding the action limit mandates air sampling, medical examination, and employee training. The sample results should be able to prove that the exposure is at least less than 50% of the PEL or the TLV. A good industrial hygiene practice could be that samples reported as "none detected" (at a specified mass) should be less than 25% of the TLV and preferably less than 10% of the TLV for the exposure to be "acceptable." If a "none detected" (at a specified mass) result is more than 25% of the TLV, a good industrial hygiene practice would be to resurvey the work area.

Example 2

The ACME Toxicology Company is testing the effects of inhalation of hydrogen chloride gas on laboratory mice. The Director of Toxicology wants an independent verification of the hydrogen chloride (HCl) concentration present in an animal exposure chamber. The animals are exposed to HCl concentrations (50, 100, 200, and 300 ppm) for 15 minutes at each concentration.

Solution 2

NIOSH method number 7903 (9) describes the air sampling and analysis protocol for hydrogen chloride gas. NIOSH gives the following sampling information on hydrogen chloride:

Range studies: 0.14–14 mg/m^3; or 0.5–200 μg/sample
Estimated LOD: 2.0 μg/sample;   1 ppm = 1.49 mg/m^3
Air sample flow rate: 0.2–0.5 lpm   1993–94 ACGIH TLV-TWA 7.5 mg/m^3
Sampling media: Orbo 24 solid sorbent tubes

To provide the verification required by ACME's Director of Toxicology, calculate the pump flow rate needed to collect a sample mass that is between 0.5 μg/sample and 200 μg/sample. A sample less than 0.5 μg is below the LOD, whereas a 200 μg sample is 400 times the LOD. The air sample must be collected during the 15 minute exposure period. Assume that the chamber concentration is 300 ppm (447.6 mg/m^3) for the total 15 minute exposure period. Let X be the air sample volume needed to quantify the airborne concentration:

$$(447.6 \text{ mg/m}^3)(1000 \text{ }\mu\text{g/mg})(X) = 200 \text{ }\mu\text{g}$$

$$4.48 \times 10^5 \text{ }\mu\text{g/m}^3 = 200 \text{ }\mu\text{g}/X$$

$$X = 0.000448 \text{ m}^3 = 0.448 \text{ l}$$

Conclusion: If the chamber concentration is 300 ppm (447.6 mg/m^3), then collect an air sample with a total volume not to exceed 0.448 liter.

Sampling at 0.5 liter per minute (lpm)   Total time of sampling @ 0.5 lpm: (min/0.5 l)(0.448 l) = 0.896 min
The sampling time is too short to assess the exposure.

Sampling at 0.2 liter per minute (lpm)   Total time of sampling @ 0.2 lpm: (min/0.2 l)(0.448 l) = 2.24 min
By lowering the flowrate to 0.2 lpm, more time is available to assess the exposure and set up the sampling train and to change the sampling tubes.

Final recommendation: Collect 7 tubes at 0.2 lpm (for 2.1 minutes each) for 14.7 minutes out of the total 15 minutes exposed.

Example 2A

What mass of hydrogen chloride gas is collected during a 2.24 minute sample if the exposure chamber concentration is 50 ppm?

Solution 2A

$$50 \text{ ppm} \left(\frac{\text{mg/m}^3}{1.49 \text{ ppm}} \right)(\text{ }\mu\text{g}/10^{-3} \text{ mg})(0.2 \text{ lpm})(2.24 \text{ min})(\text{m}^3/1000 \text{ l}) = 33 \text{ }\mu\text{g}$$

The quantity 33 μg is 16.5 times the LOD, an acceptable mass for the laboratory to analyze.

Example 3

The Commissioners for Labor and Industries and Public Health for the Commonwealth of Massachusetts want to study lead exposure of workers deleading residential property.

Solution 3

To determine lead exposure of workers, the air sampling time to produce a sufficient mass for a reliable exposure result must be calculated. The OSHA PEL for lead is 0.05 mg/m^3, and the ACGIH TLV is 0.15 mg/m^3. NIOSH method number 7082 (9) describes the evaluation of inorganic lead metals and lead salts with a $+2$ and $+4$ valence state. NIOSH gives the following sampling information on lead:

Range studied: 0.13–0.4 mg/m^3; or   10–200 μg/sample
Estimated LOD: 2.6 μg/sample;   1 ppm = N/A
Air sample flow rate: 1–4 lpm   PEL 0.05 mg/m^3
Sampling media: 0.8 μm cellulose ester membrane

To develop an air sampling protocol for lead, assume that the worker may be exposed to from 0.25 to 2.0 times the PEL; then calculate the air sample volume, flowrate, and sampling time.

OSHA PEL (mg/m^3)	Fraction of TLV	Mass conc. (mg/m^3)
0.05	0.25	0.0125
0.05	0.50	0.025
0.05	0.75	0.0375
0.05	1.0	0.05
0.05	1.5	0.075
0.05	2.0	0.10

Let X equal the air sample volume needed to quantify the airborne lead concentration. To collect a mass of 20 μg (about eight times the LOD) when the exposure is 0.25 of the TLV:

$$0.0125 \; (\text{mg/m}^3)(1000 \; \mu\text{g/mg})(X) = 20 \; \mu\text{g}$$

$$12.5 \; \mu\text{g/m}^3 = 20 \; \mu\text{g}/x$$

$$X = 1.6 \text{ m}^3 = 1600 \text{ l}$$

Conclusion: If the worker's exposure is 0.0125 mg/m^3 (0.25 times the TLV), collect an air sample with a total volume not to exceed 1600 liters.

Sampling at 4.0 liters per minute (lpm)   Total sampling time at 4.0 lpm:
(min/4.0 l)(1600 l) = 400 min
The sampling time to collect a 1600 liter air sample is adequate to assess the deleader's exposure during an eight-hour work shift.

Sampling at 1.0 liters per minute (lpm)   Total sampling time at 1.0 lpm:
$(\text{min}/1.0 \text{ l})(1600 \text{ l}) = 1600$ min
The sampling time is too long to assess a deleader's eight-hour exposure.
    If the exposure is at the PEL (0.05 mg/m^3), calculate X, the air sample volume needed:

$$0.05 \, (\text{mg/m}^3)(1000 \, \mu\text{g/mg})(X) = 20 \, \mu\text{g}$$

$$12.5 \, \mu\text{g/m}^3 = 20 \, \mu\text{g}/X$$

$$X = 0.4 \text{ m}^3 = 400 \text{ l}$$

Conclusion: If the worker's exposure is at the PEL, 0.05 mg/m^3, collect an air sample with a total volume not to exceed 400 liters.

Sampling at 4.0 liters per minute (lpm)   Total sampling time at 4.0 lpm:
$(\text{min}/4.0 \text{ l})(400 \text{ l}) = 100$ min
The sampling time is adequate to assess the deleader's exposure. Multiple samples must be collected during the eight-hour workday. If only one sample is collected, then only $4 \times 20 \, \mu\text{g}$ will be collected. This is within the analytical range of the method.

Sampling at 1.0 liters per minute (lpm)   Total sampling time at 1.0 lpm:
$(\text{min}/1.0 \text{ l})(400 \text{ l}) = 400$ min
The sampling time is adequate to assess a deleader's eight-hour exposure.
Conclusion: If the worker's exposure is 0.05 mg/m^3, collect an air sample with a total volume not to exceed 400 liters. This will collect only 20 μg per sample. The air sampling time can be increased and thus more mass collected as long as the range of the method is not exceeded. The range for this method is 10 to 200 μg/sample.

Final recommendation: Collect one filter sample at 1.0 lpm for 480 minutes.

Example 3A

Fill in the blanks in the table below.

OSHA PEL (mg/m^3)	Fraction of TLV	Mass conc. (mg/m^3)	Air sample volume (l)	Air sampling flowrate (lpm)	Time (min)	Notes
0.05	0.25	0.0125	1600	4	400	Acceptable
0.05	0.25	0.0125	1600	1	1600	Not acceptable
0.05	0.50	0.025				
0.05	0.75	0.0375				
0.05	1.0	0.05	400	1	400	Acceptable
0.05	1.0	0.05	400	4	100	Acceptable
0.05	1.5	0.075				
0.05	2.0	0.10				

Example 3B

If the air sample flow rate is 4 liters per minute and a single sample is collected for 480 minutes, what is the mass of lead collected if the exposure is at the PEL?

Solution 3B

$$(0.05 \text{ mg/m}^3)(\text{m}^3/1000 \text{ l})(4 \text{ l/min})(480 \text{ min})(1000 \text{ } \mu\text{g/mg}) = 96 \text{ } \mu\text{g}$$

The quantity 96 μg is within the range of the method (10–200 μg).

Example 4

Calculate the UCL for a measured air concentration (MAC) of toluene (125 mg/m^3). The TWA-TLV is 188 mg/m^3, and NIOSH lists the s_r as 0.052.

Solution 4

For one sample there is no distribution. If many air samples (minimum 6, generally 6 to 18) are collected, the exposure data will be lognormally distributed (18, 19, 20). Using a one-tailed statistical test, the upper 95% confidence limit (UCL) of a measured air concentration (MAC) sample result can be calculated:

$$\text{UCL} = \text{MAC} + 1.645(s_r)(\text{applicable standard})$$

$$\text{UCL} = \text{MAC} + 1.645(s_r)(\text{applicable standard})$$

$$\text{UCL} = 125 \text{ mg/m}^3 + 1.645(0.052)(188 \text{ mg/m}^3)$$

$$\text{UCL} = 125 \text{ mg/m}^3 + 16.1 \text{ mg/m}^3 = 141 \text{ mg/m}^3$$

The results could be as high as 141 mg/m^3 when the measured air concentration is 125 mg/m^3.

BIBLIOGRAPHY

1. Lewis, R. J., Sr., *Sax's Dangerous Properties of Industrial Materials*, Eighth Edition. Van Nostrand Reinhold, New York (1994).
2. National Institute for Occupational Safety and Health, *Pocket Guide to Chemical Hazards* (DHHS/NIOSH Pub. No. 90-117). U.S. Government Printing Office, Washington, DC (1990).

3. Powell, Charles, Evaluation of exposure to chemical agents. In *Patty's Industrial Hygiene and Toxicology*, Vol. III, *Theory and Rationale of Industrial Hygiene Practice*, ed. Cralley, J. V. and Cralley, L. J., Second Edition. John Wiley & Sons, New York (1985), pp. 319–358.

4. National Institute for Occupational Safety and Health, *Registry of Toxic Effects of Chemical Substances (RTECS)*, ed. Sweet, D.V. (DHHS/NIOSH Pub. No. 87-114). U.S. Government Printing Office, Washington, DC (1984).

5. Keith, L. H., Crumett, W., Deegan, J., Jr., Libby, R. A., Taylor, J. K., and Winter, C., Principles of environmental analysis. *Analytical Chemistry* 55:2210–2218 (1983).

6. Gilbert, R. O., *Statistical Methods for Environmental Pollution Monitoring*. Van Nostrand Reinhold, New York (1986).

7. American Conference of Governmental Industrial Hygienists, *Air Sampling Instruments*, Eighth Edition. American Conference of Governmental Industrial Hygienists, Cincinnati, OH (1994).

8. Occupational Safety and Health Administration, *OSHA Analytical Methods*. American Conference of Governmental Industrial Hygienists, Cincinnati, OH (1985).

9. National Institute for Occupational Safety and Health, *Manual of Analytical Methods*, ed. Eller, P. E., Third Edition (DHHS/NIOSH Pub. No. 84-100). U.S. Government Printing Office, Washington, DC (1984, revised 1987).

10. U.S. Environmental Protection Agency, *EPA Compendium of Methods for the Determination of Toxic Organic Compounds in Ambient Air*. Washington, DC (1984).

11. American Society for Testing and Materials, *D-22 Committee Book of ASTM Standards*, Part 23, Industrial Water; Atmospheric Analysis. ASTM, Philadelphia, PA (annual issue).

12. World Health Organization, *Environmental and Health Monitoring in Occupational Health*, Technical Report Series No. 535. Geneva (1973).

13. American Public Health Association Intersociety Committee, *Methods of Air Sampling and Analysis*, Second Edition. APHA, Washington, DC (1977).

14. American Conference of Governmental Industrial Hygienists, *Threshold Limit Values and Biological Indices 1993–1994*. American Conference of Governmental Industrial Hygienists, Cincinnati, OH (1993).

15. National Institute for Occupational Safety and Health, *Proficiency Analytical Testing (PAT) Program* (DHEW/NIOSH Pub. No. 77-173). U.S. Government Printing Office, Washington, DC (1977).

16. American Industrial Hygiene Association, *Quality Assurance Manual for Industrial Chemistry* (AIHA 104-BP-88) (1994).

17. Nakasone, R. I., Thomas, J. F., and Graham, R. B., United States Air Force, Occupational and Environmental Health Laboratory (USAF OEHL), *Recommended Sampling Procedures*. Brooks Air Force Base, TX (1985).

18. National Institute for Occupational Safety and Health, *Occupational Exposure Sampling Strategy Manual*, by Leidel, N. A., Busch, K. A., and Lynch, J. R. (HEW/NIOSH Pub. No. 77-173). U.S. Government Printing Office, Washington, DC (1977).

19. U.S. Environmental Protection Agency, *Quality Assurance Handbook for Air Pollution Measurement System*, Vol. I, *Principles*, EPA-600/9-76-00J. Research Triangle Park, NC (1976).

20. Hawkins, N. C., Norwood, S., and Rock, J. C., *A Strategy for Occupational Exposure Assessment*. American Industrial Hygiene Association, Fairfax, VA, (1991).
21. Wallace, L. A., et al., The TEAM study: personal exposures to toxic substances in air, drinking water, and breath of 400 residents of New Jersey, North Carolina and North Dakota. *Environmental Research* 43:290–307 (1987).

PROBLEM SET
Problem 1

Table 7-1 contains the laboratory results of a volatile organics survey using gas chromatography and mass spectroscopy (GC/MS) performed in Rooms 1 through 5 of an elementary school. The samples were collected on Supelco Carbotrap 300 solid sorbent tubes (10). The air sample volumes are included on the last line of the table. Develop a table of results (Table 7-2) in $\mu g/m^3$, and explain the calculations.

TABLE 7-1.

| Compound | MW | Sample Results (ng) | | | | | DL (ng) |
		Rm 1	Rm 2	Rm 3	Rm 4	Rm 5	
Chloromethane		25U	25U	25U	25U	25U	25
Vinyl chloride		25U	25U	25U	25U	25U	25
Bromomethane		25U	25U	25U	25U	25U	25
Chloroethane		25U	25U	25U	25U	25U	25
Ethene, 1,1-dichloro-	97	33	36	25	36	20J	25
Carbon disulfide		25U	25U	25U	25U	25U	25
Acetone		100U	100U	100U	100U	100U	100
Vinyl acetate		50U	50U	50U	50U	50U	50
Methylene chloride	84.9	105	130	65	119	40	25
trans-1,2-Dichlorethene		25U	25U	25U	25U	25U	25
Ethane, 1,1-dichloro-		25U	25U	25U	25U	25U	25
cis-1,2-Dichloroethene		25U	25U	25U	25U	25U	25
Chloroform	119.4	25U	25U	25U	25U	25U	25
Ethane, 1,2-dichloro-		25U	25U	25U	25U	25U	25
Butanone, 2-(MEK)		100U	100U	100U	100U	100U	100
Ethane, 1,1,1-trichloro	133	318	290	312	405	167	25
Carbon tetrachloride		20J	21J	20J	20J	16J	25
Benzene	78.1	201	206	162	225	115	25
Trichloroethene	131.4	50	57	20	59	35	25
Dibromomethane		25U	25U	25U	25U	25U	25
Bromodichloromethane		25U	25U	25U	25U	25U	25
Propane, 1,2-dichloro-		25U	25U	25U	25U	25U	25
cis-1,3-Dichloropropene		25U	25U	25U	25U	25U	25
trans-1,3-Dichloropropene		25U	25U	25U	25U	25U	25
Ethane, 1,1,2-trichloro-		25U	25U	25U	25U	25U	25
Dibromochloromethane		25U	25U	25U	25U	25U	25

TABLE 7-1. *Continued*

Compound	MW	Sample Results (ng)					DL (ng)
		Rm 1	Rm 2	Rm 3	Rm 4	Rm 5	
Pentanone, 4-methyl-2-(MIBK)		50U	50U	25U	25U	25U	50
Chlorobenzene		25U	25U	25U	25U	25U	25
Toluene	92.1	479	527	239	584	333	25
Tetrachloroethene	167.9	143	154	140	137	118	25
Hexanone, 2-(MBK)		50U	50U	50U	50U	50U	50
Ethylbenzene	106.2	85	92	58	106	52	25
Xylene (*meta, para*)	106.2	146	160	106	183	91	25
Xylene (*ortho*)	106.2	110	122	87	144	68	25
Styrene		29	26	14J	23J	15J	25
Bromoform		25U	25U	25U	25U	25U	25
Propane, 1,2,3-trichloro-		25U	25U	25U	25U	25U	25
Ethane, 1,1,2,2-tetrachloro-		25U	25U	25U	25U	25U	25
Dichlorobenzene (*meta*)		25U	25U	25U	25U	25U	25
Dichlorobenzene (*para*)	147	12J	13J	10J	30	9J	25
Dichlorobenzene (*ortho*)		25U	25U	25U	27	25U	25
AIR SAMPLE VOLUME (l)		36.0	35.4	36.6	34.8	32.5	—

DL = detection limit; ng = nanograms; *MW* = molecular weight.
U = undetected. The value is the LOD for that compound.
J = estimated value. The value is below the LOD.

TABLE 7-2.

Compound	Sample Results ($\mu g/m^3$)					Mean	Note
	Rm 1	Rm 2	Rm 3	Rm 4	Rm 5		
Ethene, 1,1-dichloro-	0.9	1.0	0.7	1.0	—	1.10	—
Methylene chloride	2.9	3.7	1.8	3.4	1.2	3.15	—
Chloroform	—	—	—	—	—	8	—
Ethane, 1,1,1-trichloro	8.8	8.2	8.5	11.6	5.1	8.6	52
Benzene	5.6	5.8	4.4	6.5	3.5	5.5	20
Trichloroethene	1.4	1.6	0.5	1.7	1.1	1.2	3.6
Toluene	13.3	14.9	10.8	16.8	10.2	14.1	27–62
Tetrachloroethene	4.0	4.4	3.8	3.0	3.6	4.2	10
Ethylbenzene	2.4	2.6	1.6	3.0	1.6	2.2	13
Xylene (*meta, para*)	4.1	4.5	2.9	5.3	2.8	3.6	21
Xylene (*ortho*)	3.1	3.4	2.4	4.1	2.1	2.7	7.8
Styrene	0.8	0.7	—	—	—	0.75	5.7
Dichlorobenzene (*para*)	—	—	—	0.9	—	0.9	42
Dichlorobenzene (*ortho*)	—	—	—	0.8	—	0.8	0.4
AIR SAMPLE VOLUME (l)	36.0	35.4	36.6	34.8	32.5	—	—

Mean = mean of the reported sample results.
Note: The data in this column were abstracted from a comprehensive study on volatile organic compounds in indoor air (21).

8

Exposure Assessment

Outcome Competencies *After studying this chapter you will be able to:*
- *Compute time weighted average–threshold limit values* (TWA-TLV).
- *Critique time weighted average–threshold limit values* (TWA-TLV).
- *Compute time weighted average–short-term exposure limits* (TWA-STEL).
- *Critique time weighted average–short-term exposure limits* (TWA-STEL).
- *Compute time weighted average–ceiling limits (TWA-C).*
- *Critique time weighted average–ceiling limits (TWA-C).*

1. INTRODUCTION

Industrial hygienists collect samples as a part of their professional responsibility to evaluate the workplace for contaminants that can adversely affect workers' health. The concentration of contaminants in the workplace and their exposure potential are the basis for exercising industrial hygiene judgment. Because the literature contains many protocols for industrial hygiene sampling and analysis, the hygienist needs guidance in selecting exposure assessment methods that are appropriate from a medical/legal standpoint. The NIOSH *Manual of Analytical Methods* and the *OSHA Analytical Methods* are published to meet this need (2, 8).

Air samples are required in order to quantitatively determine an index of employee exposure to airborne contaminants. The objectives of personal air sampling are to:

- Determine if there are any adverse exposures.
- Identify conditions that may yield potential adverse health effects.
- Identify unsatisfactory conditions.
- Investigate employee complaints.
- Document compliance with applicable federal, state, and local regulations.
- Establish a baseline profile of employee exposure.
- Predict the health effects of an exposure by comparing the sampling results with occupational health standards (PELs, TLVs, RELs, WEELs, internal corporate standards, etc.).
- Maintain an exposure history for retrospective epidemiological studies.

The objectives of area air sampling are to:

- Investigate bulk air or area contaminants.
- Determine the effectiveness of engineering or administrative controls.
- Evaluate the effectiveness of dilution ventilation.
- Determine the adequacy of the outdoor air volume in an indoor air quality survey.

Air sampling and analysis methods are highly specific and are selected according to the type of contaminant and the process. Reference must be made to the appropriate NIOSH (2), OSHA (8), or other recognized air sampling method for each contaminant. The sampling time must conform to the averaging time used in the applicable standard.

2. TIME WEIGHTED AVERAGE CALCULATIONS

Time weighted average calculations apportion a measured exposure to the interval of time during which the exposure occurred. A worker may have an elevated exposure during one time interval and a lower exposure in the next time interval. The purpose of time weighting the average is to give a more representative measure of exposure then just a simple mathematical average. This technique is not intended as a means to expose a worker to an unacceptably high concentration during one time interval and not expose the worker during another time interval.

The time weighted average (TWA) can be calculated by using the following relationship:

$$\text{TWA} = \Sigma C_i t_i / \Sigma t_i$$

where C_i is the concentration occurring during the ith sampling interval, and t_i is the sampling time for the interval.

By weighting the exposure concentration, C_i, for the ith sampling period, t_i, it is possible to determine a worker's TWA exposure to a chemical or an agent. The TWA concentration then can be compared to a workplace standard such as those promulgated by OSHA (PELs) or recommended by NIOSH (RELs), ACGIH (TLVs), or AIHA (WEELs). The averaging time selected for the calculation depends on the particular chemical and the applicable standard to which the exposure is to be compared. For example, ACGIH (3), OSHA (4), NIOSH (5), and AIHA (6) define several standards, each with a requisite averaging time:

- ACGIH: *Threshold Limit Value–Time Weighted Average (TLV-TWA)*: Averaging time is 480 minutes (eight hours) for a forty hour week.
- OSHA: *Permissible Exposure Limits–Time Weighted Average (PEL-TWA)*: Averaging time is 480 minutes (eight hours) for a forty hour week.
- NIOSH: *Recommended Exposure Limit–Time Weighted Average (REL-TWA)*: Averaging time is up to ten hours for a forty hour week.
- AIHA: *Workplace Environmental Exposure Levels–Time Weighted Average (WEEL-TWA)*: Averaging time is up to eight hours for a forty hour week.

The TLV-TWA, PEL-TWA, REL-TWA, or WEEL-TWA is given by $\Sigma C_i t_i / \Sigma t_i$, where:

C_i = airborne concentration of the ith species in the specified averaging time period (an eight hour period for the TLVs, PELs, and WEELs; up to a ten hour period for the RELs)

t_i = specified averaging time period (an eight hour period for the TLVs, PELs, and WELs; up to a ten hour period for the RELs)

Short-term limits are as follows:

- ACGIH: *Threshold Limit Value–Short-Term Exposure Limit (TLV-STEL) (3)*: The STEL is a 15 minute TWA to which workers can be exposed continuously and for a short period of time without suffering from: irritation, chronic or irreversible tissue damage, or narcosis of sufficient degree to increase the likelihood of accidental injury, impaired self-rescue, or materially reduced work efficiency, provided that the daily TLV-TWA is not exceeded, and averaging time is 15 minutes.
- OSHA: *Permissible Exposure Limit–Short-Term Exposure Limit (PEL-STEL) (4)*: The STEL is a 15 minute TWA exposure that shall not be exceeded at any time during a workday

unless another time limit is specified in the standard, below the limit. If another time period is specified, the time weighted average exposure over that time period shall not be exceeded at any time during the working day, and the averaging time is 15 minutes.

- NIOSH: *Recommended Exposure Limit–Short-Term Exposure Limit (REL-STEL)* (5): The STEL is a 15 minute TWA exposure that should not be exceeded at any time during a workday. The averaging time is 15 minutes.
- AIHA: *Workplace Environmental Exposure Levels–Time Weighted Average (WEEL-short-term TWA)*: The short-term TWA averaging time for the applicable agent is specified in the documentation.

The TLV-STEL, PEL-STEL, REL-STEL, or WEEL short-term TWA, is given by $\Sigma C_i t_i / \Sigma t_i$, where:

C_i = airborne concentration of the ith species in the 15 minute period

t_i = 15 minute STEL averaging period.

Ceiling limits include the following:

- *Threshold Limit Value–Ceiling (TLV-C)* (3): The standard is an instantaneous value, and no averaging time can be specified. If an instantaneous reading instrument is not available, then the averaging time can be considered to be the 15 minute STEL.
- OSHA: *Permissible Exposure Limit–Ceiling (PEL-C)* (4): The ceiling is the employee's exposure that shall not be exceeded during any part of the workday. If instantaneous monitoring is not feasible, then the ceiling shall be assessed as a 15 minute time weighted average exposure that shall not be exceeded at any time over a working day.
- NIOSH: *Recommended Exposure Limit–Ceiling (REL-C)* (5): The REL-C should not be exceeded at any time during a workday.
- AIHA: *Workplace Environmental Exposure Levels–Ceiling (WEEL-C)* (5): The WEEL-C should not be exceeded at any time during a workday.

Difficult decisions about averaging times still occur, such as:

- Novel workshifts, longer than eight hours (e.g., 10 hours/day, 4 days per week).
- Novel workshifts, shorter than eight hours (e.g., 6 hours/day, 6 days per week).
- Lunch or rest breaks that are completed in the work area.

Extensive discussions on novel work schedules appear elsewhere (9). The sampling duration depends on several variables, including the:

- Limitations imposed by sampling and analytical equipment and methods (pumps, LOD, LOQ).
- Purpose of the sample (eight hour TLV-TWA, TLV-STEL, TLV-C, or compliance sampling).
- Nature of the operation.
- Confidence desired in the results.

Understanding each variable helps the hygienist decide how long to collect a sample.

3. SAMPLING FOR EIGHT HOUR EXPOSURES

The recommended sampling method to evaluate eight hour exposures is to monitor the worker over the entire workday and compare the measured exposure to an eight hour TWA standard. However, many industrial operations last less than eight hours or are sporadic or episodic. Industrial hygienists may air-sample while the work is performed and assume zero exposure during periods of "no exposure." This approach is acceptable as long as one can assure that the remainder of the workday actually will be at "no exposure" and does not involve other contaminant exposures. For example, skin absorption is possible if the ACGIH TLVs, OSHA PELs, or NIOSH RELs have a "skin" notation next to the chemical name. Air sampling may not necessarily identify the hazard. This is especially true with high molecular weight, low vapor pressure liquids (e.g., oils, glycol ethers, "heavy aromatic naphtha," etc.).

Pump Flowrate and Sample Collection Time

The pump flowrate range is the minimum to maximum rate (e.g., liters per minute) that can be used to collect an air sample. The sampling time is the period that the sampling equipment is in operation. The product of the air sample pump flowrate and the sample duration is the air sample volume. The use of dimensional analysis will enable the calculation of volume sampled, given the air sampling flowrate and the sampling time. Recall the discussion of units in Chapter 2. There is a straightforward means to produce the units of interest in exposure monitoring; the basic approach to handling units also can be applied to this situation. Once the final form of the units is established, it is necessary to configure the input units to achieve the desired final units.

(Pump flowrate, Q)(Collection time)(Units conversion factor)(F_{TP})

= Sample volume (1)

where:

Pump flowrate is the calibrated volume flow of the pump (mlpm, lpm, etc.).

Volume sampled (liters) is the product of the air flowrate (lpm) and time.

Collection time is the duration of the air sampling.

Units conversion is needed to convert milliliters or liters to cubic meters and time to minutes, etc.

F_{TP}, the temperature and pressure correction factor, adjusts the sample volume to NTP.

The F_{TP} correction equals one [1] if the conditions are close to NTP (see Chapter 6); for example:

$$(100 \text{ ml/min})(10 \text{ min})(1/1000 \text{ ml})(1) = 1 \text{ liter}$$
$$(0.100 \text{ l/min})(10 \text{ min})(1) = 1 \text{ liter}$$

A calibrated volume flowrate standard (soap bubble flowmeter, electronic bubble meter, etc.) always is used to calibrate air sampling pumps. Pump calibration is discussed elsewhere (1). The flowrate is calculated in units of liters per minute (lpm):

[Soap bubble volume (cc)/time](Units conversion)(F_{TP} correction)

$$= \text{Pump flowrate (lpm)}$$

For example:

$$(100 \text{ cm}^3/5.3 \text{ sec})(60 \text{ sec/min})(1 \text{ l}/1000 \text{ cm}^3) = 1.1 \text{ lpm}$$

Given that the pump flowrate is calibrated (0.1 lpm) and the minimum sample volume necessary to reach the limit of detection (LOD) is 1.0 liter, the minimum sampling time can be calculated:

[Sample volume (l)][1/Pump flowrate (lpm)] = Collection time (min)

For example:

$$(1 \text{ l})(\text{min}/0.1 \text{ l}) = 10 \text{ min}$$

Air sampling pump flowrates for various chemicals are listed by NIOSH (2) and OSHA (8). Any flowrate within the range is acceptable if the LOQ mass is collected. Flowrates outside this range could result in the loss of sample mass due to breakthrough or result in collection of less than the LOD mass (see Chapter 7).

Recommended Sample Volume

The sample volumes listed by NIOSH (2) and OSHA (8) are the volumes the hygienist should try to collect during the sampling period. If an air sample is collected to assess an eight hour exposure, the hygienist should have sufficient time to collect the listed volume during the eight hour work shift. Chapter 7 describes the use of LOD and LOQ to assure the collection of a mass that the laboratory can analyze. The following examples explain how to select sampling parameters.

Example 1

NIOSH method 1500 (2) describes the evaluation of hydrocarbons and gives the following information on toluene:

Range studied: 548–2190 mg/m^3; or   1.13–4.51 mg/sample
Estimated LOD: 53 μg/sample;   1 ppm = 3.77 mg/m^3
Air sample flow rate: ≤ 0.2 lpm   1993–94 ACGIH TLV-TWA 188 mg/m^3
Air sampling media: 100 mg/50 mg coconut shell charcoal

The work process lasts 1 hour, and there is no exposure for the remaining 7 hours. The NIOSH recommended sample volume, 2 liters, is collected. At the conditions stated above, what is an appropriate sampling protocol for toluene?

Solution 1

Compute the pump flowrate by using dimensional analysis (divide the recommended volume by the expected sample time):

$$\text{Recommended volume/Sample time} = \text{Pump flowrate}$$

$$2\,1/60 \text{ min} = 0.033 \text{ lpm}$$

For this example, the pump should be calibrated to a flowrate of 0.033 lpm to collect 2 liters in 60 minutes. This is within the recommended air sample flowrate of less than 0.2 lpm. Obviously the pump selected must be able to sample at the computed flowrate.

Assume that a worker's job routine requires handling toluene for only one hour each day. For the remainder of the day the worker is in another area of the facility in an administrative capacity and *not exposed to any other chemicals*. Because the hygienist knows that the worker is not exposed to toluene or other contaminants for the rest of the workday, the eight hour time weighted average exposure is computed as follows:

$$\text{eight hour TWA} = \Sigma C_i t_i / \Sigma t_i$$

$$\text{eight hour TWA} = \left[(C_1 \times t_1) + (C_2 \times t_2) \right] / \left[(t_1 + t_2) \right]$$

where:

C_1 = contaminant concentration (mg/m^3 or ppm) during the air sampling period

t_1 = time (hours) of the air sampling period (one hour in this example)

C_2 = concentration during the seven nonexposure hours (zero in this example)

t_2 = time in hours of the nonexposure period (seven hours in this example)

Eight hours is the averaging time because the hygienist wishes to compare the exposure to an eight hour time weighted average (i.e., the threshold limit value, the permissible exposure limit, or the recommended exposure limit). (Note: Dimensional analysis requires that the time unit in the numerator be the same as the time unit in the denominator.)

The eight hour time weighted average exposure is calculated as follows:

$$\text{eight hour TWA} = \Sigma C_i t_i / \Sigma t_i \quad \text{where } i = 1, 2$$

$$\text{eight hour TWA} = \left[(C_1)(1\ \text{hr}) + (0 \times 7\ \text{hr}) \right] / 8\ \text{hr} = \Sigma C_i 1\ \text{hr} / 8\ \text{hr}$$

The analytical laboratory reports a mass of 2.25 mg in a 2 liter sample. This is within the acceptable analytical range (1.13–4.51 mg/sample) and 42 times the limit of detection. Based on the laboratory result, C_1 is 1 125 mg/m^3, and C_2 is known to be zero.

$$\text{eight hour TWA} = \left[(1\ 125\ \text{mg/m}^3)(1\ \text{hr}) + 0(7\ \text{hr}) \right] / 8\ \text{hr} = 141\ \text{mg/m}^3$$

Example 2

Given:

The LOD for toluene is 0.053 mg (53 μg).

The minimum–maximum pump flowrate listed by NIOSH is 0.02–0.2 l/min.

The recommended sample volume listed by NIOSH (2) is 2 liters.

The work process is scheduled to last eight hours.

What would be the appropriate sampling protocol for toluene at these conditions?

There is no single answer to this problem. The objectives of this air sampling program will determine how many air samples will be collected and the appropriate flowrates and sample volumes. If the objective is to determine the average concentration during each of the eight hours, then eight individual one hour samples are collected. The mass collected must exceed the limit of quantification. Unless the study has specific objectives, a minimum number of samples are used to obtain the eight hour time weighted average concentration.

Solution 2

To collect only a minimum number of samples, it is necessary to determine the longest sampling time possible per sample by dividing the listed sample volume by the slowest pump flowrate. The slowest pump rate listed by NIOSH (2) may not be the slowest flowrate the pump can sample, or it may be beyond the air sampling pump's operating limit. Check the operating manual for the specific pump selected for use.

$$(\text{Recommended volume})(1/\text{Pump flowrate})$$

$$= \text{Sample collection time} = (2 \text{ l})(\text{min}/0.02 \text{ l}) = 100 \text{ min}$$

As the actual work time is eight hours (480 min) and the longest sampling time is 100 min, several samples will be needed to cover an eight hour period. Care must be exercised to oversample and collect a mass sufficient to cause breakthrough to the backup section of the sorbent tube. If after 240 minutes the worker leaves the work area for a lunch break, the day can be considered two periods of 240 minutes each. The sampling schedule is outlined in Table 8-1.

Sampling for 100 minutes at 0.02 lpm will collect the recommended sample volume of 2 liters. However, tubes 3 and 6 will be collecting samples for only 40 minutes each. Will this sample time be sufficient to evaluate the time weighted average concentration? If enough mass is collected on tubes 3 and 6 and the analytical result is greater than the LOQ, they can be used in computing the exposure. However, if the analytical results for the two tubes are "none detected" (i.e., less than the LOD), is there sufficient information to compute the exposure? To make this determination, calculate the LOD concentration for toluene. Sample volume can be computed by multiplying

TABLE 8-1.

Sampling period	Tube Number	Time (min)
0800–0940	1	100
0940–1120	2	100
1120–1200	3	40
0100–0240	4	100
0240–0420	5	100
0420–0500	6	40
TOTAL		$\Sigma t_i = 480$ min

the sampling time by the flowrate. During the 40 minutes of sampling, 0.8 liter is collected:

$$(\text{Sampling time})(\text{Flowrate}) = \text{Volume collected}$$

$$(40\ \text{min})(0.02\ \text{lpm}) = 0.8\ l$$

Compute the LOD concentration by dividing the LOD mass by the volume collected in 40 minutes. The volume used to compute the concentration is corrected to NTP (see Chapter 6).

$$[\text{LOD}/\text{Sample volume in 40 min}(F_{TP})](\text{Unit conversion factor})$$

$$= \text{LOD concentration (Chapter 7)}$$

$$(0.053\ \text{mg}/0.8\ l)(1000\ l/\text{m}^3)(1.0) = 66.3\ \text{mg/m}^3$$

The resulting 66 mg/m^3 is 35% of the TLV-TWA for toluene (66.3 mg/m^3 divided by 188 mg/m^3 = 35.2%). This exceeds the preferred 10% to 25% of the TLV-TWA when "none detected" is the sample result. Therefore, the 40 minute collection time for tubes 3 and 6 may not provide sufficient information if the analytical results are "none detected." Compute the TWA:

eight hour TWA $= \Sigma C_i t_i / \Sigma t_i$ where $i = 1, 2, 3, 4, 5, 6$.

$$\text{TWA} = \frac{[(C_1 t_1) + (C_2 t_2) + (C_3 t_3) + (C_4 t_4) + (C_5 t_5) + (C_6 t_6)]}{480\ \text{min}}$$

where:

C_1 to C_6 = concentration (mg/m^3 or ppm) during the six air sampling periods (i.e., the six analytical results reported by the laboratory, one for each time interval, t_i, where $i = 1, 2, 3, 4, 5, 6$) (see Table 8-2)

TABLE 8-2.

Sampling period	Tube number	Time (t_i) (min)	Concentration (mg/m^3)	$C_i t_i$ (mg/m^3)min
0800–0940	1	100	$C_1 = 312$	31 200
0940–1120	2	100	$C_2 = 302$	30 200
1120–1200	3	40	$C_3 < 66$	2 640
0100–0240	4	100	$C_4 = 292$	29 200
0240–0420	5	100	$C_5 = 272$	27 200
0420–0500	6	40	$C_6 < 66$	2 640
TOTALS		$\Sigma t_i = 480$		$\Sigma C_i t_i = 123\,080$

t_1 to t_6 = time (minutes) of the six air sampling periods

480 min = total exposure and averaging time to compare to an eight hour standard

Note: The time unit in the denominator must be the same as the time unit in the numerator.

Calculate the eight hour time weighted average:

$$\text{eight hour TWA} = \Sigma C_i t_i / \Sigma t_i$$

$$\text{eight hour TLV-TWA} =$$

$$\frac{[(C_1 100) + (C_2 100) + (C_3 40) + (C_4 100) + (C_5 100) + (C_6 40)]}{480 \text{ min}}$$

Because the analytical result for C_3 and/or C_6 is "none detected," the LOD concentration of 66 mg/m^3 is used for these two samples:

$$\text{eight hour TWA} =$$

$$\frac{[(312 \times 100) + (302 \times 100) + (66 \times 40) + (292 \times 100) + (272 \times 100) + (66 \times 40)]}{480 \text{ min}}$$

$$\text{eight hour TWA} = 123\,080 (\text{mg/m}^3)(\text{min})/480 \text{ min}$$

$$\text{eight hour TWA} = 256 \text{ mg/m}^3$$

If the two 40 minute samples produced an insignificant result, the eight hour result still exceeds the eight hour standard. Appropriate industrial hygiene interventions must be implemented.

Example 3

What is an appropriate sampling protocol for the conditions stated in Example 2 if, after the work process has proceeded for 60 minutes, the hygienist is informed that the work will last another 20 minutes? The hygienist has two options, break up the sampling period and use two tubes (one for 60 minutes, the other for 20 minutes), or continue sampling using the same tube for the full 80 minute work process.

Solution 3, Option 1 (Use two tubes: one for 60 min; one for 20 min)

If this option is selected, the question is essentially the same as that asked in Example 2: Will a 60 minute and 20 minute sample be sufficient to evaluate the workplace even if the analytical results are less than the LOD? Assuming the worst-case situation that the sample is below the LOD, the LOD concentration must be computed for each sample tube. First, compute the volume of air collected during the 60 minute sample.

The suitability of a 60 minute sample time will be computed. The LOD concentration is computed for the tube used for 60 minutes. Multiply the pump flowrate (0.033 lpm) by the sampling time to obtain the volume collected:

$$(\text{Sampling time})(\text{Flowrate}) = \text{Volume collected}$$

$$(60 \text{ min})(0.033 \text{ l/min}) = 1.98 \text{ l}$$

Therefore, in 60 minutes, 1.98 liters is collected. The LOD concentration is calculated by dividing the LOD by the volume collected in 60 minutes:

$$(\text{LOD for the sample})/[\text{Volume}(F_{TP})](\text{Conversion factor})$$

$$= \text{LOD concentration}$$

$$(0.053 \text{ mg}/1.98 \text{ l})(1000 \text{ l/m}^3) = 26.7 \text{ mg/m}^3$$

The quantity 26.7 mg/m^3 is 14% of the TLV-TWA for toluene (26.7 mg/m^3 divided by 188 mg/m^3 = 14.2%). This is less than 25% of the TLV-TWA and is useful when "none detected" is the sample result. Therefore, the 60 minute collection time should provide sufficient information even if the analytical result is "none detected."

The pump flowrate used is 0.033 lpm, and sampling is at NTP. Multiply the pump flowrate by the sampling time to obtain the volume collected:

$$(\text{Sampling time})(\text{Flowrate}) = \text{Volume collected}$$

$$(20 \text{ min})(0.033 \text{ l/min}) = 0.66 \text{ l}$$

Therefore, in 20 minutes, 0.66 liter will be collected. The LOD concentration is computed by dividing the LOD by the volume collected in 20 minutes:

$$(\text{LOD/Sample volume in 20 min})(\text{Conversion factor})$$

$$= \text{LOD concentration}$$

$$(0.053 \text{ mg}/0.66 \text{ l})(1000 \text{ l/m}^3) = 80.3 \text{ mg/m}^3$$

The resulting 80 mg/m^3 is approximately 43% of the TLV-TWA for toluene (80.3 mg/m^3 divided by 188 mg/m^3 is 42.6%). This is greater than 25% of the TLV-TWA and may not be useful when "none-detected" is the analytical result. Eighty minutes is a more suitable sample time (see Solution 3, Option 2 following). If the 60 minute and 20 minute samples are used, the eight hour exposure can be computed:

$$\text{eight hour TWA} = \Sigma C_i t_i / \Sigma t_i \quad \text{where: } i = 1, 2, 3$$

$$\text{eight hour TWA} = [(C_1)(t_1) + (C_2)(t_2) + (C_3)(t_3)]/480 \text{ min}$$

where:

C_1 = LOD concentration for the 60 minute sample (26 mg/m³)
C_2 = LOD concentration for the 20 minute sample (80 mg/m³)
C_3 = concentration for the 400 minute period when the task is not
performed (assumed to be 0 mg/m³)
t_1 = sample time for the first sample (60 minutes)
t_2 = sample time for the second sample (20 minutes)
t_3 = nonexposure time of the day (400 minutes)

Thus 480 minutes is the duration in minutes over which the concentration is averaged.

The eight-hour TWA would be computed as follows:

eight hour TWA $= (C_1 t_1 + C_2 t_2 + C_3 t_3)/(t_1 + t_2 + t_3)$

eight hour TWA =

$$\frac{\left[(26 \text{ mg/m}^3)(60 \text{ min}) + (80 \text{ mg/m}^3)(20 \text{ min}) + (0 \text{ mg/m}^3)(400 \text{ min})\right]}{(480 \text{ min})}$$

eight hour TWA $= \left[(1560 + 1680) \text{ min mg/m}^3\right]/(480 \text{ min})$

$= (3160 \text{ min mg/m}^3)/(480 \text{ min})$

eight hour TWA $= 6.6 \text{ mg/m}^3$

The resulting 6.6 mg/m³ is less than 4% of the TLV-TWA for toluene (6.6 mg/m³ divided by 188 mg/m³ = 3.5%). This example indicates that the inhalation hazard had been essentially eliminated if the laboratory results came back "none detected."

Solution 3, Option 2 (Use one tube for the full 80 minutes)

The work situation may be such that it is impossible to use a new tube at the end of the 60 minute sampling period. Is it possible to use the same tube to collect more than the recommended volume? In this example, the recommended sample volume is 2 liters. If one tube is used for 80 minutes and the pump flowrate is 0.033 liter per minute, 2.6 liters will be collected. As this exceeds the recommended volume, will there be breakthrough? The answer to this question depends on the solvent capacity of the sorbent material. The media's solvent capacity is the maximum amount of contaminant that can be "held" (adsorbed) by the sorbent before breakthrough begins. Although solvent capacity values for media can be found in the literature for specific chemicals, they represent data observed under specific sampling conditions. Since the media's solvent capacity for a chemical depends on many factors such as moisture, temperature, the presence of other contaminants, and pump flowrate, it is essentially impossible to adopt a specific number for the media capacity. *Therefore, if the tube can be changed when the recommended volume is collected, change it.*

If the tube cannot be changed when the recommended volume is collected, there is a risk of sample breakthrough. If breakthrough occurs, the laboratory will notify the hygienist after the fact. The sample still may be useful if the concentration in the backup section is less then 25% of the concentration in the front section. The concentration in the backup section can be added to that in the front section and an exposure calculated. The best approach is to explain the time limitation to the worker before the work begins. If the work exceeds the time limitation, the worker will have to be available so that the sample tube can be changed. A detector tube can be used to estimate the approximate concentration in a range from $\pm 35\%$ to $\pm 50\%$. The estimated concentration then provides a guide in calculating the appropriate air sampling time.

Example 4

Assume that the concentration for the 80 minute period is at the PEL of 188 mg/m^3. If the air sample flowrate is 0.022 liter per minute, how much mass will be collected? Does the mass collected exceed the range of the analytical method specified by NIOSH?

Solution 4

$$(188 \text{ mg/m}^3)(0.033 \text{ l/min})(80 \text{ min})(\text{m}^3/1000 \text{ l}) = 0.5 \text{ mg}$$

The resulting 0.5 mg is 9 times the LOD (0.5 mg/0.053 mg = 9.4).

Example 5

An air sample for tetrahydrofuran (THF) is collected for 15 minutes. The air sample flowrate is 0.15 liter per minute. The laboratory reports that breakthrough occurred. There was 4.5 mg of THF on the front section of the charcoal tube and 1.3 mg on the backup section of the charcoal tube. What is the short-term exposure during the 15 minute time period? NIOSH method 1609 (2) describes the evaluation of THF and gives the following information on THF:

Range studied: 323–1240 mg/m^3; or   0.5–13.0 mg/sample
Estimated LOD: 50 μg/sample;   1 ppm = 2.95 mg/m^3
Air sample flowrate: 0.01–0.2 lpm   1993–94 ACGIH TLV-TWA 590 mg/m^3
                                          1993–94 ACGIH TLV-STEL 737 mg/m^3

Solution 5

$$(\text{Sampling time})(\text{Flowrate}) = \text{Volume collected}$$

$$(15 \text{ min})(0.15 \text{ lpm}) = 2.3 \text{ l}$$

The breakthrough concentration is computed by dividing the sum of the mass reported for the two sections of the charcoal tube by the volume collected in 15 minutes:

$$(\text{Breakthrough mass}/\text{Sample volume in 15 min})(\text{Conversion factor})$$

$$= \text{Breakthrough concentration}$$

$$[(4.5 \text{ mg} + 1.3 \text{ mg})/2.3 \text{ l}](1000 \text{ l/m}^3) = 2522 \text{ mg/m}^3$$

At a minimum the THF concentration is 2522 mg/m^3. This is approximately 3.4 times the STEL-TLV for THF (737 mg/m^3) (computed by dividing 2522 mg/m^3 by 737 mg/m^3). Therefore, something must be done quickly (respiratory protection) during this short-term operation while workers are awaiting a permanent process change or engineering control. This exposure would be unacceptable even if the eight hour TWA were less than the TLV-TWA of 590 mg/m^3.

4. SAMPLING FOR SHORT-TERM EXPOSURES

Short-term exposure limit (STEL) air sampling is essentially the same as eight hour time weighted average exposure air sampling except that the volume of air is collected for a 15 minute period. The following example discusses how STEL sampling parameters are computed.

Pump Flowrate

The air sampling pump flowrate for STEL sampling is the maximum flowrate listed for the chemical in the sampling method (e.g., NIOSH, OSHA, etc.). For example, for perchloroethylene, the pump flowrate range is listed by NIOSH (2) as 0.02 to 0.2 l/min. To collect a STEL sample for perchloroethylene, use the maximum air sampling flowrate of 0.2 liter per minute. This will minimize the possibility of collecting less than the LOD mass. If " < LOD" is reported, the LOD concentration can be used to estimate whether the STEL is exceeded.

Sample Volume

The sample volume for STEL sampling is the maximum pump flowrate the method allows, multiplied by the sampling interval (15 minutes). If a STEL air sample is collected at 0.2 liter per minute for a 15 minute sampling period, the sample volume is computed as follows:

$$(\text{Maximum flowrate allowed})(15 \text{ min}) = \text{STEL volume collected}$$

$$(0.2 \text{ l/min})(15 \text{ min}) = 3 \text{ l}$$

Example 6

If the result of a STEL sample analysis for perchloroethylene (tetrachloroethylene) (PCE) is less than the LOD, what is the LOD concentration if a 3 liter sample is collected in 15 minutes? NIOSH method 1003 for halogenated hydrocarbons (2) describes the evaluation of perchloroethylene (PCE) and gives the following information on PCE:

Range studied: 61–12887 mg/m³; or   0.4–12.0 mg/sample
Estimated LOD: 10 μg/sample;   1 ppm = 6.78 mg/m³
Air sample flowrate: 0.01–0.2 lpm   1993–94 ACGIH TLV-TWA 170 mg/m³
   1993–94 ACGIH TLV-STEL 685 mg/m³

Solution 6

The NIOSH recommended sample volume for perchloroethylene is 10 liters. The recommended sample volume primarily applies to eight hour sampling. In STEL sampling, the maximum volume that can be collected in 15 minutes may not equal the listed recommended eight hour sample volume. This does not normally present a problem as the LOD concentration will indicate a very low percent of the STEL even if "none detected" is the analysis result. This is explained in the following example.

The LOD concentration is computed by dividing the LOD mass by the volume collected in 15 minutes:

$$[\text{LOD mass/Volume collected}(F_{TP})](\text{Unit conversion factor})$$

$$= \text{LOD concentration}$$

$$[0.01 \text{ mg}/3.0 \text{ l}(1)](1000 \text{ l/m}^3) = 3.3 \text{ mg/m}^3$$

The quantity 3.3 mg/m³ is 0.48% of the TLV-STEL for perchloroethylene (3.3 mg/m³ divided by 685 mg/m³ is 0.48%). This is less than 10% of the TLV-STEL when "none detected" is the sample result. Therefore, the 15 minute STEL sample will provide information to evaluate the workplace even if the analytical result is " <LOD." This calculation is useful in assisting the hygienist to establish an air sampling protocol. Using NIOSH recommended air sampling and analysis techniques, a " <LOD" laboratory result still may be useful.

5. SAMPLING INSTANTANEOUS (CEILING LIMIT) EXPOSURES

Evaluations of exposures to materials with ceiling limits present measurement problems when real-time or near real-time survey instruments are not available. Industrial hygienists must use ingenuity and experience to develop exposure estimates from samples collected over short-time periods that are longer than the instantaneous period required by the ceiling value definition. The following section will focus on how to compute ceiling limit sampling parameters when near real-time survey instruments are unavailable.

Pump Flowrate

The pump flowrate for ceiling limit sampling is defined as the maximum flowrate listed for the chemical by NIOSH (2), OSHA (8), and so on. For example, for methyl ethyl ketone peroxide (MEKP), the pump flowrate range is listed as 0.1 to 1.0 l/min. To collect a ceiling limit sample for MEKP, use 1.0 l/min. This will maximize the possibility of collecting more than the LOD mass.

Sample Volume

Collect the sample volume over 15 minutes just as with STEL sampling. To obtain the sample volume, multiply the maximum pump flowrate by the sampling duration, 15 minutes. For MEKP, the sample volume is computed as 15 liters:

$$(\text{Maximum flowrate})(15 \text{ min}) = \text{Ceiling volume collected}$$

$$(1.0 \text{ l/min})(15 \text{ min}) = 15 \text{ l}$$

General Considerations

Ceiling limit air sampling presents special problems; so the following protocol is recommended:

a. Observe the work process to develop an estimate of when peak exposure may occur.
b. Estimate how long the peak exposure lasts.
c. Collect Sample 1 approximately 30 minutes prior to the peak exposure. This is essentially a "pre-peak background" average concentration.
d. Collect Sample 2 for 15 minutes including the peak exposure period.

   e. Collect Sample 3 after Sample 2 is completed. This is a "post-peak background" average concentration. Collect the sample for approximately 30 minutes.

   f. Use the results of Sample 1 and Sample 3 as a baseline to graphically compute the estimated peak concentration value.

Graphically, the sampling periods are shown in Figure 8-1. However, the results of Sample 2 are an average over the 15 minute sampling period where the peak exposure occurred. To estimate the peak exposure, assume that it occurred during the 15 minute sampling period for Sample 2 and that the peak is less than 15 minutes (e.g., the peak lasted 5 minutes). The concentration at the beginning of the peak exposure rises from the pre-peak baseline of Sample 1 (1 mg/m^3) to the peak exposure value and then decays to the post-peak background of Sample 3 (2 mg/m^3), as shown in Figure 8-2.

To estimate the peak concentration, it is necessary to compute the height of the triangle in Figure 8-2 so that the area under the curve [$C_i t_i =$ (exposure concentration)(time) in mg-minutes/m^3] is the same as the area under the curve found in Sample 2 in Figure 8-1. A careful industrial hygiene assessment of the work process may enable the hygienist to define the duration of the peak exposure. For example, if the peak is 5 minutes in duration, the pre-peak exposure can be assumed to be the same as Sample 1 (1 mg/m^3), and the post-peak exposure can be assumed to be the same as Sample 3 (2 mg/m^3). This enables a better definition of the base of the

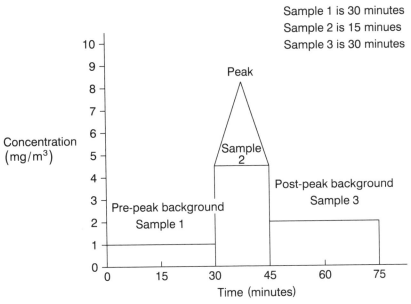

Figure 8-1. Graphical representation of TLV-ceiling sampling.

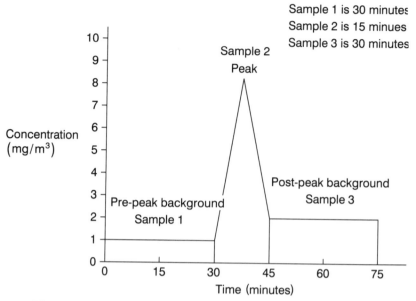

Figure 8-2. Graphical representation of actual ceiling exposure.

triangle so that the peak value (i.e., the height of the triangle) can be calculated. The next example illustrates this concept in detail.

Example 7

What is the estimated peak MEKP concentration if a sample is collected at 1.0 l/min for 15 minutes and the estimated period that the peak concentration occurred is 5 minutes? The pre-peak and post-peak air sampling results are shown in Figure 8-3.

- The TLV-ceiling limit for MEKP is 1.5 mg/m^3
- The LOD for MEKP is 0.001 mg
- Sample 1 concentration is 0.20 mg/m^3
- Sample 3 concentration is 0.4 mg/m^3
- Sample 2 analytical result is 0.010 mg

Solution 7

The sampling results are shown in Figure 8-3. The average concentration in Sample 2 is calculated as:

$$[\text{Mass collected/Volume collected in 15 min}(F_{TP})](\text{Units conversion factor})$$

$$= (0.010 \text{ mg/15 l})(1000 \text{ l/m}^3)(1) = 0.66 \text{ mg/m}^3$$

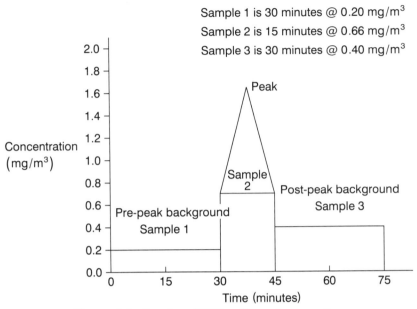

Figure 8-3. Results of TLV-ceiling value sampling.

Knowing that the average concentration during the peak exposure period (Sample 2) was 0.66 mg/m³ is of little help in evaluating the peak exposure concentration. However, the datum can be used to *estimate* the peak-exposure concentration. First, compute the area under the concentration versus time graph ($C_i t_i$ in mg-min/m³) collected during the 15 minute period of the peak exposure. The average concentration over the 15 minute period was 0.66 mg/m³; so the area under the Sample 2 curve is:

$$(\text{Concentration})(\text{Time}) = (C_i t_i) = \text{Area under Sample 2 curve}$$

$$(0.66 \text{ mg/m}^3)(15 \text{ min}) = 10 \text{ mg-min/m}^3$$

It is not known what the actual shape of the peak exposure curve is; however, the area under the curve is 10 mg-min/m³ (Figure 8-4A). Assume that a reasonable curve shape for the exposure is a triangle. Knowing the area of the triangle enables the peak concentration to be estimated. From on-site observation it appears that the peak concentration probably occurred over a 5 minute period (from 35 minutes to 40 minutes) during the 15 minutes that Sample 2 was collected. Further, assume that the concentration rises from the baseline concentration of Sample 1 up to a peak value, and then decays to the baseline concentration of Sample 3. What was the peak exposure concentration?

To answer the question, assume that the actual concentration rises from 0.2 mg/m³ up to the peak concentration and decays to 0.4 mg/m³ over the

Pre-peak background = 5 minutes @ 0.20 mg/m^3

During peak = 5 minutes @ 0.66 mg/m^3

Post-peak background = 5 minutes @ 0.40 mg/m^3

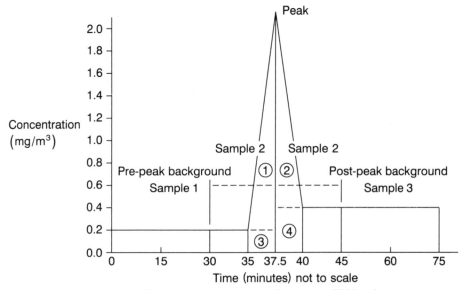

Figure 8-4A. Graphical integration to determine TLV-ceiling.

5 minute period (Figure 8-4B). This assumption "concentrates" the exposure into a 5 minute time interval and gives a worst-case estimate of the ceiling value. The area under the curve can be integrated by dividing it into two triangles (1 and 2) and two rectangles (3 and 4).

The total area of the two triangles (1 and 2) and the two rectangles (3 and 4) in Figure 8-4B must equal 10 mg-min/m^3. The total area is computed as follows:

Total area = (Area triangle 1) + (Area triangle 2) + (Area rectangle 3)

+ (Area rectangle 4)

Total area = $\left[1/2(\text{Base})(\text{Height}) + 1/2(\text{Base})(\text{Height})\right]$

+ $\left[(\text{Base})(\text{Height}) + (\text{Base})(\text{Height})\right]$

Total area = $\left[1/2(B_1)(H_1) + 1/2(B_2)(H_2)\right] + \left[(B_3)(H_3) + (B_4)(H_4)\right]$

Sample 1 (pre-peak background) 5 minutes @ 0.20 mg/m³

Sample 2 (peak value) @ 3.3 mg/m³

Sample 3 (post-peak background) 5 minutes @ 0.40 mg/m³

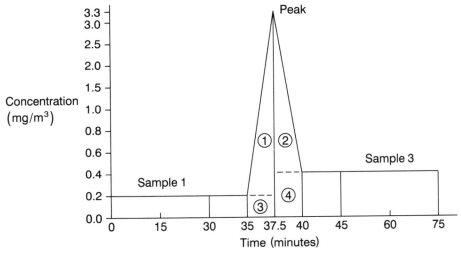

Figure 8-4B. Graphical integration to determine TLV-ceiling.

(B_1) = Base of triangle 1 = 2.5 min (B_2) = Base of triangle 2 = 2.5 min

(B_3) = Base of rectangle 3 = 2.5 min (B_4) = Base of rectangle 4 = 2.5 min

(H_1) = Height of triangle 1 = (H_2) + 0.2 mg/m³ (H_2) = Height of triangle 2

(H_3) = Height of rectangle 3 = 0.2 mg/m³ (H_4) = Height of rectangle 4 = 0.4 mg/m³

Area of triangle 1 = $[1/2(B_1)(H_1)]$ = (1.25 min)$[(H_2) + 0.2$ mg/m³$]$

Area of triangle 2 = $[1/2(B_2)(H_2)]$ = (1.25 min)(H_2)

Area of rectangle 3 = $[(B_3)(H_3)]$ = (2.5)(0.2)mg-min/m³

Area of rectangle 4 = $[(B_4)(H_4)]$ = (2.5)(0.4)mg-min/m³

10 mg-min/m³ = (1.25 min)$[(H_2) + 0.2$ mg/m³$]$ + $[(1.25$ min)$(H_2)]$ + ...

.... + (2.5)(0.2)mg-min/m³ + (2.5)(0.4)mg-min/m³

10 mg-min/m³ = (2.5 min)(H_2) + 1.7 mg-min/m³

Solving for H_2 gives the height of the triangle in Figure 8-4B:

$$H_2 = 3.3 \text{ mg/m}^3$$

The estimated peak concentration (H) of 3.3 mg/m^3 exceeds the TLV-ceiling value of 1.5 mg/m^3. Therefore, until a continuous real-time analysis is obtained, the work process is assumed to exceed the TLV-ceiling, and protective equipment must be used while workers are awaiting the installation of engineering controls.

6. EVALUATION OF THE SAMPLING DATA

This section provides only a cursory introduction to the evaluation of industrial hygiene air sampling data. Although most industrial hygiene air sampling data are lognormally distributed, the problems in this section are solved by assuming the data are normally distributed. This is an oversimplification, and a rigorous analysis of sampling data should use lognormal statistics rather than normal statistics. The reader is referred to the statistics references in this chapter and to the Chapter 7 Bibliography for other appropriate references. These references contain many pertinent references to specific statistical methods related to lognormally distributed data (10–14).

Industrial hygienists use professional judgment in the evaluation of sampling data results and workplace conditions. The data should be examined for unusual deviations, and further sampling may be required to explain such deviations. The justification for using the results should be documented in the inspection report. Confidence in a measurement increases with the number of times the measurement is made, as any single measurement (sample) could be in error for any one of a number of reasons:

- An interruption in the operation.
- A sampling error (flowrate or sampling time).
- A faulty analysis.
- Intentional sabotage.

If only one sample is taken, there is nothing against which to judge whether the result is reasonable. Duplicate samples are an obvious solution. If their results are close (within ±25%), the hygienist can have confidence in them. If they are quite different when they should be similar, that may be an indication that something is wrong. There is no guarantee that any one sample, however carefully taken, represents the true exposure. Another possible alternative is to take consecutive samples of approximately equal length if the process is at a steady state.

After the laboratory results are received and the measured air concentration (MAC) is calculated, a decision has to be made about whether the worker exposure is above or below the standard. A "one-sided confidence limit test" will predict a worker's exposure with 95% confidence; the relative standard deviation (s_r) must be known or determined. The relative standard deviation is the estimated standard deviation (s) divided by the mean of a series of measurements (12):

s_r = estimated standard deviation/mean of a series of measurements

The upper confidence limit (UCL) will predict how high the reported concentration can be at the maximum coefficient of variation. The UCL is calculated from:

UCL = measured air concentration (TWA) + 1.645(s_r)(standard)

The lower confidence limit (LCL) will predict how low the reported concentration can be at the maximum coefficient of variation. The LCL is calculated from:

LCL = measured air concentration (TWA) − 1.645(s_r)(standard)

If the MAC does not exceed the standard and the UCL of that exposure also does not exceed the standard, then the hygienist can be 95% sure that the worker is not overexposed (the employer is in compliance). If the MAC exceeds the standard and the LCL of that exposure also exceeds it, then the hygienist can be 95% sure that the worker is overexposed (the employer is not in compliance). If the MAC does not exceed the standard, but the UCL of that exposure does exceed it, the hygienist cannot be 95% confident that the worker is not overexposed (the employer *may not* be in compliance). Similarly, if the MAC exceeds the standard but the LCL of that exposure is below it, the hygienist cannot be 95% confident that the worker is not overexposed (the employer *may not* be in compliance).

Example 8

Given that the measured air concentration (MAC) of trichloroethylene is 33 mg/m^3, the method s_r is 0.25, and the ACGIH TWA-TLV is 50 mg/m^3, how high could the measured air concentration be even though great care is taken in collecting and analyzing the sample?

$$UCL = MAC(TWA) + 1.645(s_r)(TLV)$$

$$UCL = 33 \text{ mg/m}^3 + 1.645(0.25)(50 \text{ mg/m}^3)$$

$$= (33 + 20.6) \text{ mg/m}^3 = 53.6 \text{ mg/m}^3$$

If the TLV-TWA is 50 mg/m^3 and the air sampling result is 33 mg/m^3, there remains a 5% chance that the worker is overexposed, which is due to variation in sampling and analytical errors.

Example 9

Given that the measured air concentration (MAC) of asbestos in air is 0.17 fibers/cc, the method s_r is 0.183, and the OSHA-PEL is 0.2 fiber/cc, how low could the measured air concentration be even though great care is used in collecting and analyzing the sample?

$$LCL = MAC(TWA) - 1.645(s_r)(OSHA\ PEL)$$

$$LCL = 0.17\ f/cc - 1.645(0.183)(0.2\ f/cc)$$

$$LCL = (0.17 - 0.06)\ f/cc = 0.11\ f/cc$$

If the OSHA PEL is 0.2 f/c and the air sampling result is 0.17 f/cc, there remains a 5% chance that the worker is below the standard, due to variation in sampling and analytical errors.

BIBLIOGRAPHY

1. DiNardi, S. R., et al., Industrial hygiene laboratory procedures. Unpublished.

2. National Institute for Occupational Safety and Health, *Manual of Analytical Methods*, Third Edition. U.S. Government Printing Office, Washington, DC (1984, revised 1987).

3. American Conference of Governmental Industrial Hygienists, *Threshold Limit Values and Biological Indices 1993–1994*. American Conference of Governmental Industrial Hygienists, Cincinnati, OH (1993).

4. Occupational Safety and Health Standards for General Industry, 29 CFR Part 1910.1000(a)(5).

5. National Institute for Occupational Safety and Health, *Pocket Guide to Chemical Hazards* (DHHS/NIOSH Pub. No. 90-117). U.S. Government Printing Office, Washington, DC (1990).

6. Ronald Conrad, Personal communication.

7. Nakasone, R. I., Thomas, J. F., and Gramham, R. B., United States Air Force, Occupational and Environmental Health Laboratory (USAF OEHL), *Recommended Sampling Procedures*. Brooks Air Force Base, TX (1985).

8. Occupational Safety and Health Administration, *OSHA Analytical Methods*. American Conference of Governmental Industrial Hygienists, Cincinnati, OH (1985).

9. Brief, R. S., and Scola, R. A., Occupational exposure limits for novel work schedules, *American Industrial Hygiene Association Journal* 36: 467 (June 1975).

10. Gilbert, R. O., *Statistical Methods for Environmental Pollution Monitoring*. Van Nostrand Reinhold, New York (1986).

11. National Institute for Occupational Safety and Health, *Proficiency Analytical Testing (PAT) Program* (DHEW/NIOSH Pub. No. 77-173). U.S. Government Printing Office, Washington, DC (1977).

12. National Institute for Occupational Safety and Health, *Occupational Exposure Sampling Strategy Manual*, by Leidel, N. A., Busch, K. A., and Lynch, J. R.

(HEW/NIOSH Pub. No. 77-173). U.S. Government Printing Office, Washington, DC (1977).

13. U.S. Environmental Protection Agency, *Quality Assurance Handbook for Air Pollution Measurement System,,* Vol. 1, *Principles,* EPA-600/9-76-00J. Research Triangle Park, NC (1976).

14. Hawkins, N. C., Norwood, S., and Rock, J. C., *A Strategy for Occupational Exposure Assessment.* American Industrial Hygiene Association, Fairfax, VA (1991).

PROBLEM SET
Problem 1

Trichloroethylene (TCE) has a limit of detection of 100 μg detected by gas chromatography. What is the minimum sample volume required to have a limit of detection concentration of 10% of the TLV-TWA?

Solution 1

Range studied: 150–4700 mg/m³; or   0.5–16.0 mg/sample
Estimated LOD: 10 μg/sample;   1 ppm = 5.37 mg/m³
Air sample flowrate: 0.01–0.2 lpm   1993–94 ACGIH TLV 269 mg/m³
    1993–94 ACGIH STEL 537 mg/m³

The objective of this solution is to calculate the minimum volume of air that must be sampled to collect a mass of sample sufficient to meet the limit of detection of 100 μg. The ACGIH TLV-TWA is 269 mg/m³, and the LOD from the NIOSH *Manual of Analytical Methods* is 10 μg. 10% TLV-TWA = 26.9 mg/m³. An alternative expression of 10% of the TLV-TWA is:

$$(26.9 \text{ mg/m}^3)(1 \ \mu g/10^{-3} \text{ mg})(\text{m}^3/1000 \text{ l}) = (26.9 \ \mu g/l).$$

The stated concentration of the contaminant is 26.9 μg/l or 26.9 mirograms of contaminant for each liter of air sampled.

$$(100 \ \mu g)(1 \text{ l}/26.9 \ \mu g)$$

$$= 3.7 \text{ l of air sampled to collect the LOD concentration}$$

Sampling 4 liters of air collects 29.1 μg of TCE per sample (10% TLV), which is 3.1 μg above the LOD.

Problem 2

Given the following exposures to individual contaminants and their respective TLV's, what is the worker's combined exposure if the contaminants are considered additive?

Contaminant solvent	Exposure (C_i) (mg/m³)	TLV (T_i) (mg/m³)
X	100	500
Y	200	500
Z	300	500

Solution 2

The ACGIH (3) gives the TLV for mixtures as:

$$\text{TLV}_{\text{MIX}} = \Sigma[C_i/T_i]$$

where:

C_i = observed atmospheric concentration of the ith component
T_i = corresponding TLV of the ith component

If $\Sigma C_i/T_i > 1$, the TLV_{MIX} is considered to be exceeded.

$$\text{TLV}_{\text{MIX}} = [(100/500) + (200/500) + (300/500)] = 1.2$$

Therefore, the TLV for the mixture is exceeded.

Problem 3

A worker is exposed for only 30 minutes per eight hour workday to a concentration of 50 ppm of X. The TLV-TWA of X is 25 ppm, and the STEL is 60 ppm. Evaluate the exposure.

Solution 3

$$\text{TLV-TWA} = (C_1 t_1 + C_2 t_2)/(t_1 + t_2)$$

where:

C_1 = airborne concentration of the chemical species during t_1
t_1 = interval of time of the exposure during the workday
C_2 = airborne concentration of the chemical species during t_2
t_2 = interval of time of the exposure during the workday

This 480 minute workday is a simple workday. During a simple workday, the worker:

- Is only exposed for the interval of time of the air sampling, eight hours in this example.
- Takes refreshment breaks in a location remote from the workplace.
- Takes meal breaks in a location remote from the workplace.

In this example the only exposure that the worker receives is limited to a 30 minute period during the entire shift:

$$\text{TLV-TWA} = (C_1 t_1 + C_2 t_2)/(t_1 + t_2)$$

$$\text{TLV-TWA} = [(50 \text{ ppm})(30 \text{ min}) + (0)(450 \text{ min})]/480 \text{ min} = 3.1 \text{ ppm}$$

The eight hour TLV-TWA is not exceeded.

The TLV-STEL cannot be calculated in this example because the sampling time exceeds the 15 minute STEL time limit.

If a worker takes breaks in the work area that is contaminated similarly to the workplace, then a sampling strategy must be developed to assess the exposure. Under these conditions the TLV-TWA must be appropriately calculated. More appears on this topic later.

Problem 4

Given a TLV-TWA of 0.025 mg/m^3 and a limit of detection of 0.1 mg, calculate the air sampling time required to determine an exposure concentration at 20% of the TLV if the sampling pump flowrate is set at 4 lpm.

Solution 4

$$\text{TLV} = 0.025 \text{ mg/m}^3; \text{LOD} = 0.1 \text{ mg}$$

$$20\% \text{ of the TLV} = 0.2(0.025 \text{ mg/m}^3) = 0.005 \text{ mg/m}^3$$

Calculate the minimum time to collect a sufficient mass of material to exceed the LOD, given the air sampling flowrate of 4.0 lpm.

$$\text{Time required} = (0.1 \text{ mg})(m^3/0.005 \text{ mg})(1000 \text{ l/m}^3)(1 \text{ min}/4 \text{ l})$$

$$\text{Time required} = 5000 \text{ minutes} = 83 \text{ hours or } 10.4 \text{ workdays!}$$

What will you recommend to your client?

Problem 5

Given a sampling rate of 2 lpm for 6 hours, collection of 9.2 mg, and a TLV of 10 mg/m^3, evaluate a worker's exposure compared to the TLV-TWA.

Solution 5

Because the TLV is 10 mg/m^3 and the breathing zone is sampled for 6 hours, it is possible that there may be an overexposure. The only way to determine if the eight hour time weighted average–threshold limit value is

TABLE 8-3.

t_i (min)	C_i (mg/m³)	$C_i t_i$ (mg/m³)(min)
$t_1 = 360$	$C_1 = 12.8$	4 608
$t_2 = 120$	$C_2 = 0$	0
$\Sigma t_i = 480$ min		$\Sigma C_i t_i = 4\ 608$ (mg/m³)(min)

exceeded is to sample for the full eight hour shift. If the work practice and the process are the same throughout the shift, then an overexposure is likely, based on professional judgment. If the worker is away from the site for the remaining 2 hours of the shift, an exposure of zero can be assumed, and a TWA concentration can be determined. To help solve this problem, organize the data as outlined in Table 8-3.

$$\text{TLV-TWA} = \Sigma C_i t_i / \Sigma t_i = 4\ 608\ (\text{mg/m}^3)(\text{min}) / 480\ \text{min}$$

$$\text{TLV-TWA} = 9.6\ \text{mg/m}^3$$

Given the range of variation in sampling and analysis, there is a likelihood that an overexposure exists. Without knowledge of the C_V for the procedure, professional judgment indicates an overexposure.

Problem 6

Victoria Woodhull, a thirty-five-year-old single parent, works for the Lizard Lick urethane foam manufacturing plant in Bug Tussle, Nebraska. The OSHA compliance person visited the plant one hot and sultry day in August. The ambient temperature was 102°F, and the relative humidity was 97.2%. Fortunately the plant was air-conditioned. Victoria works on the polymerization line where toluene-2,4-diisocyanate (CAS 584-84-9) is polymerized to produce urethane foam, which is subsequently sold to the Acme Speaker Company to be used as acoustic/decorative panels for the new model Acme BOOM/EM speakers.

Ms. Woodhull comes to work every day at 6:30 A.M. and leaves at 3:45 P.M. to pick up her son Giovanni and her little brother Josh at day care. She has 12 minute coffee breaks every day at 9:00 A.M. and at 2:00 P.M. and a lunch break from 11:00 A.M. to 12:10 P.M. The hygienist plans to monitor Victoria with impingers filled with 10 ml of Mercalli reagent and a Gillian personal air sampling pump. The sampling flowrate was calibrated at 1.0 lpm using a soap bubble flowmeter. She is monitored during the first part of the shift, which occurs before her coffee break, while the reactor is sealed and pressurized to 2.78 atmospheres. After her break she empties the reactor and opens it up for cleaning for one-half hour. The reactor then is sealed, pressurized to 3.0 atmospheres, and allowed to run until the second shift empties and cleans it. During the remainder of her shift Ms. Woodhull works in the area of the reactor performing routine housekeeping chores.

Determine Ms. Woodhull's eight hour time weighted average exposure to TDI.

Solution 6

The objectives of this problem are to:

1. Collect sufficient air samples in the breathing zone to fully characterize exposure.
2. Continuously monitor the air for TDI.
3. Monitor changes in the work process.
4. Monitor changes in the surrounding work area.

To compute the time weighted average concentration the hygienist must recognize that individual differences in workplace exposures exist. In this case the worker presumably is exposed to very little if any TDI during the first part of her shift. Based on previous experience, the hygienist will assume that the exposure before the reactor is opened is essentially zero, and that the exposure during entry and cleaning of the reactor is potentially above the TLV. However, this may not always be the case, and the hygienist must sample this exposure period using a recognized NIOSH sampling and analytical method. The ACGIH threshold limit values for TDI are listed below. Compliance with these standards dictates the sampling and analytical techniques to be employed in this survey.

ACGIH TWA-TLV	ppm	$\mu g/m^3$
8 hour TLV-TWA	0.005	0.036
TWA-STEL	0.02	0.14

During the time that the reactor is opened and being cleaned, it is possible for the exposure to exceed the STEL, and appropriate sampling must be utilized to assess this exposure. The next issue to consider is that of sampling the worker during her coffee breaks and lunch break. The only way to deal with this matter is to observe the work practice at this particular plant. Under the best of circumstances, the worker leaves the work area for breaks and her lunch period. If the hygienist observes that this is the case, then sampling may not be necessary, and the exposure can be considered to be zero. Assumptions about exposure cannot be made without direct observation.

Some assumptions to consider in evaluating exposure are as follows:

6:30–9:00   During this time the reactor is sealed and pressurized. "Sealed" means that no TDI escapes from the reactor. However, monitoring will indicate a reactor leak or the presence of other sources of isocyanates

9:01–9:12   During this time Ms. Woodhull is on break, and she goes to the break room and drinks six cups of coffee. If we choose to monitor her during this period, we can determine if she is at risk of TDI exposure in the workroom.

9:13–9:43   During this period the reactor is opened, and she cleans it. This period is essential to monitor because it will most likely pose the greatest exposure. Two samples can be taken during this time interval to determine STEL concentrations.

9:44–11:00   The reactor is sealed and pressurized. This monitoring time is important because it would indicate her exposure level after the reactor is sealed. It could indicate whether or not she is at risk after the reactor is opened to the air.

11:01–12:10 This is her lunch break, and she leaves the plant.

12:11–2:00   This is the period after her lunch break and up to the beginning of her afternoon break.

2:01–2:13   This is her afternoon break, which is important because it means a change in her work location.

2:14–3:45   This is the last time period before leaving, and it is important to monitor her.

With a complete exposure profile it is possible to evaluate exposure over the full shift and to determine how her exposure changes during the entire shift.

NIOSH method 5521 describes the evaluation of toluene-diisocyanate (TDI). The NIOSH *Manual of Analytical Methods* gives the following information on TDI:

Range studied: 0.039–0.53 mg/m^3; or   0.3–25 μg/sample
Estimated LOD: 0.1 μg/sample;   1 ppm = 7.12 mg/m^3
Air sample flow rate: 0.2–1.0 lpm   1993–94 ACGIH TLV-TWA 5.0 μg/m^3
Air sampling media: $\underline{\text{N}}$-[(4-nitrophenyl)methyl]-propylamine on glass wool
Samples unstable; refrigerate at 4°C as soon as possible

Organize the data as shown in Table 8-4.
The sample identification includes the following:

PLANT'S NAME: LIZARD LICK
  URETHANE FABRICATORS   BUG TUSSLE, NEBRASKA
EMPLOYEE'S NAME: EMPLOYEE'S NUMBER:
  VICTORIA WOODHULL   095/35/2376
PUMP SERIAL NUMBER: 8723   SAMPLING TEMPERATURE: 24.5°C
R.H. 37%   ATMOSPHERIC PRESSURE: 765.2 mm Hg

LOCATION: LINE 23, SHIFT-1
TECHNICIAN: SRD
LABORATORY: NERI, CONNECTICUT
DATE COLLECTED: 07/03/94
DATE SENT TO LABORATORY: 07/03/94
AIR BILL NUMBER: 9743711
DATE RECEIVED BY THE LABORATORY: 07/05/94
DATE OUT OF THE LABORATORY: 08/12/94
DATE RECEIVED FROM THE LABORATORY: 08/13/94
CHAIN OF CUSTODY

TABLE 8-4.

Ending time	Start time	Time, t_i (min)	Flow-rate (lpm)	Total volume (l)	Lab mass (μg)	Conc. μg/m^3	Time*Conc. (μg/m^3)(min)
9:00	6:30	180	1	180	0.2	1.1	200
9:12	9:01	11	0	0	—	0	
9:27	9:13	14	1	14	ND	< 7.1	99.4
9:43	9:27	16	1	16	0.3	18.8	300.8
11:00	9:44	76	1	76	ND	< 1.3	98.8
12:10	11:01	69	1	69	ND	< 1.4	96.6
2:00	12:11	109	0	0	—	0	
2:13	2:01	12	0	0	—	0	
3:45	2:14	91	1	91	0.3	3.3	300.3

$\Sigma t_i = 480$ min $\Sigma C_i t_i = 1\,096\,(\mu g/m^3)(min)$

Calculation of TWA-TLV is as follows:

$$\text{TWA-TLV} = \Sigma C_i t_i / \Sigma t_i = 1\,096\,(\mu g/m^3)(min)/480 \text{ min}$$

$$\text{TWA-TLV} = 2.2 \ \mu g/m^3$$

The LOD mass was used to compute the concentration for the three samples with ND concentration. The TWA-TLV exposure is less than 2.3 μg/m^3 or 46% of the TWA-TLV.

Problem 7

Evaluate a worker's daily eight hour exposure to trichloroethylene if the worker spends 30 minutes where the concentration is 300 ppm, $4\frac{1}{2}$ hours at 200 ppm, and 3 hours at 50 ppm.

Solution 7

The help solve this problem, organize the data as outlined in Table 8-5.

TABLE 8-5.

t_i (min)	C_i (ppm)	$C_i t_i$ (ppm min)
$t_1 = 30$	$C_1 = 300$	9,000
$t_2 = 270$	$C_2 = 200$	54,000
$t_3 = 180$	$C_3 = 50$	9,000
$\Sigma t_i = 480$ min		$\Sigma C_i t_i = 72\,000$ ppm min

Recall: TLV-TWA $= \Sigma C_i t_i / \Sigma t_i$, where C_i is the airborne concentration of the ith species and t_i is the ith sampling time interval. In this problem i varies from $i = 1$ to $i = 3$; hence:

$$\text{TLV-TWA} = \Sigma C_i t_i / \Sigma t_i = (C_1 t_1 + C_2 t_2 + C_3 t_3)/(t_1 + t_2 + t_3)$$

$$\text{TLV-TWA} = (72\,000 \text{ ppm min})/(480 \text{ min}) = 150 \text{ ppm}$$

TLV-TWA = 50 ppm, PEL = 50 ppm, NIOSH: a suspected human carcinogen.

Problem 8

Evaluate John Smith's TWA exposure to airborne asbestos fibers given the information in the following air sampling data sheet (with data organized in Table 8-6):

John Smith   1st shift: 7 A.M.–3 P.M.
     Vermiculite bagger on bagging station
Toad Suck, Arkansas   Total workday in minutes: 480 min
Normal break time allowed: 60 minutes out of the work area
Location: Furnace D-16   L-ore #3   Product: masonry fill

TABLE 8-6.

Pump on	Pump off	t_i Time monitored (min)	t_i Breaks monitored (min)	t_i Time excl. breaks (min)	C_i Lab results f/cc	$C_i t_i$
0700	0800	60	0	60	0.03	1.80
0801	0903	62	0	62	0.01	0.62
0903	1049	106	17	89	0.08	7.12
1050	1230	100	30	70	0.14	9.80
1231	1345	74	0	74	0.05	3.70
1346	1504	78	15	63	0.03	1.89
	Σt_i	480	62	418		$\Sigma C_i t_i = 24.93$ (f/cc)(min)

Solution 8

Total hours worked – normal breaks

(no exposure, he is out the work area) = 418 min

Total hours worked – Normal breaks = Exposure time = 480 min.

Exposure time is the time exclusive of breaks over which the worker is monitored = t_i.

TWA = $\Sigma C_i t_i / \Sigma t_i$, where $i = 1, 2, 3, 4, 5, 6$

TWA = $\Sigma C_i t_i / \Sigma t_i = [24.93 \ (f/cc)(min)]/480 = 0.052 \ f/cc$

TWA = $\Sigma C_i t_i / \Sigma t_i = [24.93 \ (f/cc)(min)]/418 = 0.06 \ f/cc$

Do the calculation *both* ways, $t_i = 418$ minutes and t_i 480 minutes, and make a recommendation based on the results of the TWA-TLV calculation.

Problem 9

Given the concentration and time time exposure as 150 ppm for 2 hours, 75 ppm for 1.5 hours, 125 ppm for 2.5 hours, 350 ppm for 0.75 hour, and 175 ppm for 75 minutes, what is the TWA?

Solution 9

The best approach to solving this problem is to organize the data as in Table 8-7.

TABLE 8-7.

t_i (min)	C_i (ppm)	$C_i t_i$ (ppm min)
$t_1 = 120$	$C_1 = 150$	18,000
$t_2 = 75$	$C_2 = 90$	6,750
$t_3 = 125$	$C_3 = 150$	18,750
$t_4 = 45$	$C_4 = 350$	15,750
$t_5 = 75$	$C_5 = 175$	13,125
$t_6 = 40$	$C_6 = $ none	break period
$\Sigma t_i = 480$ min $= t$		$\Sigma C_i t_i = 72\ 375$ ppm min

Recall: TLV-TWA $= \Sigma C_i t_i / \Sigma t_i$, where C_i is the airborne concentration of the ith species and t_i is the ith sampling time interval. In this problem i varies from $i = 1$ to $i = 6$; hence:

$$\text{TLV-TWA} = \sum C_i t_i \Big/ \sum t_i$$

$$\text{TLV-TWA} = (C_1 t_1 + C_2 t_2 + \cdots C_6 t_6)/(t_1 + t_2 + \cdots t_6)$$

$$\text{TLV-TWA} = (72\,375 \text{ ppm min}/480 \text{ min}) = 151 \text{ ppm}$$

$$\text{TLV-TWA} = 151 \text{ ppm}$$

Because the chemical is not specified, no comment can be made on exposure above or below an occupational exposure limit (OEL).

9

Dilution Ventilation and Simple Models in Air

Outcome Competencies   *After studying this chapter you will be able to:*

- *Define dilution ventilation and local exhaust ventilation.*
- *Calculate the quantity of air flowing through a space.*
- *Determine the generation rate of hydrogen gas from a battery charger.*
- *Calculate the concentration of gas in a space under various conditions.*
- *Derive a dilution ventilation model to control evaporation from a tank.*
- *Compute the airflow volume needed to dilute an evaporated liquid.*
- *Explain the mixing factor in a space.*
- *Develop dilution ventilation models to predict contaminant concentration.*
- *Contrast the results of different dilution ventilation design decisions.*
- *Define mass balance.*
- *Evaluate mass balance models to predict contaminant concentration.*
- *Derive mass balance models to predict contaminant concentration.*
- *Define the relationship between contaminant generation and volume.*
- *Define air changes per hour.*

213

- *Define contaminant generation and infiltration rates.*
- *Calculate the result of exponential decay on contaminant concentration.*
- *Derive the ASHRAE indoor air quality model to predict ventilation rate.*
- *Recognize the operation of HVAC systems.*
- *Derive the recirculation fraction (RF) model to predict ventilation rate.*
- *Evaluate the RF model's ability to predict ventilation rate.*
- *Derive the outdoor air fraction (OAF) model to predict ventilation rate.*
- *Evaluate the OAF model's ability to predict ventilation rate.*

1. MODELING

Modeling makes possible the simulation of a system, process, or workplace by using mathematical techniques. The mathematical techniques are an equation or a set of equations that predict changes in a system as various parameters in that system change. Some models are used to calculate the concentration of power plant effluents downwind and in the area surrounding the plant. Known as atmospheric dispersion models, they contain many mathematical terms. Some dispersion models require main frame computers to manipulate dozens of input variables. There are mathematical techniques (pharmacokinetic models) used to predict the fate of drugs in patients and solvent exposure among workers. Mathematical models are used to predict the environmental fate of chlorofluorocarbons (CFCs) in the ozonosphere and to predict the impact of greenhouse gases on global warming. Modeling contaminant concentrations permits hygienists to estimate possible exposures so that appropriate air monitoring can be developed. Modeling may be used to estimate past exposures (retrospective exposure assessment). Retrospective modeling techniques can be applied to epidemiological studies to classify an individual as exposed or not exposed.

Several simple models are developed in this chapter to predict contaminant concentration in traditional workplaces and carbon dioxide concentration in nontraditional workplaces. A carbon dioxide model is useful in diagnosing building-related occupant complaints (sometimes called the tight building syndrome). Some examples are included to demonstrate the use of various models.

Modeling the concentration of gases and vapors or any contaminant in the air of traditional and nontraditional workplaces requires an understanding of the similarity and differences between the two types of ventilation used to control contaminants in the indoor environment. When considering ventilation as a solution to control contaminants, the designer must clearly understand that differences exist between local exhaust and dilution ventilation. The designer is obligated to choose a system that protects the worker's breathing zone. A frequent error made by ventilation designers is to use dilution ventilation as the technique of choice to control hazardous exposures.

- *Dilution ventilation* improves air quality in a space by diluting low concentrations of contaminants in that space with uncontaminated air, thus reducing the contaminant concentrations below a given level.
- *Local exhaust ventilation* removes a contaminant at the source, before it reaches the worker's breathing zone.

Dilution ventilation serves many useful purposes in nontraditional workplaces (e.g., commercial and public buildings, offices, and schools). It is primarily used to control nuisance odors, trace quantities of volatile organic compounds, tobacco combustion products, and carbon dioxide, after source control, elimination, substitution, and isolation are implemented.

The American Society for Heating Refrigeration and Air Conditioning Engineers (ASHRAE) recommends dilution ventilation rates to control the accumulation of indoor air pollutants in Standard 62-1989 (2). Carbon dioxide is a surrogate for efficient and effective dilution ventilation. The assumption is that if carbon dioxide is kept within the limits proscribed by ASHRAE, the dilution ventilation also is controlling many other possible indoor air pollutants.

Dilution ventilation almost never is used to protect a workers' breathing zone. ASHRAE 62-1989 has limited usefulness in traditional workplaces (plants, foundries, etc). Dilution ventilation is not a substitute for a correctly designed local industrial exhaust ventilation system in the tradition workplace. Dilution ventilation may not assure worker protection and typically requires larger air volumes and may be more costly to operate than the local exhaust ventilation system. The control of occupational exposures using dilution ventilation appears to be simple and straightforward to the uninformed. The volume of air needed to dilute contaminants to a predetermined level (TLV, PEL, REL, WEEL, LEL, LFL, etc.) may be calculated by using equations derived later in this chapter. Relying on dilution ventilation to accomplish occupational health objectives is strongly discouraged because it may result in adverse health consequences for workers and citations from OSHA. A more detailed critique of the differences between dilution and local ventilation is critical but is outside the scope of this book (6).

2. DILUTION VENTILATION I

Many techniques exist to generate models that predict the concentration of contaminants in air. A dilution ventilation model can be developed to predict concentration variation based on the concentration equations in Chapter 5. A portion of Table 5-3 is included here as Table 9-1.

TABLE 9-1. Concentration of Gases, C_k, in a Multicomponent Mixture, ppm

Basis	Unit	Symbol, k	Formula
Volume	ppm	ppm	$(V_A/\Sigma V_i)10^6$
Pressure	ppm	ppm	$(P_A/\Sigma P_i)10^6$
Flowrate	ppm	ppm	$(Q_A/\Sigma Q_i)10^6$
Mass	ppm	ppm	$(m_A/\Sigma m_i)10^6$
Molecules	ppm	ppm	$(N_A/\Sigma N_i)10^6$
Mole	ppm	ppm	$(n_A/\Sigma n_i)10^6$

Note: Subscript A replaces subscript j of Chapter 5.

A dilution ventilation model can be developed from the relationship $C_{\text{PPM}} = (Q_A/\Sigma Q_i)10^6$. The model is used for calculation of the concentration of a gas or a vapor generated at a volume flowrate Q_A into a dilution air flowrate Q_B. One possible application of this technique is to model concentration as demonstrated in Example 1.

Example 1

A battery charging space in a manufacturing facility has seven battery chargers for lifting and moving equipment. There were concerns about the level of hydrogen gas emitted from the batteries during the charging cycle. A study of the area was performed to determine if the level of hydrogen gas could create a fire or explosion hazard. The battery charging area is approximately 20 feet wide and 60 feet long with a ceiling height of 20 feet. What is the concentration range of hydrogen gas?

Solution 1

One approach to solving this problem is to calculate the expected concentration range of hydrogen gas at the best and worst situations.

Given:

1. The charging area is 20 feet wide by 60 feet long by 20 feet high.
2. Hydrogen has a Lower Explosive Limit (LEL) of 4% (100% of the LEL is 4%).
3. The National Fire Protection Association (NFPA) and the Occupational Safety and Health Administration (OSHA) allow up to a 1% hydrogen gas concentration (25% of the LEL) in air before corrective action is taken. This is the upper limit of hydrogen gas concentration that will be allowed in the area.

Assumptions:

1. Measure the normal dilution ventilation or effective ventilation rate (EVR) in the battery charging area on a typical day (best case condition), and:

2. Assume that the mechanical ventilation systems are shut down and the battery charging stations are left *on* (worst-case condition).
3. The room air is moving through the space, diluting the hydrogen produced by the charging batteries.
4. Hydrogen is lighter than air and will rise to the ceiling. Therefore, the volume of air available for dilution is located next to the ceiling and is only a fraction (F) of the actual room volume available.

To solve this problem, the hydrogen gas generation rate must be known. Information on the generation rate of hydrogen from charging batteries is available from the manufacturer (1) and depends on the finish rate. The finish rate at which the batteries are charging near the end of the cycle. It is at this point that the hydrogen gas emission reaches a maximum. In both cases, assume that all the battery charging stations are operating and all batteries are above the 80% recharge status at the finish rate of 2.37 volts, and that they will remain at the finish rate charge for three hours. This gives the maximum hydrogen emission. The hydrogen gas concentration, in percent, can be calculated as described in Chapter 5:

$$ C_\% = \left[Q_A / (Q_A + Q_B) \right] 100 = \left[Q_{H_2} / (Q_{EDV} + Q_{H_2}) \right] 100 $$

where:

Q_{EDV} = the effective dilution air volume flowrate moving through the area

Q_{H_2} = hygrogen gas volume flowrate generated by the batteries at the finish rate

Calculation of the Effective Dilution Ventilation Rate (Q_{EDV})

The effective dilution ventilation flowrate (Q_{EDV}) is defined as the product of the air velocity through the space and the cross-sectional area of the space. The effective dilution ventilation flowrate (Q_{EDV}) is calculated by measuring the air velocity (V) throughout the entire cross-sectional area (A) of the battery charging station at different elevations (cross-sectional area). The effective dilution ventilation flowrate (Q_{EDV}) of the air moving through the area is:

$$ Q_{EDV} = (\text{Cross-sectional area})(\text{Measured velocity}) = (A)(V) $$

The locations for the air velocity measurements throughout the battery charging station are indicated in Figure 9-1. The average of the measured velocity is used to calculate the effective dilution ventilation flowrate (Q_{EDV} in cfm) for the air moving through this location. Measurements were made 12 feet above the floor and 4 feet from the 20-foot-high ceiling (16 feet above the floor). The measured average flowrate was 25 feet per minute (fpm)

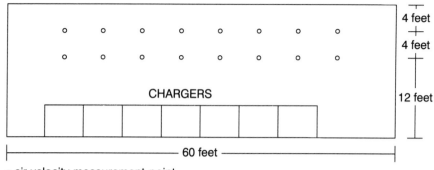

o air velocity measurement point

Figure 9-1. Cross section of the battery charging station.

throughout the area with a general direction away from the charging area toward the loading dock doors (south). Assume that one-third of the 60-foot-long area has air moving through (the other two-thirds being dead still air). This is the mixing fraction and can range from zero to one ($F \leq 1$). This assumption will yield a maximum hydrogen concentration in air. Using a mixing factor of 0.33 implies that the hydrogen is mixing into one-third of the space, or into a space 20 feet wide by 20 feet high [0.33(60) = 20 feet].

$$Q_{EDV} = (\text{air velocity})(\text{cross-sectional area})$$

$$Q_{EDV} = (25 \text{ fpm})(20 \text{ feet})(20 \text{ feet}) = 10{,}000 \text{ cfm}$$

The effective dilution ventilation flowrate, Q_{EDV} is 10,000 cfm through the charging station.

Calculation of the Hydrogen Emission Rate (Q_{H_2})

Most of the outgassing from a lead-acid battery occurs after the battery reaches the 80% recharge state. Emission of hydrogen gas from battery charging occurs at a nearly steady rate and can be calculated based on the finish rate of the charging batteries and the number of cells in the battery. According to the manufacturer (1), the following model gives the rate of hydrogen emission from a charging battery:

$$Q_{H_2} = \text{Cubic feet of hydrogen produced per minute}$$

$$Q_{H_2} = 0.00027(\text{finish rate})(\text{number of cells})$$

The manufacturer gives the finish rate for these batteries as 2.37 volts. The number of charging batteries varies according to usage and needs at the facility. This particular facility has the capacity to charge six batteries per charger with seven chargers total. There are 18 cells per battery or 756 cells total [(42 batteries)(18 cells/battery) = 756 cells].

The hydrogen emission is:

$$Q_{H_2} = \text{cubic feet of hydrogen produced per minute}$$

$$Q_{H_2} = 0.00027(\text{finish rate})\text{number of cells}$$

where:

FR = finish charging rate of the battery (volts)
n_{cell} = number of cells in the battery (no units)
Q_{H_2} = cubic feet of hydrogen per minute = 0.00027(2.37)(756)
Q_{H_2} = 0.484 cfm

Q_{H_2} is the hydrogen volume flowrate into the battery charging location for a three hour period at the end of the charging cycle. This is the time it takes for the batteries to go from 80% to 99 + % charge. Under best-case conditions, hydrogen is diluted by mixing it into the room volume assisted by the effective dilution ventilation in a given period of time.

$$[(Q_{EDV})(\text{time}) = \text{volume}].$$

Case 1—Best-Case Condition: Normal Ventilation in Battery Charging Area

The effective dilution ventilation flowrate (Q_{EDV}) through the location is 10,000 cfm. Adding the room volume and the effective dilution ventilation volume yields the total amount of dilution air volume available to reduce the hydrogen gas concentration:

$$C_\% = \text{Hydrogen gas concentration } (\%)$$

$$C_\% = \frac{\text{volume of hydrogen}}{\text{room volume} + Q_{EDV} \ (\text{time})} 100$$

Assume that the hydrogen concentrates in the top 10 feet of the ceiling area, and the volume of the battery charging station is 24,000 cubic feet (20 feet wide by 20 feet high by 60 feet long). This means that hydrogen gas will collect in one-half the charging station volume. The reduced volume is the mixing fraction (F) times the room volume. When the mixing fraction is one-half, ($F = 0.5$) is used:

$$\text{H}_2 \text{ concentration } (\%) = \frac{(Q_{H_2} \text{ emitted})(3 \text{ hr})}{F(\text{Room volume}) + Q_{EDV}(3 \text{ hr})} 100$$

$$\text{H}_2 \text{ concentration } (\%) = \frac{(0.495 \text{ cfm})(180 \text{ min})}{0.5(24,000 \text{ cf}) + (10,000 \text{ cfm})(180 \text{ min})} 100$$

$$\text{H}_2 \text{ concentration } (\%) = 0.005\%$$

This level of hydrogen gas (0.005%) is insignificant. The normal ventilation rate in the area is sufficient to keep the level of hydrogen well below 25% of the LEL or 1% hydrogen:

$$\text{Fraction of the LEL} = (0.005\%/4\%) = 0.0013 \text{ of the LEL}$$

Case 2—Worst-Case Condition: No Ventilation in the Battery Charging Area

Calculate the expected concentration of hydrogen for a period when all mechanical ventilation systems are shut down and only outdoor air infiltration–induced air changes exist. Assume an infiltration rate (IR) through the area for this condition. A conservative estimate of the infiltration rate in a tight building is 0.1 air changes per hour (acph). Calculate the effective infiltration ventilation flowrate (Q_{EIV}) through the location by multiplying the number of air changes per hour by the volume of the space; this number is the volume of dilution air available per hour if the mixing is complete:

$$Q_{EIV} \text{ worst case} = (\text{infiltration rate, acph})(\text{room air volume})$$

$$Q_{EIV} \text{ worst case} = (0.1 \text{ air change per hour})(24,000 \text{ cf}) = 2,400 \text{ cfm}$$

$$Q_{EIV} \text{ worst case} = (7,200 \text{ cf})(3 \text{ hours})(\text{time battery is at finish rate})$$

As in the first case (Case 1), a conservative assumption that the hydrogen concentrates in the top 10 feet of the ceiling area will be used. Use only one-half the charging location volume ($F = 0.5$) for dilution calculations:

$$\text{H}_2 \text{ concentration } (\%) = \frac{Q_{\text{H}_2}}{FV + (Q_{EIV})} 100$$

$$\text{H}_2 \text{ concentration } (\%) = \frac{[(0.000027)(FR)(n_{cell})t]}{[FV + (Q_{EIV})(t)]} 100$$

where:

F = fraction of the space available for dilution (no units)
V = volume of the space (cubic feet)
Q_{EIV} = effective infiltration ventilation air flowrate (cfm)
t = time increment (minutes)

$$\text{H}_2 \text{ concentration } (\%) = \frac{[(Q \text{ of H}_2 \text{ emitted})(3 \text{ hours})]}{[F(\text{Room volume}) + IR(\text{Room volume})]} 100$$

$$\text{H}_2 \text{ concentration } (\%) = \frac{(0.495 \text{ cfm})(180 \text{ minutes})}{(0.5)(24,000 \text{ cf}) + (7,200 \text{ cf})} 100 = 0.46\%$$

$$\text{Fraction of the LEL} = (0.46\%/4\%) = 0.115 \text{ of the LEL}$$

This level of hydrogen (0.46%) is not significant ($< 12\%$ of the LEL). The normal infiltration into the area is sufficient to keep the level of hydrogen below one-half of one percent of the LEL for hydrogen. This is about one-half of the allowable 25% of the LEL.

It is prudent to install a hydrogen gas alarm system for this area, set at 10% of the lower explosive limit (10% of the LEL is 0.4% H_2). The alarm can be connected (interlocked) to shut down the chargers when the hydrogen reaches 10% of the LEL.

Even during the worst-case assumption when all mechanical ventilation systems are not operating and all battery charging stations are charging at the finish rate, the level of hydrogen is still within acceptable limits ($< 12\%$ LEL). Later in this chapter a dilution ventilation model will be used to determine the hydrogen level.

Summary of Results

Effective Dilution Ventilation Flowrate Method:

Q_{H_2} (cfm)	Dilution fraction (F)	Room volume (cfm)	Effective volume (cf)	Q_{EDV} (cfm)	H_2 concentration (%)	LEL fraction
0.495	0.5	24,000	12,000	10,000	0.005	0.0013

Effective Infiltration Ventilation Flowrate Method:

Q_{H_2} (cfm)	Dilution fraction (F)	Room volume (cfm)	Effective volume (cf)	Infiltra. volume (cf)	H_2 concentration (%)	LEL fraction
0.0495	0.5	24,000	12,000	7,200	0.46	0.115

Example 2

The Technical Committee on Road Tunnels of the Permanent International Association of Roads Congress (PIARC) describes a dilution ventilation model for carbon monoxide in highway tunnels. This model appears in an article "Road tunnel ventilation design and application," *ASHRAE Journal* (October 1991), pp. 40–51. The dilution ventilation (fresh air requirement) for the dilution of carbon monoxide in tunnels is given by the model:

$$Q_{CO} = q^0 CO(f_V)(f_I)(f_H)(D_V)(L)10^3/(3600)(CO_{lim})$$

where:

Q_{CO} = required fresh air quality (m^3/s km, lane)
$q^0 CO$ = basic value of CO emission rate per passenger car (pc) = (m^3/h, pc)
f_V = speed factor (—)
f_I = gradient factor (—)

$$f_H = \text{altitude factor } (—)$$
$$D_V = \text{number of passenger cars (pc/km, lane)} = M_v/V$$
$$V = \text{mean driving speed (km/h)}$$
$$CO_{lim} = \text{maximum permissible carbon monoxide concentration (ppm}$$
$$CO)$$
$$L = \text{total length of the tunnel}$$

Explain the development of this model.

3. DILUTION VENTILATION II

Another dilution ventilation model can be developed to calculate the concentration of contaminants in air resulting from the evaporation of a mass of solvent into a space. The model is based on the equations that express the concentration in parts per million (ppm) as a function of volume per time $(Qt = v)$:

$$C_{PPM} = (V_A/V_B)10^6$$

where:

V_A = contaminant volume calculated from the ideal gas equation
V_B = volume of air needed to dilute a specific contaminant to a selected occupational exposure limit concentration in ppm (i.e., TLV, PEL, LFL, LEL, etc.)

Substituting V_A from the ideal gas equation yields:

$$C_{PPM} = (V_A/V_B)10^6 = (mRT/MPV_B)10^6$$

Solving for V_B:

$$V_B = (mRT/PMC_{PPM})10^6$$

Recall the definition of density:

$$\rho = m/V$$

where:

$m = \rho_L V_L = m_L$ (mass of liquid)
$\rho_L = SG(\rho_w) = $ (specific gravity of liquid)(water density 70°F)

Then:

$$V_B = (\rho_L V_L RT/PMC_{PPM})10^6$$

The volume flowrate of air, Q_B, necessary to dilute a contaminant released from a tank can be calculated. The contaminant evaporation rate must be known or measured in volume per time (e.g., liters per minute, grams per minute in the SI system; pints per minute or pounds per minute in the English system). The air volume (ft^3) needed to effect this dilution must be delivered during the same time interval that the evaporation occurs (e.g., minutes). In a specified time interval $(V_A/V_B)10^6$ becomes $(Q_A/Q_B)10^6$ $(Qt = V)$.

$$V_B/\text{minute} = Q_B = (\rho_L V_L/\text{minute})(RT/PMC_{\text{PPM}})10^6$$

$$Q_B = (SG\rho_w V_L/\text{minute})(RT/PMC_{\text{PPM}})10^6$$

$$W = V_L/\text{min, the liquid volume released per time interval}$$

$$\text{(liters per minute, pints per minute, etc.)}$$

$$Q_B = (SG\rho_w W)(RT/PMC_{\text{PPM}})10^6$$

The units must be converted so that the final equation gives an air volume flowrate in cubic meters per second or cubic feet per minute. To accomplish this, substitute values for all the variables in the equation for Q_B. Substituting in values for the constants:

For the English system:

$Q_B = (SG\rho_w W)(RT/PMC_{\text{PPM}})10^6$
ρ_w = density of water, 1.0 gram per cubic centimeter
T = 70°F (industrial ventilation standard temperature) or 21.1°C = 294.3 K
P = 1 atmosphere (29.921 inches of mercury)
W = liquid volume released, pints per minute
R = 0.08205 liter atmosphere per mole degree K (Any R value can be used, but all the units must be converted to cubic feet/minute, or liters per second.)
SG = specific gravity, which is dimensionless
M = molecular weight
C_{PPM} = occupation exposure limit concentration in parts per million

This yields:

$Q_B =$

$$\frac{(SG)\left(\rho_w \frac{g}{cc}\right)\left(W\frac{\text{pints}}{\text{min}}\right)\left(\frac{0.08205\,l\,\text{atm}}{\text{mole K}}\right)(294.3\,\text{K})\left(\frac{1000\,cc}{l}\right)\left(\frac{1\,\text{gal}}{8\,\text{pints}}\right)\left(\frac{3.785\,l}{\text{gal}}\right)\left(\frac{\text{ft}^3}{28.32\,l}\right)}{(1\,\text{atm})\left(M\frac{g}{\text{mole}}\right)(C_{\text{PPM}})}10^6$$

$$Q_B = 403.41\frac{(SG)(W)}{(M)(C_{\text{PPM}})}10^6\ \text{(English system)}$$

where:

Q_B = cubic feet per minute (cfm)
403.41 = a units conversion factor in the English system
SG = specific gravity, which is dimensionless
W = liquid volume released in pints per minute
M = molecular weight of the released material
C_{PPM} = occupational exposure limit concentration in parts per million

If the liquid volume generation rate is in pounds per minute, the unit conversion factor changes from 403.41 to 387:

$$Q_B = (387)\left[(SG)(W)/(M)(C_{PPM})\right]10^6$$

where:

387 = a unit conversion factor in the English system
SG = specific gravity, which is dimensionless
W = liquid volume released in pounds per minute
M = molecular weight of the released material
C_{PPM} = occupational exposure limit concentration in parts per million

For the SI system:

$$Q_B = (SG\rho_w W)(RT/PMC_{PPM})10^6$$

ρ_w = density of water, 1.0 gram per cubic centimeter
T = 25°C (industrial hygiene standard temperature) = 298.15 K
P = 1 atmosphere (760 millimeters of mercury)
R = 0.08205 liter atmosphere per mole degree K (Any R value can be used, but all the units must be converted to cubic feet/minute, or liters per second.)
SG = specific gravity, which is dimensionless
W = liquid volume released in liters per minute
M = molecular weight (gram molecular weight)

This yields:

$$Q_B =$$

$$\frac{(SG)\left(\rho_w \dfrac{g}{cc}\right)\left(W\dfrac{l}{min}\right)\left(\dfrac{0.08205\ l\ atm}{mole\ K}\right)(298.15\ K)\left(\dfrac{1000\ cc}{l}\right)\left(\dfrac{m^3}{1000\ l}\right)}{(1\ atm)\left(M\dfrac{g}{mole}\right)(C_{PPM})}10^6$$

$$Q_B = 24.45\frac{(SG)(W)}{(M)(C_{PPM})}10^6 \text{ (SI system)}$$

where:

Q_B = cubic meters per minute
24.45 = a units conversion factor in the SI system
SG = specific gravity, which is dimensionless
W = liquid volume released in liters per minute
M = gram molecular weight of the released material
TLV = threshold limit value concentration in parts per million

These models assume that the mixing is ideal and that the mixing factor K is 1. For situations where the mixing factor is not the ideal value ($K > 1$), then Q_B calculated must be multiplied by the appropriate mixing factor, which can range from 1 to 10. The problem in developing this model is converting the units to comply with the units needed to produce the conversion constant; otherwise calculation errors will result.

Example 3

A tank of perchloroethylene (1,1,2,2-tetrachloroethylene, $Cl_2\text{-}C = C\text{-}Cl_2$), produces noncombustible vapors and is in use during an eight hour shift. The operator must add in 4.35 pounds of solvent to replace the evaporated material. Calculate the volume flowrate of dilution ventilation needed to keep the evaporated solvent at the TLV in the room.

Solution 3

$$Q_B = (387)[(SG)(W)/(M)(TLV)]10^6$$
$$W = (4.35\text{lb}/8\text{ h})(1\text{ hr}/60\text{ min}) = 0.0091\text{ lb/min}$$
$$SG = 1.62$$
$$TLV = 25\text{ ppm}$$

Molecular weight of tetrachloroethylene,

$$Cl_2\text{-}C = C\text{-}Cl_2 = 12.011(2) + 35.45(4) = 165.82\text{ g/mole}$$

$$Q_B = (387)[(1.62)(0.0091)/(163.82)(25)]10^6$$

$$Q_B = 1,378\text{ cfm, if the mixing is perfect } (K = 1)$$

$$Q_B = 13,780\text{ cfm if the mixing is poor } (K = 10)$$

NIOSH lists perchloroethylene (perc) as a suspected carcinogen. The hygienist should minimize the workplace exposure concentration and the number of workers exposed. In fact, the hygienist should substitute another solvent for perchloroethylene, e.g., methylchloroform, $H_3C\text{-}CCl_3$ ($SG = 1.34$). However, the latter solvent produces a combustible vapor and may adversely affect the ozone layer. An aqueous solvent also should be considered as a means of minimizing the exposure. Whatever solvent is used, local exhaust ventilation should be used to control the contaminant at the source instead of relying on dilution ventilation. Local exhaust ventilation will protect the workers and their breathing zone and will conserve energy.

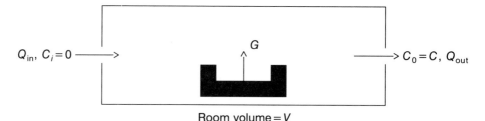

Room volume = V

Figure 9-2. Mixing in a typical work room.

4. CONCENTRATION VARIATION WITH TIME: PART I

Figure 9-2 is a schematic of a process emitting a solvent vapor or gas into a ventilated space.

The labels in Figure 9-2 are defined as indicated below:

- C_i is the airborne concentration of the contaminant entering the space,
- $C_i = 0$ in this example.
- C_0 is the airborne concentration of the contaminant leaving the space.
- G is the generation rate of contaminant from the tank into the space.
- Q_{out} is the rate of ventilation adjusted for incomplete mixing; $Q_{out} = Q_{in}/K$.
- K is the mixing factor, which may vary from 1 to 10, and is a dimensionless constant. K equal to 1 is perfect mixing, and K equal to 10 is poor mixing. The mixing factor varies with each space and may be estimated or measured using tracer dilution techniques (described later in this chapter). The mixing factor depends on several parameters, including indoor/outdoor temperature, wind speed and direction, barometric pressure, the presence and location of air-moving devices, etc.
- V is the volume of the space or room.

It is possible to calculate the airborne concentration of the evaporated contaminant, given some boundary conditions. The contaminant accumulation rate in a space depends upon the generation rate, the removal rate due to ventilation, and the removal rate due to any "sinks" for the material in the space. Assume that there are no sinks for the contaminant, as the walls are nonporous, ceramic-tile-covered concrete blocks. The mass balance is:

Contaminant accumulation rate = Generation rate − Removal rate

Another way to express this situation is as concentration per unit time:

Concentration/Unit time = Generation rate/Volume − Dilution rate

The concentration per unit time is the mass concentration of the material generated per unit time, t; the dimensions are $mg/m^3/s = mg/m^3s$. The generation rate per volume is the rate at which the material is being added into the volume, V; the dimensions are $mg/s/m^3 = mg/m^3s$.

The dilution rate is the rate at which the material at concentration C (mg/m^3) is diminished by flowing into a space of volume V (m^3), and further diminished by the flow out of the space, Q_{out} (m^3/s). Q_{out} is Q_{in}/K, the air volume into the space adjusted for incomplete mixing. The dimensions are mg/m^3s:

$$(Q_{out}C_0)/V = \left[(m^3/s)(mg/m^3)\right]/m^3 = mg/m^3s$$

Dimensional analysis shows there is comparability of the units and indicates the following:

$$\text{Concentration/Unit time} = \text{Generation rate/Volume} - \text{Dilution rate}$$

$$C/t = G/V - Q_{out}C_0/V$$

$$mg/m^3/s = (mg/s)/m^3 - \left[(m^3/s)(mg/m^3)\right]/m^3$$

$$mg/m^3s = (mg/m^3s) - (mg/m^3s)$$

This indicates that the C/t mass balance relationship is valid:

$$C/t = G/V - Q_{out}C_0/V$$

This equation for the variation of concentration with respect to time, C/t, can be simplified. Assume the special case where the generation rate $(G) = 0$; for example, a spill occurs in a space and all the contaminant evaporates. There is no more vapor generated; so the generation rate is zero $(G = 0)$. Then:

$$C/t = -Q_{out}C_0/V$$

After a small increment of time the concentration will change, and the change can be expressed quantitatively by establishing a differential equation from the C/t equation. If the time increment is small (dt), then the corresponding concentration increment is also small (dC). This assumption leads to a simple first order differential equation:

$$dC = -(Q_{out}C/V)\,dt$$

To solve this equation, separate the variables and integrate the resulting equation between the specified integration limits:

$$\int_{C_i}^{C} dC/C = -(Q_{out}/V)\int_{t_i}^{t} dt$$

This gives:

$$\ln(C/C_i) = -Q_{out}/V(t - t_i) = -Q_{out}/V(\Delta t)$$

$$(\Delta t) = -\ln(C/C_i)/Q_{out}/V = -(V/Q_{out})\ln(C/C_i)$$

where $Q_{out} = Q_{in}/K$.

Example 4

If the initial concentration of a pollutant $C_i = 100$ ppm, how long will it take to change the initial concentration to 0.25 ppm when the ventilation rate $Q_{in} = 3000$ cfm, and the room volume (V) is 30,000 ft^3? (Assume ideal mixing.)

Solution 4A

To solve this problem determine Δt in the following equation:

$$(\Delta t) = -\frac{V}{Q_{out}}\ln(C/C_i) = -\frac{KV}{Q_{in}}\ln(C/C_i)$$

Assume ideal mixing; $K = 1$ and $Q_{out} = Q_{in}/K = Q_{in}$.

$$\Delta t = -\frac{(30,000 \text{ ft}^3)}{(3000 \text{ ft}^3/\text{min})}\ln(0.25 \text{ ppm}/100 \text{ ppm})$$

$$\Delta t = 30,000/3,000(5.99)\text{min} = 59.9 \text{ min}$$

In 60 minutes the concentration decreases from 100 ppm to 0.25 ppm at the stated conditions.

Solution 4B

Assume incomplete mixing, that is, $K = 10$. To solve this problem determine Δt in the following equation:

$$(\Delta t) = -\frac{KV}{Q_{in}}\ln(C/C_i)$$

Assume incomplete mixing; $K = 10$ and $Q_{out} = Q_{in}/K = 3000$ cfm/10 = 300 cfm.

$$\Delta t = -\frac{(30,000 \text{ ft}^3)}{(300 \text{ ft}^3/\text{min})}\ln(0.25 \text{ ppm}/100 \text{ ppm})$$

$$\Delta t = 30,000/300(5.99)\text{min} = 599 \text{ min}$$

In 600 minutes the concentration decreases from 100 ppm to 0.25 ppm at the stated conditions.

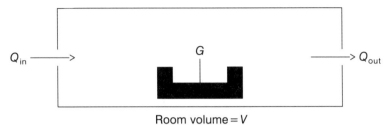

Room volume = V

Figure 9-3. Mixing in a typical work room.

5. CONCENTRATION VARIATION WITH TIME: PART II

Figure 9-3 is a schematic of a process emitting a solvent vapor or gas into a ventilated space.

The labels in Figure 9-3 are defined as they were in Figure 9-2, as indicated below:

- C_1 is the airborne concentration of the contaminant at time equal one.
- C_2 is the airborne concentration of the contaminant at time equal two.
- G is the generation rate of contaminant from the tank into the space.
- Q_{out} is the rate of ventilation adjusted for incomplete mixing; $Q_{out} = Q_{in}/K$.
- K is the mixing factor and may vary from 1 to 10, and is a dimensionless constant. K equal to one is perfect mixing, and K equal to 10 is poor mixing. The mixing factor varies with each space and may be estimated or measured using tracer dilution techniques (described later in this chapter). The mixing factor depends on several parameters, including indoor/outdoor temperature, wind speed and direction, barometric pressure, the presence and location of air-moving devices, etc.
- V is the volume of the space or room.

Here too it is possible to calculate the airborne concentration of the evaporated contaminant, given some boundary conditions. Recall that the contaminant accumulation rate in a space depends upon the generation rate, the removal rate due to ventilation, and the removal rate due to any "sinks" for the material in the space. Again assume that there are no sinks for the contaminant as the walls are nonporous, ceramic-tile-covered concrete blocks. The mass balance is:

Contaminant accumulation rate = Generation rate − Remove rate

Expressed as a concentration per unit time, this mass balance is:

Concentration/Unit time = Generation rate/Volume − Dilution rate

As in the earlier analysis, concentration/unit time is the mass concentration of the material generated per unit time, t (dimensions of $mg/m^3/s = mg/m^3s$). The generation rate per volume is the rate at which the material is being added into the volume V (dimensions of $mg/s/m^3 = mg/m^3s$). The dilution rate is the rate at which the material at concentration C (mg/m^3) is diminished by flowing into a space of volume V (m^3) and further diminished by the flow of air out of the space, Q_{out} (m^3/s):

$$(Q_{out}C)/V = [(m^3/s)(mg/m^3)]/m^3 = mg/m^3s$$

Dimensional analysis shows there is comparability of the units and indicates the following:

$$C/t = G/V - Q_{out}C/V$$

$$mg/m^3/s = (mg/s)/m^3 - [(m^3/s)(mg/m^3)]/m^3$$

$$mg/m^3s = (mg/m^3s) - (mg/m^3s)$$

This indicates that the C/t mass balance relationship is valid:

$$C/t = G/V - Q_{out}C/V$$

This problem assumes that G is a constant. For example, when an empty tank is filled, the generation rate goes from zero to a constant value. The generation rate remains constant while the tank has liquid in it. Assume that the generation rate is independent of the liquid level in the tank. As the liquid in the tank evaporates, the generation rate remains constant. Another example of a constant generation rate is a welder cutting a coated metal producing a heavy metal fume at a constant rate. The generation rate will go to zero only when the liquid in the tank evaporates completely or the welder stops welding.

After a small increment of time (dt) the concentration will change (dC). This can be expressed quantitatively by establishing a differential equation from the C/t equation above when the time increment is small (dt) and the corresponding concentration increment is also very small (dC). In Part I above, the equation for the variation of concentration with respect to time,

C/t, was simplified by assuming the special case where the generation rate (G) was zero. In this model the generation rate will be a constant.

$$C/t = G/V - Q_{out}C/V = (G - Q_{out}C)/V$$

$$C = (G - Q_{out}C)t/V$$

$$t/V = C/(G - Q_{out}C)$$

After an increment of time, dt, the concentration will change by dC:

$$dt/V = dC/(G - Q_{out}C)$$

To solve the equation, separate the variables and integrate the resulting equation between the specified limits:

$$\int_{C_1}^{C_2} dC/(G - Q_{out}C) = (1/V)\int_{t_1}^{t_2} dt$$

This gives:

$$(1/Q_{out})\ln[(G - Q_{out}C_2)/(G - Q_{out}C_1)] = -(1/V)(t_2 - t_1)$$

where:

C_1 = airborne concentration of the contaminant at time equal to one

C_2 = airborne concentration of the contaminant at time equal to two

G = generation rate of contaminant from the tank into the space

Q_{out} = rate of ventilation adjusted for incomplete mixing

$Q_{out} = Q_{in}/K$

Let $Q_{out} = Q' = Q_{in}/K$ adjusted for incomplete mixing.

Example 5

You are asked by a group of artists about the hazardous emissions from welding and cutting metal sculptures. The question is whether artists are adversely affected while welding within an enclosed area. The artists work in an enclosed space, out of the elements and the prying eyes of art critics. This can pose a health risk to workers on the project. The company has a contract to repair a large fabricated metal sculpture covered with an architectural coating reported to contain 0.5 to 1.7 ppm of mercury and 3.2% lead. During the project various pieces of steel plates must be cut from the structure and replaced. Before the project begins, the client wants to know if the hazard will be sufficient to require the workers to wear respirators to control mercury in addition to lead exposure. Based on the results of this model, you will recommend whatever is necessary to control the mercury during the project. This may include hydroblasting the coating off the sculpture before the cutting process begins, with recommendations up to and including the use of supplied air respirators. The 1993–1994 ACGIH TWA-TLV for eight hours is 0.05 mg/m^3 or 50 μg/m^3.

Solution 5

The solution to this problem requires information on the following:

1. Length of the weld or cut to be made by the welders.
2. Area on either side of the weld or cut that is heated by the torch.
3. Thickness of the paint on the surface of the metal to be heated.
4. Mass of mercury generated by the welding process.
5. Time it takes to perform the individual welding operations.
6. Amount of dilution air provided.
7. Volume that welders occupy within the containment.
8. Volume of the containment.
9. Duration of exposure during the day.
10. Initial concentration of mercury at the start of a work shift.

Total Mass of Mercury Liberated during Torch Cutting   The welders cut sections of steel plates that are about three feet (36 inches) by five feet (60 inches) because they are easily handled. This represents a cut line that is about 200 inches long (36 + 36 + 60 + 60 = 192 inches). If cutting with the oxyacetylene torch affects an area that is about two inches wide (one inch on either side of the cut line), the volume of paint volatilized can be calculated. The resulting mass of mercury liberated can be calculated. The cut is along a line that is about 200 inches long by 2 inches wide, or 400 square inches (in^2). The paint thickness can be measured with a magnetic thickness gauge or can be estimated from the paint manufacturer's technical product bulletin on rust-preventive architectural coatings. If the paint is 0.002 inch thick, the total volume of paint that burned off the surface is:

$$(400 \text{ in}^2)(0.002 \text{ in}) = 0.8 \text{ in}^3 \text{ of paint burned off during a 200-inch-long cut}$$

This is extremely conservative because only the first piece of steel plate removed requires a cut that is 200 inches long. If the second piece is above or below the previous piece, the cut line is reduced by 60 inches. If the second piece is to the right or left of the previous piece, the cut line is reduced by 36 inches. Subsequent cuts within a given section are reduced in length as adjacent pieces are removed, so that the mass of mercury burned off the steel plates is reduced. Assuming 200 inches of cutting overestimates the mass of mercury released. Using the worst-case result, the average mercury metal concentration in the architectural coating is 1.7 ppm, and the volume of mercury contained in the paint and released per cut is:

$$(0.8 \text{ in}^3)(1.7 \text{ parts}/10^6) = 1.4 \times 10^{-6} \text{ in}^3 \text{ Hg}$$

This 1.4×10^{-6} in^3 Hg (assumed to exist as mercury metal in the paint) is equal to 2.3×10^{-8} liter of mercury metal liberated per 200-inch-long cut.

This is the volume of mercury metal present in the paint before cutting; it is not the volume of vapor released during the cutting process. The cutting process reduces organic and inorganic forms of mercury to elemental mercury. That calculation will follow.

Airborne Mercury Vapor Concentration   The density of mercury metal is 13.5 g/cm^3. Since density is mass per unit volume ($\rho = m/V$), then $m = pV$. The volume of mercury metal present in the paint burned off by the welders is 2.3×10^{-8} liter. The mass of mercury present in the paint and released during the cutting of the 3 foot by 5 foot section of steel plates can be calculated:

$$m = \rho V = (13.5 \text{ g/cm}^3)(2.3 \times 10^{-8} \text{ l})(1000 \text{ cm}^3/\text{l}) = 0.0003 \text{ g Hg}$$

There is 0.0003 gram (0.3 mg) of mercury in the paint on the section of steel sculpture being cut. Using an oxyacetylene torch, it takes approximately 10 minutes to make a 200-inch-long cut. Mercury vapor is generated during this 10 minute cutting interval. The generation rate of mercury vapor (G in mg/minute) is: 0.30 mg of mercury released per welder per 10 minutes, or 0.03 mg of mercury released per welder per minute. If there is more than one welder cutting, the generation rate G increases by the number of welders actually cutting (i.e., nG). Assuming poor mixing, the mixing factor is ten ($K = 10$).

The effect of dilution ventilation on the contaminant concentration can be calculated using the equation derived above in this section:

$$(1/Q_{\text{out}})\ln[(G - Q_{\text{out}}C_2)/(G - Q_{\text{out}}C_1)] = -(1/V)(t_2 - t_1)$$

Correcting for the numbers of welders (n) and recalling that $Q_{\text{out}} = Q' = Q_{\text{in}}/K$ (adjustment for incomplete mixing) yields:

$$(1/Q')\ln[(nG - Q'C_2)/(nG - Q'C_1)] = -(1/nV)(t_2 - t_1)$$

where:

$Q' = Q_{in}/K =$ effective ventilation rate, corrected for incomplete mixing, (cfm) $= Q_{out}$

$K =$ mixing factor (dimensionless)

$n =$ number of welders cutting

$G =$ rate of generation of the contaminant vapor (mg/min/welder)

$V =$ volume of the enclosure (cubic feet, ft^3)

$C_1 =$ airborne concentration of the contaminant at time equal to one

$C_2 =$ airborne concentration of the contaminant at time equal to two

$t_1 =$ first time interval, i.e., 0 minutes, beginning of the work shift

$t_2 =$ second time interval, i.e., 480 minutes, after the workday starts

The initial concentration of mercury is zero ($C_1 = 0$) at time t_1 ($t_1 = 0$); the equation becomes:

$$\ln[(nG - Q'C_2)/(nG)] = (Q't_2)/nV$$

or:

$$(nG - Q'C_2)/(nG) = \exp(-Q't_2/nV)$$

$$(nG - Q'C_2) = (nG)\exp(-Q't_2/nV)$$

$$(-Q'C_2) = (ng)\exp(-Q't_2/nV) - nG$$

$$(Q'C_2) = nG - (nG)\exp(-Q't_2/nV)$$

$$(Q'C_2) = [1 - \exp(-Q't_2/nV)](nG)$$

$$C_2 = [1 - \exp(-Q't_2/nV)](nG)/(Q')$$

The model predicts the concentration for a given ventilation rate, Q', corrected for incomplete mixing, time, and volume. Several assumptions about the variables used in the model will be made and the resulting impact evaluated before an attempt is made to model the concentration. Assuming that a mixing factor simplifies the model, let K be ten ($K = 10$, poor mixing):

$$Q' = Q/K = Q/10.0 = 0.10Q$$

The model becomes: $(C_2) = [1 - \exp(-0.1Qt_2/nV)](nG)/(0.1Q)$.

Other reasonable assumptions can be made to simplify the model; these assumptions must reflect what is expected to occur in the workplace. The variables to evaluate are:

- Time t_2—Select a typical workday of 480 minutes, and the resulting concentration is the workers' eight hour average exposure.
- Volume V—Select a typical volume (in cubic feet) that a worker is constrainted to work within, and the result is the volume available to dilute the contaminant. This requires making a field visit to a similar work site to estimate the "typical volume."

Two sets of assumptions are presented below to determine the effects of the exponential on the model. Given reasonable "real world" assumptions, the exponential term in the model may not be important and the model will be simplified.

Given: $\exp(-0.100t_2/nV)$.
Let:

$t = 480$ minutes, the dilution of the welders' exposure (8 hours) to mercury vapor
$V = 200$ ft^3/welder (4 feet by 5 feet by 10 feet)
$n = 10$ welders cutting within the space
$nV = 2000$ ft^3 (10×200 ft^3)

$$\exp(-0.10Qt_2/nV) = \exp\left[-0.1Q(480 \text{ min})/(2000 \text{ ft}^3)\right]$$

$$= \exp(-0.024Q)$$

The following table lists the results of the calculation of the value of the exponential as Q varies from 1 to 1200 cfm:

$(Q$, cfm)	1.0	10	75	100	150	200	600	1200
$\exp(-0.024Q)$	0.9736	0.7866	0.17	0.09	0.02	0.0082	10^{-7}	10^{-13}

For a Q greater than 100 cfm, the exponential essentially goes to zero. The model used to predict the mercury vapor concentration inside the contaminant when ten welders ($n = 10$) are cutting inside a volume of 2000 cubic feet ($nV = 2000$ ft^3) for 8 hours without stopping then reduces to the following equation:

$$C_2 = (nG)/(0.10Q) \quad (\text{in mg/ft}^3)$$

$$C_2 = 353(nG)/(Q) \quad (\text{in mg/m}^3)$$

where:

C_2 = mercury vapor concentration after 480 minutes
G = 0.03 mg of mercury vapor/welder cutting casing/minute
n = 10 welders cutting (WC) on one level
Q = 1200 cfm to 6800 cfm ventilation rate

$$C_2 = 353\, nG/Q \quad \text{(in mg/m}^3\text{)}$$

C_2 (mg/m^3)	G (mg/min)	n (WC)	Q (cfm)	C_2/ACGIH TLV
0.09	0.03	10	1200	1.8
0.06	0.03	10	1700	1.2
0.03	0.03	10	3400	0.6
0.01	0.03	10	6800	0.2

Recommendations: The model predicts that ten welders generating 0.3 mg/min/welder require at least 6800 cfm to maintain the mercury concentration at 0.01 mg/m^3 or 0.2 times the ACGIH TLV. This is equivalent to 680 cfm per welder.

Given: $\exp(-0.10Qt_2/nV)$.
Let:

t = 480 minutes, the duration of the welders' exposure (8 hours) to mercury vapor
V = 2000 ft^3/welder (20 feet by 10 feet by 10 feet)
n = 3 welders cutting within the space
nV = 6000 ft^3 (3 × 2000 ft^3)

$$\exp(-0.10Qt_2/nV) = \exp\left[-0.1Q(480 \text{ min})/(6000 \text{ ft}^3)\right] = \exp(-0.008Q)$$

The table below list the results of the calculation of the value of the exponential as Q varies from 1 to 1200 cfm.

(Q, cfm)	1.0	10	75	100	150	200	600	1200
$\exp(-0.008Q)$	0.9992	0.9231	0.5488	0.4493	0.3012	0.2019	0.0082	0.0001

For a Q greater than 600 cfm, the exponential essentially goes to zero. The model used to predict the mercury vapor concentration inside the containment, when three welders (n = 3) are cutting inside a volume of 6000 cubic feet (nV = 6000 ft^3) for 8 hours without stopping reduces to the following equation:

$$C_2 = \frac{nG}{0.10Q} \quad \text{(in mg/ft}^3\text{)} = 353\frac{nG}{Q} \quad \text{(in mg/m}^3\text{)}$$

where:

C_2 = mercury vapor concentration after 480 minutes
G = 0.03 mg of mercury vapor/welder cutting/minute
n = 3 welders cutting (WC) on one level
Q = 1200 cfm to 6800 cfm ventilation rate

$$C_2 = \frac{353(nG)}{Q} \quad (\text{in mg/m}^3)$$

C_2 (mg/m^3)	G (mg/min)	n (WC)	Q (cfm)	C_2/ACGIH TLV
0.03	0.03	3	1200	0.6
0.02	0.03	3	1700	0.4
0.009	0.03	3	3400	0.18
0.005	0.03	3	6800	0.10

Recommendations: The model predicts that three welders generating 0.3 mg/min/welder require at least 3400 cfm to maintain the concentration at 0.009 mg/m^3 or 0.18 times the ACGIH TLV. This is equivalent to 1133 cfm per welder.

6. CONCENTRATION VARIATION WITH VOLUME

In Section 4, the generation rate was zero ($G = 0$), and the concentration varied with the volume. Under these conditions a first order differential equation emerged. Similarly, a first order differential equation relating the change in concentration to an incremental volume change can be developed:

$$dC = -(Q_{\text{out}}C)\,dV$$

This equation can be used to solve many dilution ventilation problems. The terms in the equation are defined as: C = contaminant concentration, V = container volume, and dV = the increment of volume removed and the amount of diluent air or gas added to maintain a constant pressure.

Since V, the container volume is constant, and the volume flowrate Q_{out} is constant, the differential equation can be solved by separating the variables and integrating:

$$dC/C = -(Q_{\text{out}}/V)\,dV = -(1/V)Q_{\text{out}}\,dV$$

$$\int_{C_0}^{C} dC/C = \int_{V_w}^{V} dV/V = (-1/V)\int_{V_w}^{V} dV$$

$$\ln(C/C_0) = -(V - V_w)$$

where:

$$C/C_0 = \exp - (V - V_w) = \exp(V_w - V) = \exp(-V_w/V)$$

$$C = C_0 \exp(-V_w/V)$$

with C = resultant concentration, C_0 = initial concentration, V = volume of the chamber, and V_w = volume of the sample withdrawn or added.

Example 6

Calculate the concentration of sulfur hexafluoride trace gas remaining in a 900 m^3 house, after three hours, if the initial concentration is 2.0 ppb and the infiltration rate is 0.2 air changes per hour (acph).

Solution 6

The infiltration rate is the number of air changes per hour or the rate that air leaks into and out of a building in one hour. Infiltration rate has units similar to frequency (e.g., 1/second or cycle/second). "Air change" is occupying a space in the numerator to keep the unit of infiltration rate from appearing as 1/hour, which really is much easier to understand. The total volume of SF$_6$ free air that will "leak" or infiltrate into the house in three hours is:

$$(0.2 \text{ air change/hour})(3 \text{ hours})(900 \text{ m}^3) = 540 \text{ m}^3 = V_w$$

Therefore, 540 m^3 of SF$_6$-free dilution air enters the house. If the trace gas is diluted by infiltration and not adsorbed to the walls and furniture, the change in concentration will follow first order decay kinetics:

$$C = C_0 \exp - (V_w/V) = 2.0 \text{ ppb} \exp(-540 \text{ m}^3/900 \text{ m}^3)$$

$$C = 2.0 \exp(-0.6) = 2 \, (0.55) \text{ ppb} = 1.1 \text{ ppb}$$

Example 7

How many chamber volumes are required to purge a vessel and change the concentration of a gas in that vessel to: (A) 1% of its original concentration? (B) 0.1% of its original concentration?

Solution 7

$$V_w = \text{number of chamber volumes}$$
$$V = \text{volume used to purge a volume}$$
$$V_w/V = \text{dilution ratio}$$

This is another example of a first order dilution problem where:

$$C = C_0 \exp(-V_w/V)$$

Solving this equation for V_w/V by taking the natural logarithm of both sides yields:

$$V_w/V = \ln[C_0/C]$$

(A) If $C_0 = 100$ (arbitrary units) and $C = 1\%$ of $C_0 = 1$ (arbitrary units):

$$V_w/V = \ln(100/1) = 4.6 \text{ chamber volume}$$

$$V_w = 4.6V$$

(B) If $C_0 = 100$ (arbitrary units) and $C = 0.1\%$ of $C_0 = 0.1$ (arbitrary units):

$$V_w/V = \ln(100/0.1) = 6.9 \text{ chamber volume}$$

$$V_w = 6.9V$$

Example 8

A spill occurs in an enclosed room and the maximum concentration of the spilled material reaches 18,000 ppm and the TLV-ceiling value (TLV-C) is 1 ppm.
(A) How many room air changes would be needed to change the concentration to the TLV-C?
(B) If a 500 cfm exhaust is operating in the area (10 feet by 12 feet by 18 feet), how long will it take to reduce the concentration from 18,000 ppm to 1 ppm with perfect mixing?
(C) If a 500 cfm exhaust fan is operating in the area (10 feet by 12 feet by 18 feet), how long will it take to reduce the concentration from 18,000 ppm to 1 ppm with poor mixing?

Solution 8A

This is a first order dilution problem where:

$$C = C_0 \exp(-V_w/V)$$
$$V_w/V = \ln(C_0/C), \text{ with } C_0 = 18\,000 \text{ ppm and } C = 1 \text{ ppm}$$
$$V_w/V = \ln(18\,000/1) = 9.8$$
$$V_w = 9.8V$$

The value of $V_w = 9.8V$ is the number of room volumes or air changes needed to provide a first order dilution from $18\,000$ ppm to 1 ppm. This solution assumes that the mixing factor $K = 1$. The mixing factor is an indication of how active or well mixed the air in the room is.

Solution 8B

Assume that a 500 cfm fan is exhausting air out of the building to the ambient air, and that 500 cfm of outdoor (diluent) air is entering the space (if this does not occur the room will depressurize or, in the extreme case, collapse) (the room is 10 feet by 12 feet by 18 feet). How long would it take to change the concentration to 1 ppm with good mixing (i.e., the mixing factor K is 1)?

$$\ln(C/C_i) = -\frac{Q}{V}(t - t_i) = -\frac{Q}{V}\Delta t$$

$$\ln(1/18000) = -\frac{(500 \text{ ft}^3/\text{min})\,\Delta t}{(10 \text{ ft})(12 \text{ ft})(18 \text{ ft})}$$

$$-9.8 = -0.23\Delta t, \qquad \Delta t = 43 \text{ min}$$

It requires 43 minutes to change the concentration from 18 000 ppm to 1 ppm.

Solution 8C

How long will it take to change the concentration to 1 ppm with poor mixing (i.e., the mixing factor K is 10)? The time to bring the concentration to 1.0 ppm from 18 000 ppm will be ten times greater than it is if the mixing factor is one ($\Delta t = 430$ minutes).

Example 9

A sterilizer contains 5000 mg/l ethylene oxide. How many chamber volumes of air must be purged through the sterilizer to lower the ethylene oxide concentration to 0.5 ppm?

Solution 9

This is a first order dilution problem where:

$$C = C_0 \exp(-V_w/V)$$
$$V_w/V = \ln(C_0/C)$$

Calculate C_0, the initial concentration of ethylene oxide in parts per million: Molecular weight of $C_2H_4O = 42.04$ g/mole

$$C_{\text{PPM}} = C_{M/V}(RT/MP)10^6$$

$$C_{\text{PPM}} = \frac{(5000 \text{ mg/l})(0.08205 \text{ l atm/mole K})(298.15 \text{ K})}{(42.04 \text{ g/mole})(1 \text{ atm})}10^6$$

$$C_{\text{PPM}} = 2910 \text{ ppm}$$

$$C_0 = 2910 \text{ ppm and } C = 0.5 \text{ ppm}$$

$$V_w/V = \ln(2910/0.5) = 8.7$$

$$V_w = 8.7V$$

If the chamber volume (V) is known, then a dilution ventilation fan can be sized to the chamber to provide the needed dilution if and only if the mixing factor is one $(F = 1)$. Mixing factors can vary widely and depend on the sterilizer and the way it is packed with products. A further complication is that ethylene oxide remains adsorbed to the products placed in the sterilizer. To promote desorption, it is common either to heat the products or to allow room temperature aeration for an extended period (e.g., 6 or more days in a ventilated storage area).

7. VENTILATION TO MAINTAIN ACCEPTABLE INDOOR AIR QUALITY

Ventilation with fresh outside air is the primary method used to maintain an adequate indoor air quality (IAQ) in nontraditional workplaces (schools, offices, shopping malls, etc.). The assumption is that indoor air contains the typical contaminants [e.g., particles, odors, low levels of volatile organic compounds (VOCs), formaldehyde, and an accumulation of carbon dioxide] that result from the collection of people and the usual array of plants, pets, human activities, furnishings, and so forth, within a space. After source control/elimination, the way to improve indoor air quality is to dilute indoor air pollutants with fresh outdoor air. The outdoor quality must be acceptable; for example, it must meet or exceed the United States Environmental Protection Agency (USEPA) ambient air quality standards (3).

As people breathe, they exhale carbon dioxide, but the accumulation of carbon dioxide is not sufficient to cause an adverse health effect. More specifically, it does not approach the OSHA PEL or the ACGIH TLV. The indoor carbon dioxide concentration can be used as an easily measured surrogate or indicator of the amount of outdoor air (dilution air) introduced to the space. ASHRAE 62-1989 recommends that carbon dioxide levels be maintained below 1000 ppm. There is another requirement in the standard, that the outdoor air be delivered to the occupied space. Many reports exist of IAQ-related complaints when the carbon dioxide concentration is between 750 ppm and 1000 ppm. This may have to do with the sources and types of contaminants or the quality of the mixing that the air undergoes on its way through the space. It is important that one review Standard 62 before emerging as an "IAQ expert." The objective of this section is to describe the development of simple models, not to produce IAQ specialists.

8. INDOOR AIR QUALITY MODELS FOR VENTILATION

The ASHRAE Indoor Air Quality Standard (62-1989) recommends specific outdoor air ventilation rates for a wide array of indoor spaces. Ventilation rates are expressed as outdoor air volume per person in cubic feet per minute (cfm/person). ASHRAE assumes "typical" office occupancy rates of 7 people/1000 GSF (GSF, gross square feet and includes aisles, etc.). This is equivalent to 142 GSF/person. The ASHRAE recommended outdoor air ventilation rate is based on a steady state model that predicts the carbon dioxide concentration difference (ΔCO_2) between indoor carbon dioxide concentration $[C_{CO_2}(\text{INDOORS})]$ and ambient background carbon dioxide concentration $[C_{CO_2}(\text{OUTDOORS})]$. The definition of the carbon dioxide concentration difference (indoor concentration minus outdoor concentration) depends on the difference between the generation rate (GR) of carbon dioxide and the removal rate (RR) of carbon dioxide, divided by the ventilation (VR) of outdoor air into the space:

$$(\Delta CO_2) = \left[C_{CO_2}(\text{INDOORS})\right] - \left[C_{CO_2}(\text{OUTDOORS})\right] = (GR - RR)/VR$$

The information about the difference between carbon dioxide indoors and outdoors can be developed into a steady state model that predicts the relationship between outdoor air volume (in cfm) and the increment of carbon dioxide concentration (in ppm) over the ambient (outdoor) carbon dioxide concentration. Assume that the generation rate of carbon dioxide for a "typical" office worker is 32 grams of a carbon dioxide per hour. This rate varies with age and physical activity levels.

In developing the model it is essential to know that the steady state model predicts the carbon dioxide concentration difference (ΔCO_2) between indoor carbon dioxide $[C_{CO_2}(\text{INDOORS})]$ and ambient background carbon dioxide concentration $[C_{CO_2}(\text{OUTDOORS})]$:

$$(\Delta CO_2) = \left[C_{CO_2}(\text{INDOORS})\right] - \left[C_{CO_2}(\text{OUTDOORS})\right]$$

where:

$C_{CO_2}(\text{INDOORS})$ = indoor CO_2 concentration (ppm)

$C_{CO_2}(\text{OUTDOORS})$ = outdoor or ambient CO_2 concentration (ppm), typically 360 ppm

ΔCO_2 = indoor to outdoor CO_2 concentration difference in ppm = ΔC

$(\Delta CO_2) = (GR - RR)/VR$

GR = CO_2 generation rate, and depends on the occupants' activity, in grams per person per hour (g/person/hr)

RR = CO_2 removal rate, which is site-specific, in grams per hour (g/hr)

(Under steady state assumptions RR goes to 0, that is, the walls, floors, and furniture are not a sink for carbon dioxide.)

VR = Ventilation rate, in outdoor air volume per person $(VR > 0)$

$$(\Delta C) = \left[C_{CO_2}(\text{INDOORS}) - C_{CO_2}(\text{OUTDOORS})\right] = (GR - RR)/VR$$

The equation is solved by using these assumptions:

$GR = 32$ g CO_2 per person per hour (typical office worker)
$RR = 0$ (steady state assumptions, RR goes to 0)
$VR =$ from 1.0 to 1000 cfm/person

$$(\Delta C) = \left[C_{CO_2}(\text{INDOORS}) - C_{CO_2}(\text{OUTDOORS}) \right]$$

$$= (GR - RR)/VR = (GR - 0)/VR = (GR)/VR$$

To convert from mg/m^3 CO_2 to ppm CO_2:

$$C_{PPM} = (V_A/V_B)10^6 = (mRT/V_B MP)10^6 = (RT/MP)(m/V_B)10^6$$

$$RT/MP = C_{PPM}(V_B/m)10^{-6} = C_{PPM}(C_{M/V})10^{-6}$$

$$RT/MP = (0.082\,05 \text{ l atm/mole K})(298.15 \text{ K})/(44.0 \text{ g } CO_2/\text{mole})(1 \text{ atm})$$

$$RT/MP = 0.555\,98 \text{ l } CO_2/\text{g} = C_{PPM}(C_{M/V})10^{-6}$$

$$C_{PPM} = C_{M/V}(0.555\,98 \text{ l/g})(1 \text{ g}/10^3 \text{ mg})(m^3/10^3\text{l})10^6$$

$$C_{PPM} = (0.556 \text{ m}^3/\text{mg})C_{M/V}$$

$$C_{M/V} = 1.7986 \text{ mg/m}^3(C_{PPM})$$

(1 mg/m^3 is equivalent to 0.556 ppm, or 1 ppm $= 1.7986$ mg/m^3.

$$(\Delta C) = \left[C_{CO_2}(\text{INDOORS}) \right] - \left[C_{CO_2}(\text{OUTDOORS}) \right] = (GR)/VR$$

$$\frac{GR}{VR} = \frac{(32 \text{ g } CO_2)(\text{min person})(1 \text{ hr})(\text{ft}^3)(10^3 \text{ l})(10^3 \text{ mg})(1 \text{ ppm})}{(\text{person hr})(VR \text{ ft}^3)(60 \text{ min})(28.32 \text{ l})(m^3)(g)(1.798 \text{ mg/m}^3)}$$

$$= \Delta C$$

$(GR)/VR = 10{,}470.5$ ppm CO_2

$$\left[C_{CO_2}(\text{INDOORS}) \right] = (GR)/VR + \left[C_{CO_2}(\text{OUTDOORS}) \right]$$

where:

$[C_{CO_2}(\text{INDOORS})] =$ carbon dioxide concentration indoors, which can be measured using appropriate analytical instruments and used to determine the ventilation rate

$(GR)/VR =$ generation rate of carbon dioxide divided by the outdoor air ventilation rate (in cfm) or 10,470.5 ppm CO_2/VR (cfm/person)

$C_{CO_2}(\text{OUTDOORS})] =$ carbon dioxide concentration outdoors, which has a reasonably constant value of 360 ppm

Substituting:

$$\left[C_{CO_2}(\text{INDOORS}) \right]$$

$$= [(10{,}470.5 \text{ ppm } CO_2)/\underbrace{VR \text{ (cfm/person)}}_{GR/VR}] + \llcorner CO_2(\text{OUTDOORS})\lrcorner$$

$$+ (360 \text{ ppm } CO_2)$$

This equation also can be solved for the ventilation rate if the indoor and outdoor carbon dioxide concentrations are known:

$$VR \text{ (cfm/person)} = \frac{10{,}470.5 \text{ ppm } CO_2}{\left[C_{CO_2}(\text{INDOORS}) \right] - \left[C_{CO_2}(\text{OUTDOORS}) \right]}$$

A table of the increment of indoor carbon dioxide concentration over the ambient background carbon dioxide concentration (360 ppm) versus the outside air ventilation rate from 1 to 1 000 (cfm/person) will help illustrate the effect of outdoor air on indoor carbon dioxide concentration (see Table 9-2). To verify the model, let the ventilation rate (VR) vary from 1 to 1 000 cfm/person:

$$VR(\text{cfm/person}) = 1, 5, 10, 15, 20, 25, 50, 75, 100, 200, 300, 400, 500, 1000$$

A plot of the outdoor air volume from 1 to 1 000 (cfm/person) versus the increment of carbon dioxide concentration over ambient background will

TABLE 9-2. Ventilation rate vs. indoor carbon dioxide concentration

VR (cfm/person)	(ΔCO_2) (ppm)	$[C_{CO_2} = (\text{INDOORS})]$ (ppm)
1.0	10,470.5	10,830.5
5.0	2094.2	2454.1
10.0	1047.0	1407.0
15.0	698.0	1058.0
20.0	523.5	883.5
25.0	418.8	778.8
50.0	209.4	569.4
75.0	139.6	499.6
100.0	104.7	464.7
200.0	52.4	412.4
300.0	34.9	394.9
400.0	26.2	386.2
500.0	20.9	380.9
1000.0	10.5	370.5

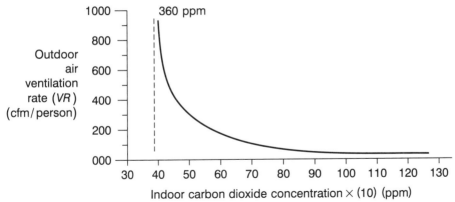

Figure 9-4. Indoor carbon dioxide concentration (ppm) versus outdoor air ventilation rate (*VR*, cfm/person).

help illustrate the effect of outdoor air on indoor carbon dioxide concentration (see Figure 9-4):

$$(\Delta CO_2) = \left[C_{CO_2}(\text{INDOORS}) \right] - \left[C_{CO_2}(\text{OUTDOORS}) \right]$$

$$\left[C_{CO_2}(\text{INDOORS}) \right] = (\Delta CO_2) + \left[C_{CO_2}(\text{OUTDOORS}) \right] = (\Delta CO_2) + 360 \text{ ppm}$$

Conclusion: Working through this IAQ model demonstrates that after the basic assumptions a predictive equation is developed. The rest of the model development is nothing more than a *units conversion* problem. The recommended outdoor air volume per person is based on the assumptions made at the beginning of the model's development.

The outdoor air that is introduced indoors mixes with the indoor air contaminants, reducing their concentration and thus improving the overall quality of the indoor air. As the indoor carbon dioxide concentration is diluted, all other indoor air pollutants (particles, gases, and vapors) also are reduced. This dilution of contaminant discussion is similar to the discussion in Chapter 5, Sections 10 and 11, on static and dynamic dilution of gases and vapors.

It is sometimes difficult or impossible to measure the outdoor air volume flowrates needed to dilute indoor carbon dioxide in an actual operating air handler. Estimates of outdoor air volumes (dilution ventilation) can be made from measurements of outdoor, indoor, and return air temperature (4) or derived from a few simple measurements of carbon dioxide. There are two techniques based on carbon dioxide measurements to estimate the quantity of outdoor air moving into an indoor space. One method depends on calculating the recirculation quotient (*RF*), which is the ratio of the

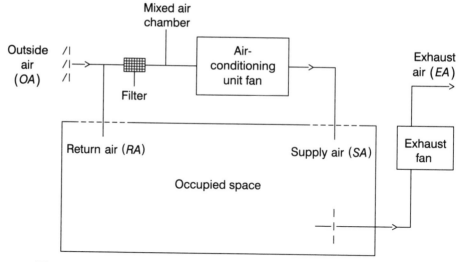

Figure 9-5. Typical heating, ventilating, air-conditioning system with partial air recirculation.

quantity of air flowing through the mixed air chamber or recirculated to the supply air volume flowing into the room. This method is described by Göthe et al. (4). The other method estimates the outdoor air volume moving into an indoor space using the method described by the USEPA (5). This approach estimates the fraction (or percent) of outdoor air that enters a space. The fraction of outdoor air (OAF) is the ratio of the flowrate of outside air to the flowrate of the supply air into a space. The outdoor air fraction (OAF or $OA\%$) method varies slightly from the recirculation quotient (RF) method. Both methods are developed later in this section. Figure 9-5 is a schematic representation of a typical ventilation system with partial recirculation.

The following terminology is useful in discussing this type of ventilation:

$$C_i = \text{carbon dioxide concentration in the } i\text{th location}$$
$$Q_i = \text{air volume flowrate in the } i\text{th location}$$

Carbon Dioxide Concentration

C_o = outside air (OA)
C_m = mixed air chamber (MA)

C_s = supply air (SA)
C_r = return in (RA)
C_e = exhaust air (EA)
C_{room} = concentration in center of room

Air Volume Flowrate

Q_0 = outside air (OA) into space
Q_m = recirculation air volume flowrate
Q_s = supply air into room
Q_r = return air from room
Q_e = exhaust air out of building

It is easy to measure the fresh air volume in the schematic pictured in Figure 9-5. Systems are rarely as simple as the schematic, and it is not always possible to find straight unobstructed locations within a system to make volume or velocity measurements. Carbon dioxide measurements are simple to make and permit the indirect measurement of the outside air fraction (*OAF* or *OA%*) (5) or the fraction of air recirculated (*RF*) (4). Both methods enable the calculation of the fresh outside air volume, with slightly different results.

The Outdoor Air Fraction Method

The USEPA (5) recommends the concentration of carbon dioxide as a surrogate for the amount of outside air that enters a space be calculated using the outside air fraction model. The model can be used to calculate the volume of outdoor air that is entering a space, based on the carbon dioxide concentration in that space. The derivation is described below. Given:

$$Q_o + Q_m = Q_s \text{ (flow balance)} \tag{1}$$

$$Q_o C_o + Q_m C_m = Q_s C_s \text{ (mass flow balance)} \tag{2}$$

$$Q_o/Q_s = OAF \text{ [fraction of outside air } (OAF)] \tag{3}$$

Solve equation (1) for Q_m:

$$Q_m = Q_s - Q_o \tag{4}$$

Substituting Q_m into equation (2) gives:

$$Q_o C_o + (Q_s - Q_o) C_m = Q_s C_s$$

$$Q_o C_o + Q_s C_m - Q_o C_m = Q_s C_s \tag{5}$$

Since $C_m \approx C_r$:

$$Q_o C_o + Q_s C_r - Q_o C_r = Q_s C_s$$

$$Q_o (C_o - C_r) = Q_s (C_s - C_r) \tag{6}$$

Solve for the fraction of outside air $Q_o/Q_s = OAF$:

$$OAF = Q_o/Q_s = (C_s - C_r)/(C_o - C_r)$$

where:

Q_o = outside air volume supplied to the space
$Q_s = Q_o + Q_m$ = supply air volume into space
Q_m = air volume recirculated through mixed air chamber (hard to measure)
C_o = carbon dioxide concentration in outside or ambient air $\equiv 360$ ppm
C_s = carbon dioxide concentration $[CO_2]$ in supply air
C_r = carbon dioxide concentration in the return air
C_m = carbon dioxide concentration in the mixed air $\equiv [CO_2]$ in return air $\equiv C_r$
C_{room} = carbon dioxide concentration in the indoor space $\equiv [CO_2]$ in return air $\equiv C_r$

The percent of the outside air (%OA) is equal to outside air fraction (OAF) times 100:

$$OA\% = (OAF)100 = (Q_o/Q_s)100$$

$$OA \text{ volume (cfm)} = (OAF) \text{ total air flow (cfm)}$$

$$\equiv [(OA\%)/100] \text{ total air flow (cfm)}$$

For example, assume that the OA% is 65% and the supply air (Q_s) to the room is measured at 1200 cfm. Based on the calculated OA%, the supply air is 65% fresh outside air and 35% recirculated; that is, of the 1200 cfm of supply air to the space, 780 cfm [780 cfm = 0.65(1200 cfm)] is fresh outdoor air and 420 cfm [420 cfm = 0.35(1200 cfm)] is recirculated. The occupancy of the space must be known or counted to determine if the space complies with the outdoor air volume per person recommended in ASHRAE 62-1989 (2).

$$\text{Outdoor air (fraction)} = (C_s - C_r)/(C_o - C_r) = OAF$$

$$\text{Outdoor air (percent)} = (C_s - C_r)/(C_o - C_r)100 = OA\%$$

where:

C_s = carbon dioxide concentration (ppm) in the supply if measured in the room
C_s = carbon dioxide concentration (ppm) in the mixed air measured in the air handler
C_r = carbon dioxide concentration (ppm) in the return air
C_o = carbon dioxide concentration (ppm) in the outside air

$$\text{Outdoor air (cfm)} = [\text{Outdoor air (fraction)}][\text{Total air flow (cfm)}]$$

$$\text{Outdoor air (cfm)} = [\text{Outdoor air (percent)}/100][\text{Total air flow (cfm)}]$$

The Recirculation Fraction Model

Göthe (4) describes a slightly different approach to calculate the outdoor air volume flowrate. The derivation below will yield the equation to calculate the fraction of outdoor air recirculated through a space based on the carbon dioxide concentration in the space. Given:

$$Q_o + Q_m = Q_s \text{ (flow balance)} \tag{1}$$

$$Q_o C_o + Q_m C_m = Q_s C_s \text{ (mass flow balance)} \tag{2}$$

$$Q_m / Q_s = RF \text{ [fraction of air flow recirculated } (RF)] \tag{3}$$

Solve equation (1) for Q_o:

$$Q_o = Q_s - Q_m$$

Substituting Q_o into equation (2) gives:

$$Q_s C_o - Q_m C_o + Q_m C_m = Q_s C_s$$

$$(C_m - C_o) Q_m = (C_s - C_o) Q_s$$

Solve for the recirculation quotient:

$$Q_m / Q_s = (C_s - C_o)/(C_m - C_o) = RF$$

where:

Q_m = air volume recirculated through the mixed air chamber (hard to measure)

$Q_s = Q_o + Q_m$ = supply air volume into space

C_o = carbon dioxide concentration in the outside or ambient air ≡ 360 ppm

C_m = carbon dioxide concentration in the mixed air ≡ $[CO_2]$ in return air ≡ C_r

C_{room} = carbon dioxide concentration in the indoor space ≡ $[CO_2]$ in return air ≡ C_r

C_s = carbon dioxide concentration $[CO_2]$ in supply air

C_r = carbon dioxide concentration in the return air

$$Q_m / Q_s = (C_s - C_o)/(C_m - C_o) = (C_s - C_o)/(C_{room} - C_o) = RF$$

$$Q_m / Q_s = (C_s - 360)/(C_{room} - 360) = RF$$

$$Q_m / Q_s = (C_s - C_o)/(C_m - C_o) \equiv (C_s - C_o)/(C_{room} - C_o)$$

The fraction of the air recirculated (RF), sometimes called the recirculation quotient (Q_m/Q_s), is used to calculate the actual volume of fresh outside air (Q_o) that is in the supply air entering the space. Q_o is the outside air volume that combines with the recirculated air (Q_m) in the mixed air chamber to produce the supply air (Q_s) entering a space. This requires measuring the supply air volume entering the room (Q_s) and then using the fraction of the air recirculated (RF) to calculated the outside air volume:

$$Q_o = Q_s - Q_m$$

For example, the recirculation fraction is 0.65, and the supply air (Q_s) to the room is measured at 1200 cfm. Based on the calculated fraction the supply air is 65% recirculated and 35% fresh outside air. That is, of the 1200 cfm of supply air to the space, 420 cfm is fresh outside air:

$$0.35(1200 \text{ cfm}) = 420 \text{ cfm}$$

Since ($Q_o = Q_s - Q_m$) is the fresh air supply volume flowrate, then the recirculated volume flowrate is 780 cfm (780 cfm = 1200 cfm−420 cfm). The occupancy of the space must be known or counted to determine if the space complies with the outdoor air volume per person recommended by ASHRAE 62-1989.

In summary:

$$RF = Q_m/Q_s = (C_s - C_o)/(C_m - C_o) \equiv (C_s - C_o)/(C_{\text{room}} - C_o)$$

where the terms are as defined above.

Example 10

During an indoor air quality survey, a hygienist measures the carbon dioxide concentration at several locations in an elementary school to determine the source of complaints about "stuffiness and stale air" from the teachers, staff, parents, and students. The results of the survey are shown in Table 9-3. With these data, calculate the volume of outside air that is

TABLE 9-3.

Space, room number	C_o Ambient CO_2 (ppm)	C_{room} Room CO_2 (ppm)	C_s Supply CO_2 (ppm)	C_r Return CO_2 (ppm)	Q_s Total supply (cfm)
216	360	1075	675	1000	1225
286	360	850	700	900	1175
306	360	725	600	700	1345
342	360	725	575	675	945

entering each space, using the recirculated fraction method. Determine if the air volume per person recommended in ASHRAE 62 is satisfied.

Solution 10

$$RF = (C_s - C_o)/(C_{\text{room}} - C_o)$$

Room 216 $RF = (675 - 360)/(1075 - 360) = 0.44 = Q_m/Q_s$
Room 286 $RF = (700 - 360)/(850 - 360) = 0.69 = Q_m/Q_s$
Room 306 $RF = (600 - 360)/(725 - 360) = 0.66 = Q_m/Q_s$
Room 342 $RF = (575 - 360)/(725 - 360) = 0.59 = Q_m/Q_s$

Recirculation air volume (Q_m) is calculated by multiplying the recirculation fraction by total air supplied to the space (Q_s); that is, $Q_m = RF(Q_s)$. Calculations of Q_m and Q_o are shown below, and the results are given in Table 9-4.
Room 216 $RF = (C_s - C_o)/(C_{\text{room}} - C_o) = 0.44$:

$$Q_m = RF(Q_s) = 0.44(1225) = 539 \text{ cfm; total supply air volume}$$

$$= Q_s = 1225 \text{ cfm}$$

$$Q_o = Q_s - Q_m = 1225 - 539 = 686 \text{ cfm} = \text{fresh air supply volume}$$

Room 286 $RF = (C_s - C_o)/(C_{\text{room}} - C_o) = 0.69$:

$$Q_m = RF(Q_s) = 0.69(1175) = 811 \text{ cfm; total supply air volume}$$

$$= Q_s = 1175 \text{ cfm}$$

$$Q_o = Q_s - Q_m = 1175 - 811 = 364 \text{ cfm} = \text{fresh air supply volume}$$

TABLE 9-4.

Space, room number	Q_s Total supply (cfm)	Recirc. fraction (RF)	Q_m Recirc. volume (cfm)	Q_o OA volume (cfm)	Number of persons	OA/person cfm/person	Actual/ ASHRAE
216	1225	0.44	539	686	31	22.1	1.11
286	1175	0.69	811	364	22	16.5	0.83
306	1345	0.66	888	457	29	15.8	0.79
342	945	0.59	558	387	22	17.6	0.88

Room 306 $RF = (C_s - C_o)/(C_{room} - C_o) = 0.66$:

$$Q_m = RF(Q_s) = 0.66(1345) = 888 \text{ cfm}; \text{ total supply air volume}$$

$$= Q_s = 1345 \text{ cfm}$$

$$Q_o = Q_s - Q_m = 1345 - 888 = 457 \text{ cfm} = \text{fresh air supply volume}$$

Room 342 $RF = (C_s - C_o)/(C_{room} - C_o) = 0.59$:

$$Q_m = RF(Q_s) = 0.59(945) = 558 \text{ cfm}; \text{ total supply air volume}$$

$$= Q_s = 945 \text{ cfm}$$

$$Q_o = Q_s - Q_m = 945 - 558 = 387 \text{ cfm} = \text{fresh air supply volume}$$

The design requires 20 cfm per person, and 1250 cfm is being delivered by the univents.

Recommendation: Based on the recirculation fraction method, the system is performing less well than expected. In most rooms (286, 306, and 342) the ratio of the actual outside air to the ASHRAE recommended outside air volume (actual/ASHRAE as seen in the last column in Table 9-4) is less than one. A repair or modification to the mechanical system may be required.

Example 11

During an indoor air quality survey a hygienist measures the carbon dioxide concentration at several locations within an elementary school to determine the source of complaints of "stuffiness and stale air" reported by the teachers, staff, parents, and students. The results of the survey are as shown in Table 9-3. With those data, calculate the volume of outside air that is entering each space, using the outdoor air fraction method. Determine if the air volume per person recommended in ASHRAE 62 is satisfied.

Solution 11

Room 216 $OAF = (C_s - C_r)/(C_o - C_r) = (675 - 1000)/(360 - 1000) = 0.51$

$$Q_s = 1225 \text{ cfm}; Q_o = OAF(Q_s) = 0.51(1225 \text{ cfm}) = 622 \text{ cfm OA (outside air)}$$

Room 286 $OAF = (C_s - C_r)/(C_o - C_r) = (700 - 900)/(360 - 900) = 0.37$

$$Q_s = 1175 \text{ cfm}; Q_o = OAF(Q_s) = 0.37(1175 \text{ cfm}) = 435 \text{ cfm OA}$$

TABLE 9-5.

Space, room number	Q_s Total supply (cfm)	Recirc. fraction (RF)	Q_m Recirc. volume (cfm)	Q_o OA volume (cfm)	Number of persons	OA/person cfm/person	Actual/ ASHRAE
216	1225	0.51	50.8	622	31	20.1	1.0
286	1175	0.37	37.0	435	22	19.7	0.99
306	1345	0.29	29.0	396	29	13.7	0.69
342	945	0.32	32.0	302	22	13.7	0.69

Room 306 $OAF = (C_s - C_r)/(C_o - C_r) = (600 - 700)/(360 - 700) = 0.29$

$Q_s = 1345$ cfm; $Q_o = OAF(Q_s) = 0.29(1345$ cfm$) = 396$ cfm OA

Room 342 $OAF = (C_s - C_r)/(C_o - C_r) = (575 - 675)/(360 - 675) = 0.32$

$Q_s = 945$ cfm; $Q_o = OAF(Q_s) = 0.32(945$ cfm$) = 302$ cfm OA

Results of the calculations are given in Table 9-5.

Recommendation: Based on the outdoor air fraction method, the system is performing less well than expected. In one-half of the rooms the ratio of the actual outside air to the ASHRAE recommended outside air volume (actual/ASHRAE as seen in the last column in Table 9-5) is less than one. A modification or repair to the mechanical system may be required.

Example 12

Summarize the results of examples 10 and 11 and compare the results of the two procedures.

Solution 12

See Table 9-6.

TABLE 9-6.

Space, room number	RF method, OA/person (cfm/person)	OA fraction method, OA/person (cfm/person)	Percent difference [(RF − EPA)/RF]100
216	22.1	20.1	−9.0
286	16.5	19.7	+19.4
306	15.8	13.7	−13.2
342	17.6	13.7	−22.2

Recommendation: Although there is not perfect agreement between the two methods, the trends that they both indicate are similar. Both indicate that the system is performing less well than expected. A repair or a modification to the mechanical system may be required.

BIBLIOGRAPHY

1. *Instructions for Installation, Operation and Maintenance of Lead-Acid Batteries in Motive Power Service*, Hobart Corporation Technical Service Bulletin 2700. (Check this out.)
2. American Society of Heating, Refrigeration and Air-Conditioning Engineers, ASHRAE 62-1989, *Ventilation for Acceptable Indoor Air Quality*. Atlanta, GA.
3. American Society of Heating, Refrigeration and Air-Conditioning Engineers, *ASHRAE Handbook of Fundamentals*. Atlanta, GA (1993).
4. Göthe, C. J., Bjurström, R., and Ancker, K., A simple method of estimating air recirculation in ventilation systems. *American Industrial Hygiene Association Journal* 49(2):66–69 (1988).
5. USEPA, *Building Air Quality, A Guide for Building Owners and Facility Managers*. (EPA-400/1-91-033, DHHS/NIOSH Pub. No. 91-114). U.S. Government Printing Office, Washington, DC (1991).
6. American Conference of Governmental Industrial Hygienists, *Industrial Ventilation; A Manual of Recommended Practice*, 21st Edition. Cincinnati, OH (1992), Chapter 2.
7. Jayjocks, M., Backpressure modeling of indoor air concentrations from volatilizing sources. *American Industrial Hygiene Association Journal* 55:230–233 (1994).

PROBLEM SET

Problem 1

Given an emission rate (m_A) from an ethylene oxide sterilizer of 0.20 gram per second into an exhaust ventilation stream (Q_B) of 2000 cfm (944 l/sec), what is the concentration of ethylene oxide emitted into the ambient air? Calculate the corresponding concentration of ethylene oxide in ppm and mg/m³ (assume NTP).

Solution 1

$$C_{PPM} = (Q_A/Q_B)10^6$$

The exhaust gas and ethylene oxide are given as flowrates. Assume that the system is observed at a point in time. The concentration equation reduces to a relationship based on volume:

$$C_{\text{PPM}} = (V_A/V_B)10^6$$

where:

> A = volume of ethylene oxide released into the exhaust gas stream
> B = volume of the air exhausted from the chamber or room
> M_A = molecular weight of ethylene oxide (C_2H_4O)
> M_A = 12.011(2) + 1.0079(4) + 15.9994(1) = 24.022 + 4.0316 + 15.9994
> M_A = 44.05 g/mole

Since the system is operating at NTP, assume:

1. That the temperature of the ventilation air and the ethylene oxide is at 25°C. Convert this to absolute or thermodynamic temperature: 273.15° + 25° = 298.15K.
2. That the system is operating at a standard atmospheric pressure of one atmosphere.

Solving the ideal gas equation for V gives:

$$V = nRT/P = mRT/MP$$

Identifying V as the volume of component A in a mixture of gases yields:

$$V_A = n_A RT/P = m_A RT/M_A P$$

Substituting this into the equation for concentration in ppm yields:

$$C_{\text{PPM}} = (V_A/V_B)10^6 = (m_A RT/M_A PV_B)10^6$$

Recall:

> $m_A = 0.2$ g/sec
> $R = 0.08205$ l atm/mole K
> $T = 298.15$ K
> $P = 1$ atm
> $M_A = 44.05$ g/mole
> $V_B = 944$ l/sec
> $C_{\text{PPM}} = (V_A/V_B)10^6 = (m_A RT/M_A PV_B)10^6 = 118$ ppm

The conversion from concentration in ppm to milligrams per cubic meter follows:

$$C_{M/V} = [(C_{\text{PPM}} M_A P)/(RT)]10^{-6}$$

$$C_{M/V} = \frac{118 \text{ ppm}(44.05 \text{ g/mole})(1 \text{ atm})}{(0.082 \text{ l atm/mole K})(298.15 \text{ K})} 10^{-6}$$

$$C_{M/V} = 213 \text{ mg/m}^3$$

Problem 2

In *Batman* the movie, the Caped Crusader must foil the Riddler and keep him and his band of criminals from stealing the "Mammoth of Moldavia." The Riddler added laughing gas into the ventilation system of the Gotham City Museum. Will the Patrons of the Arts fall asleep at the exhibit and allow the Riddler to steal the Moldavian treasure? This is a critical question, as you can avoid an ugly international incident. Make any assumptions that you wish, and use the toxicological literature to justify your calculations!

Solution 2

There is no single answer to this problem. It will make an interesting topic for discussion. The main points to discuss are the volume of gas, the volume of the room, the dilution ventilation rate, and the concentration in air that will anesthetize everyone reversibly. The movie producers did not think about all these issues before they released the gas into the museum.

Problem 3

Repeat the problem from Example 1, given the generation rate of hydrogen from a charging battery using the dilution ventilation model with a constant generation rate:

$$C_2 = [1 - \exp(-Qt_2/KV)](G)/(Q/K)$$

where G has to be in mg/sec.

$$(0.484 \text{ ft}^3/\text{min})(0.08988 \text{ g/l})(28.32 \text{ l/ft}^3)(\text{min}/60 \text{ sec})(1000 \text{ mg/g})$$

$$= 20.5 \text{ mg/sec}$$

Solution 3

Volume of the space = (20 feet wide by 10 feet high × 20 feet deep) = 4000 cubic feet

Cubic feet of hydrogen produced per minute = 0.00027 (finish rate) number of cells

G_{H_2} = cubic feet of hydrogen per minute = 0.484 cfm = Q_{H_2}

$K = 10$

t_2 = time that the batteries are charging and emitting hydrogen = 180 minutes

Given the mixing factor, volume, and time, the exponential in the model can be evaluated:

$$\exp(-0.10Qt_2/nV) = \exp[-0.1Q(180 \text{ min})/(4000 \text{ ft}^3)] = \exp(-0.0045Q)$$

The tabulation below lists the results of the calculation of the value of the exponent as Q varies from 1 to 4000 cfm:

(Q, cfm)	1.0	10	75	100	200	500	1000	4000
$\exp(-0.0045Q)$	0.9955	0.9560	0.7136	0.6476	0.4066	0.1054	0.0111	10^{-8}

For a Q greater than 1000 cfm, the exponential essentially goes to zero. The model used to predict the hydrogen gas concentration inside the battery charging area, when 754 cells are charging inside a volume of 4000 cubic feet for three hours without stopping, reduces to:

$$(C_2) = (10G)/(Q) \text{ (ppm)}$$

When the hydrogen generation rate is in cubic feet per minute (cfm), the dilution ventilation rate is in cubic feet per minute (cfm), and the mixing factor is 10 (poor mixing):

where:

C_2 = hydrogen gas concentration after 180 minutes
G = 0.484 cfm of hydrogen gas
Q = 1000 cfm to 12,000 cfm ventilation rate

Results are as follows:

Q (cfm)	G (cfm)	C_2 (%)	Fraction of LEL
1,000	0.484	0.0048	0.001
2,000	0.484	0.0024	0.0006
3,000	0.484	0.0016	0.0004
4,000	0.484	0.0012	0.0003
6,000	0.484	0.0008	0.0002
8,000	0.484	0.0006	0.0002
12,000	0.484	0.0004	0.0001

Recommendation: The model predicts that when the batteries are generating 0.484 cubic feet per minute of hydrogen, it will require at least 1,000 cfm to maintain the hydrogen concentration at 0.0048%.

Problem 4

Your client, Sal's Semiconductor Company (SSC), is in the final stages of a design for a new fabrication area. During a process review, a consultant recommended that SSC use cylinders of fluorine gas diluted to 0.125% fluorine in nitrogen (1.5 cubic feet at 2200 psi). The gas cylinder is equipped with a flow-limiting orifice with a leak rate of 0.1 standard cubic feet per minute (scfm). The cylinder is located in a high bay area (30 feet by 29 feet by 40 feet).

(A) Can the cylinder be placed in this area without being put into a ventilated and monitored toxic gas cabinet?

(B) What ventilation rate is required to keep the concentration below 0.1 (PEL)?

Solution 4A

Density of pure fluorine = 1.69 g/l at NTP
Assumption: The fluorine cylinder ruptures, and the room has no ventilation.
OSHA TWA-PEL = 0.1 ppm

$$P_S V_S / T_S = P_F V_F / T_F$$

$$V_S = V_F (P_F / P_S) / (T_S / T_F)$$

$$= 1.5 \text{ ft}^3 (2200 \text{ psi} / 14.7 \text{ psi}) / (298.15 \text{ K} / 298.15 \text{ K})$$

$$V_S = 225 \text{ ft}^3$$

The cylinder is 0.125% fluorine in nitrogen.

$$V_{\text{FLUORINE}} = 0.00125(225 \text{ ft}^3)$$

$$V_{\text{VLUORINE}} = 0.28 \text{ ft}^3$$

$$C_{\text{PPM}} = \left[0.28 \text{ ft}^3 / 30 \times 29 \times 40 \text{ ft}^3 \right] 10^6 = 8 \text{ ppm}$$

This is 800 times the acceptable concentration of 0.01 ppm fluorine!

Solution 4B

Calculate the generation rate (G) in milligrams fluorine per minute:

$$G = (0.1 \text{ ft}^3 / \text{min})(0.00125)(28.32 \text{ l/ft}^3)(1.69 \text{ g/l}) = 0.006 \text{ g/min}$$

$$G = 6.0 \text{ mg/min}$$

Use the constant generation rate model developed in this chapter:

$$(1/Q') \ln \left[(G - Q' C_2) / (G - Q' C_1) \right] = (t_2 - t_1) / V$$

where:

$Q' = Q/K$ = effective ventilation rate, corrected for incomplete mixing, (cfm) = Q_{out}

K = mixing factor (dimensionless)

Q = ventilation rate (cfm)

G = rate of generation of the contaminant gas (mg/min)

V = volume of the space (cubic feet, ft^3)

C_2 = concentration after a time interval of t_2

C_1 = concentration after a time interval of t_1

t_2 = second time interval, i.e., 480 minutes after the leak starts

t_1 = first time interval, i.e., 0 minutes, beginning of the work shift

The initial concentration of fluorine is zero ($C_1 = 0$) at time (t_1); the equation becomes:

$$\ln[(G - Q'C_2)/(G)] = -(Q't_2)/V$$

or:

$$(G - Q'C_2)/(G) = \exp(-Q't_2/V)$$

$$(G - Q'C_2) = (G)\exp(-Q't_2/V)$$

$$(-Q'C_2) = (G)\exp(-Q't_2/V) - G$$

$$(Q'C_2) = G - (G)\exp(-Q't_2/V)$$

$$(Q'C_2) = [1 - \exp(-Q't_2/V)](G)$$

$$C_2 = [1 - \exp(-Q't_2/V)](G)/(Q')$$

The model predicts the concentration for a given ventilation rate, Q', corrected for incomplete mixing, time, and volume. Several assumptions about the variables used in the model can be made and the resulting impact evaluated before an attempt is made to model the concentration. Assuming a mixing factor simplifies the model. Let K be ten ($K = 10$, poor mixing):

$$Q' = Q/K = Q/10.0 = 0.10Q$$

The model becomes: $(C_2) = [1 - \exp(-0.1Qt_2/V)](G)/(0.1Q)$. Other reasonable assumptions can be made to simplify the model. The assumptions must reflect what is expected to occur in the area. The variables to evaluate are:

- Time t_2: Select a typical workday of 480 minutes, and the result is the area concentration after eight hours.
- Volume, V: Select the volume of the high bay area (in cubic feet). The result is the volume available to dilute the fluorine.

Two sets of assumptions are presented below to determine the effects of the exponential on the model. Given reasonable "real world" assumptions, the exponential term in the model may not be important, and the model will be simplified.

Given: $\exp(-0.10Qt_2/V)$

Let: $t = 480$ minutes, the duration of the fluorine leak

$V = 84,800$ ft^3 (29 feet by 30 feet by 40 feet)

$$\exp(-0.10Qt_2/V) = \exp\left[-0.1Q(480 \text{ min})/(84,000 \text{ ft}^3)\right] = \exp(-0.0006Q)$$

The tabulation below lists the results of the calculation of the value of the exponential as Q varies from 1 to 10,000 cfm.

(Q, cfm)	1.0	10	100	1 000	5 000	10 000
$\exp(-0.0006Q)$	0.9994	0.994	0.94	0.56	0.06	0.003

Glossary

ABIH   American Board of Industrial Hygiene

Absolute pressure   Pressure is *never* less than zero. The pressure in a system can approach zero, but for the pressure to be negative it would first have to pass through zero, which is like absolute temperature on a thermodynamic scale. It is possible to approach but not reach absolute zero pressure.

Absolute zero   The temperature at which all molecular motion stops. Either $-273.15°C$ (0 K) in the SI system or $-459.67°F$ (0°R) in the English system.

Absorption   The penetration of a substance into the body of another; i.e., dissolving of a material in another.

Acceleration   Any gradual speeding up of a process. The time rate of change of velocity.

Accuracy   The measure of the correctness of data, as given by differences between the measured value and the true or specified value. Ideal accuracy is zero difference between measured and true value.

ACGIH   American Conference of Governmental Industrial Hygienists.

ACIL   American Council of Independent Laboratories.

ACS   American Chemical Society.

Adsorption   Condensation of gases, liquids, or dissolved substances on the surfaces of solids.

Aerosol   Dispersion of solid or liquid particles of microscopic size in a gaseous medium.

AIChE   American Institute of Chemical Engineers.

AIHA   American Industrial Hygiene Association.

AIME   American Institute of Mining, Metallurgical, and Petroleum Engineers.

Aliquot   Of, pertaining to, or designating an exact divisor or factor of a quantity, especially of an integer; contained exactly or an exact number of times.

Ambient   Surrounding, encircling, pertaining to the environment.

Angstrom (Å)   Unit of length equal to one hundred-millionth (10^{-8}) of a centimeter, used especially to specify radiation wavelengths. (See also **Nanometer.**)

ANSI   American National Standards Institute (formerly titled USA Standards Institute, American Standards Association).

APHA   American Public Health Association, Inc.

Aqueous   Relating to or resembling water.

ASA   Acoustical Society of America.

Asbestosis   Pneumoconiosis caused by breathing asbestos dust.

Asphyxiation, chemical   Toxic reaction wherein chemicals reaching the bloodstream react in such a way as to deprive the body of oxygen.

Asphyxiation, simple   Coating or blockage of passageways in the lungs so that oxygen cannot reach the alveoli or be absorbed into the bloodstream.

ASSE   American Society of Safety Engineers.

ASTM   American Society for Testing and Materials.

Atom   The smallest unit of an element that still maintains the physical and chemical properties of the element.

Atomic weight   The relative mass of the atom on the basis of $^{12}C \equiv 12$.

Avogadro's number   The number of molecules (6.02×10^{23} molecules/mole) contained in one gram molecular weight or one gram molecular volume (e.g., 28.001 grams of CO = 6.02×10^{23} molecules of CO).

Barometer   A long glass tube, closed at one end, evacuated, filled with mercury, and inverted in a cistern of mercury. The height of the column of mercury is a measure of atmospheric pressure.

BCSP   Board of Certified Safety Professionals of the Americas, Inc.

Bias   A systemic error inherent in a method or caused by some idiosyncrasy of the measurement system.

Billion   In the United States, 10^9; in the United Kingdom and Germany, 10^{12}.

Blank   The measured value obtained when a specified component of a sample is not present during the measurement.

Boiling point   The temperature at which the vapor pressure of a liquid equals the atmospheric pressure.

Boyle's law   At a constant temperature the volume of a given quantity of any gas varies inversely as the pressure to which the gas is subjected.

BTU (British Thermal Unit)   Amount of heat required to raise the temperature of one pound of water one degree F.

BZ   Breathing zone.

C   Ceiling value. (See also **Ceiling limit**.)

Calibrate   To check, adjust, or systematically standardize the graduations of a quantitative measuring instrument.

Carcinogen   Any cancer-producing substance.

Carcinogenic   Capable of producing cancer.

Ceiling limit, Ceiling   Control of exposure to fast-acting substances by value placing a limit on their concentration. Such substances are marked with a "C" in the TLV table. The concentration of these substances cannot at any time in the work cycle (except for a 15-minute period) exceed the TLV. (See also **Threshold limit value**.)

Charles–Gay-Lussac law   Gases increase in volume for each one degree Celsius rise in temperature. This increase is equal to approximately $1/273.15$ of the volume of the gas at $0°C$.

Chemical agent   Dust, gas vapor, or fume that acts on or reacts with the human physiologic system.

Chemical hazard   Exposure to any chemical that, in acute concentrations, has a toxic effect.

Chronic effort   Disease symptom or process of long duration, usually frequent in occurrence and almost always debilitating.

Chronic symptom   Symptom that persists over a long period.

Coefficient of variation (CV)   The sample standard deviation divided by the sample mean.

Compound   A chemical substance composed of individual molecules.

Concentration   The amount of a substance in mass, moles, volume equivalents contained in a unit volume.

Confidence interval   A range of values (an interval) that has a specified probability of including the true value of a parameter of an underlying distribution.

Confidence level   The probability that a stated confidence interval will include a population parameter.

Confidence limits   The upper and lower boundaries of a confidence interval.

Conservation of energy law   Energy can neither be created nor destroyed, and therefore the total amount of energy in the universe is constant.

Conservation of mass   In all ordinary chemical changes, the total mass of the reactants is always equal to the total mass of the products.

Contaminant   Any harmful, irritating, or nuisance material foreign to the normal atmosphere or other medium.

Continuous operation   Industrial operation where the final product is produced at or near a continuous rate.

Convection   Motion resulting in a fluid from the difference in density and the action of gravity; heat loss or gain by a body to the surrounding atmosphere.

CPS   Cycles per second. (See also **Hertz**.)

Criterion   Standard upon which a judgment or a decision may be based.

Criteria document   Publication of NIOSH-related research upon which standards can be based. Such documents contain essential parts of a standard, including environmental limits, sampling requirements, labeling, monitoring requirements, medical examinations, compliance methods, protective equipment, record-keeping requirements, and other recommendations to OSHA for establishment of a standard.

C–T   Concentration–time; two factors upon which dosage is based. (See also **Dose**.)

Dalton's law   (Dalton's law of partial pressure) At constant temperature the total pressure exerted by a mixture of gases in a definite volume is equal to the sum of the partial pressures of the individual components of the mixture.

Density   Characteristic of a material (solid, liquid, gas or vapor) given by the relationship between the mass of the material and the volume the mass occupies.

Desorption   Removal of a substance from the surface at which it is absorbed.

Dimensional analysis   A technique used to manipulate units as numbers.

Direct reading instrument   Instrument that gives a direct reading on a dial without the need for further computations or laboratory processing.

Dose   Concentration of a contaminant multiplied by the duration of human exposure ($D = C \times T$).

Dose, cumulative   Total dose resulting from repeated exposures.

Dose–effect study   Laboratory experiment in which animals are given varying doses of known or potentially harmful substances over varying periods of time, and the physical effects are measured in order to set exposure limits for these substances in the occupational environment.

Dose, permissible   Amount of radiation that may be received by an individual within a specified period with expectation of no significantly harmful result.

Dose–response curve   Graphic representation relating biologic response to concentration of contaminant and time of exposure. By multiplying these factors, dose is determined.

Dosimeter   Instrument used to detect and measure an accumulated dose of radiation. It is usually a pencil-sized chamber with a built-in self-reading meter, used for personnel monitoring.

Dosimetry   Accurate measurement of doses.

Dust   General term applied to solid particles predominantly larger than colloidal particles and capable of temporary suspension in air or other gases. Derivation from larger masses through the application of physical force usually is implied.

Dyne   Centimeter-gram-second unit of force, equal to the force required to impart an acceleration of one centimeter per second per second to a mass of one gram.

Electron   A subatomic particle that carries a negative charge.

Environmental monitoring   Program in which samples of air contaminants or energy measurements are taken, and which establishes the level of worker exposure to such agents.

Environmental quality   Any standard specifying lower limits for contaminants, chemical or physical agents, and/or resulting stresses to the human body in order to maintain a particular healthful and safe environment in which to work.

Epidemiology   Study of disease as it spreads and involves large numbers of people; the study of disease patterns in larger populations.

Equation of state   An equation that relates the pressure, P, volume, V, and thermodynamic temperature of an amount of substance. The simplest form is the ideal gas law: $PV = nRT$.

Excursion factor   Maximum extent to which a TLV can be exceeded.

Exposure limit value   General term designating any standard or measurement restricting human exposure to harmful or toxic agents.

Exposure profile   Graphic presentation of data on exposure of workers to contaminants in industry.

Extrapolation   The process of estimating unknown values from known values.

Fempto   A prefix meaning 10^{-15}.

Fibrous   Made up of fibers or fiberlike tissue.

Flash point   The temperature at which the vapor above a volatile liquid forms a combustible mixture with air.

Fog   General term applied to visible aerosols in which the dispersed phase is liquid; formation by condensation is implied.

Frequency of sound   Rate of oscillation or vibration; units: 1 cycle per second (cps) or 1 Hertz (Hz).

Fundamental units   Mass, length, and time.

Fume   Solid particles generated by condensation from the gaseous state, generally after volatilization from melted substances and often accompanied by a chemical reaction such as oxidation.

Gas   Any material that has a boiling point below 25°C and 760 mm Hg and expands to fill its container.

Gas chromatography   An analytical chemistry technique to quantitatively analyze volatile organic compounds in a sample.

Gas constant (R)   The constant factor in the equation of state for ideal gases ($R = 0.08205$ liter atmosphere/mole K).

Gaseous exchange   In the alveoli, the absorption of oxygen and concomitant removal of waste gases.

Gram mole   The amount of substance represented by one gram molecular weight or one gram molecular volume (mole).

Gram molecular weight   The sum of the individual atomic weights of all the atoms in a molecule (express mass in units of grams, g).

Hazard evaluation   Evaluation based on data concerning concentration of a contaminant and duration of exposure.

Heat   Energy transferred by a thermal process.

Hertz (Hz)   Unit of frequency equal to one cycle per second. (See also **Frequency of sound**.)

Homolog   One of a series of compounds, each of which is formed from the one before it by the addition of a constant element; any chemical structurally similar to another chemical.

Ideal gas law   An equation of state; a relationship between the pressure, volume, and thermodynamic temperature of a gas.

Impervious   Incapable of being passed through or penetrated.

Impinge   To impact, hit, strike, collide, or push against.

Impingement   Method of measuring air contaminants in which particulates are collected by their collision against some other material; also refers to the way in which particulate matter collects inside the respiratory tract.

International System of Units   Le Systeme International d'Unites, the SI system, divides units into three categories: base units, supplementary units, and derived units. The base units consist of seven well-defined and dimensionally independent quantities. These are length, mass, time, thermodynamic temperature, electric current, amount of a substance, and luminous intensity.

Industrial hygiene survey   Systematic analysis of a workplace to detect and evaluate health hazards and recommend methods for their control.

Industrial hygienist   Professional hygienist primarily concerned with the control of environmental health hazards that arise out of or during the course of employment.

Inert dust   Dust that does not chemically react with other substances.

Infrared radiation   Wavelengths of the electromagnetic spectrum that are longer than those of visible light and shorter than radio waves; infrared wavelengths measure 10^{-4} cm to 10^{-1} cm.

Ingestion   Introduction of substances into the digestive system.

Inspired air   Air drawn in during the breathing process.

Instantaneous sampling   Sampling done at one particular time either by a direct reading instrument or by trapping a definite volume of air for analysis.

IR   Infrared.

Isomer   A molecule that has the same number and kind of atoms as another molecule, but has a different arrangement of the atoms.

Isotope   Atoms of the same element that differ in atomic weight.

Joule   In the International System of Measurements, the unit of energy equal to the work done when a current of one ampere is passed through a resistance of one ohm for one second; a unit of energy equal to the work done when the point of application of a force of one Newton is displaced one meter in the direction of the force. (See also **Newton**.)

Kilocalorie   Amount of heat required to raise the temperature of 1000 grams of water one degree C.

Kilogram molecular weight   The sum of the individual atomic weights of all the atoms in a molecule (express mass in units of kilograms, kg).

Kilogram mole   The amount of substance represented by one kilogram molecular weight or one kilogram molecular volume (mol).

Kinetic energy   Energy due to motion.

Lethal concentration (LC) LC_{50} indicates atmospheric concentration of a substance at which half of a group of test animals die after a specified exposure time. LC_0 indicates atmospheric concentration at which no deaths occur.

Lethal dose (LD) LD_{50} indicates a dose that kills half of a group of test animals. LD_0 indicates a dose at which no deaths occur.

LEL   Lower explosive limit.

Level   Logarithm of the ratio of one quantity to a reference quantity of the same kind. The base of the logarithm, the reference quantity, and the kind of level must be specified.

Limit of Detection   A stated limiting value which designates the lowest concentration that can be detected and which is specific to the analytical procedure used.

Limit of Quantification   A stated limiting value which designates the lowest concentration that can be quantified with confidence and which is specific to the analytical procedure used.

Lognormal distribution   The distribution of a random variable that has the property that the logarithms of its values are normally distributed.

Manometer   A "U"-shaped tube filled with a colored liquid, used to measure pressure difference between different legs of the "U" tube. Typical liquids used are mercury, water, or various oils.

Mass spectroscopy   An analytical chemistry technique to qualitatively analyze volatile compounds in a sample.

Mean free path   The average distance traveled between collisions by the molecules in a gas or a vapor.

mg/m³   Air sampling measurement in milligrams (of contaminant) per cubic meter (of air).

Microbar   Unit of sound pressure equal to one dyne per square centimeter or 0.1 Newton per square meter.

Microwave   Any electromagnetic radiation having a wavelength in the approximate range of from one millimeter to one meter; the region of the electromagnetic spectrum between infrared and short wave radio lengths.

MIG   Metal inert gas; a type of welding.

Mist   General term applied to dispersion of liquid particles, many large enough to be individually visible to the naked eye.

Moist Air   ASHRAE defines moist air as: "A binary (or two component) mixture of dry air and water vapor. The amount of water vapor varies from zero (dry air) to a maximum which depends on temperature and pressure."

Mole   The amount of substance represented by one molecular weight or one molecular volume.

Molecule   The smallest unit of a compound that retains the physical and chemical properties of the compound.

Molecular volume   The volume occupied by one molecular weight of a gas (either kilogram molecular weight or gram molecular weight).

Monitoring   Periodic or continuous determination of the amount of contamination present in an occupied region; used as a safety measure for purposes of health protection.

Mppcf   Million particles per cubic foot (of air).

Nanometer (nm)   Unit of measurement for radiation wavelengths. One nanometer (nm) equals 10^{-6} millimeter on 10 Angstrom units. (See also **Angstrom**.)

Newton   In the meter-kilogram-second system, the unit of force required to accelerate a mass of one kilogram one meter per second per second; equal to 100,000 dynes. (See also **Dyne**.)

NFPA   National Fire Protection Association.

NIOSH   National Institute for Occupational Safety and Health, established by the Occupational Safety and Health Act under the aegis of the Department of Health and Human Services with the responsibility to conduct research and training in occupational safety and health, develop criteria, publish lists of toxic substances, and make inspections.

Normal distribution   An important symmetric continuous probability distribution characterized completely by two parameters, the mean and the standard deviation.

Noxious   Harmful to health.

NSC   National Safety Council.

NTP   Normal temperature and pressure (298.15 K and 1 atmosphere, 760 mm mercury).

Occupational Exposure Limit (OEL)   A health-based workplace standard to protect workers from adverse exposure (PELs, TLVs, RELs, WEELs, etc.).

Origin   The point on a graph that represents zero on both the vertical and the horizontal axes or lines.

Oscillate   To move back and forth in a steady uninterrupted rhythm; to vary between alternate extremes, usually within a definable period.

OSHA   Occupational Safety and Health Administration, U.S. Department of Labor.

OSHRC   Occupational Safety and Health Review Commission.

Parameter   Limit of consideration in a study or an investigation.

Partial pressure   Pressure of a gas in a mixture, equal to the pressure that it would exert if it occupied the same volume alone at the same temperature; this property is described by Dalton's law of partial pressure.

Particulate   Particle of solid or liquid matter.

Periodic motion   Any motion that is repeated at regular intervals. (See also **Oscillate**.)

Permissible concentration   Official term that replaces "Threshold Limit Value."

Permissible Exposure Limit (PEL)   An OEL promulgated by OSHA.

Personal sampler   Air sampling instrument developed in the United States for estimating exposure of individual workers to air contaminants.

Planck's constant   Constant of proportionality relating the quantum of energy that can be possessed by radiation to the frequency of that radiation; value is approximately 6.625×10^{-27} erg/sec. (See also **Quantum**.)

ppm   Air sampling measurement indicating parts (of contaminant) per million (parts of air).

Precision   A measure of the reproducibility of a measured value under a given set of conditions. Accuracy usually refers to the size of deviations from the true mean, whereas precision refers to the size of deviations from the mean observation.

Primary standard   A measurement device that can be directly traced to the National Institute for Standards and Technology (NIST). Examples of traceable primary standards for volume are soap bubble flow meters and spirometers.

Protocol   In science, the rules and outline of an experiment.

Psi   Pounds per square inch.

Qualitative   Pertaining to kind or type (name).

Quantitative   Pertaining to the amount (mass).

Quantum   Invisible unit of energy equal to the product of Planck's constant (h) and the frequency of radiation (ν). (See also **Planck's constant**.)

Recommended Exposure Limit (REL)   Used by NIOSH.

Relative humidity   Ratio, times 100, of the weight of water vapor contained in a unit volume of air and the weight it can contain at a given temperature and pressure.

Respirable   Capable of being inhaled.

Secondary Standard   A measuring device that can be traced to the National Institute for Standards and Technology (NIST) through a primary standard; a secondary standard is calibrated by using a primary standard. Wet test meters, dry gas meters and rotameters, or other variable area orifice meters, the measurement of pressure drop across an orifice plate, and a critical orifice are examples of secondary volume flowrate standard measuring devices.

Significant figures   Numerical values containing as many digits (other than location zeros) as are contained in the least exact factor used in their determination. Note: The student must not confuse significant figures with the ten to sixteen decimal places that appear on the display of scientific and engineering calculators.

Smog   Smoke and fog; applied to extensive atmospheric contamination by aerosols arising from a combination of natural and manufactured sources.

Smoke   Small, gas-borne particles created by incomplete combustion and consisting predominantly of carbon and other combustible materials.

Specific gravity   The ratio of the density of a substance to that of a reference material. In the case of a liquid the reference material is water, and for a gaseous substance the reference material is air at 25°C.

Standard   Any rule, principle, or measure established by a governing authority.

Standard atmosphere   Standard atmospheric pressure, the barometric pressure at an arbitrarily chosen standard condition (25°C and sea level).

Standard deviation   The positive square root of the variance of a distribution; the parameter measuring the spread of values about the mean.

Standard error   The standard deviation of the distribution of a sample statistic.

Temperature   That property of a body which determines the flow of heat. Heat will flow from a warm body to a cold body.

Threshold Limit Value (TLV)   Term used by the American Conference of Governmental Industrial Hygienists to designate degree of exposure to contaminants and expressed as parts of vapor or gas per million parts of air by volume at 25°C and 760 mm Hg pressure, or as approximate milligrams of particulate per cubic meter of air (mg/m^3). (See also **Permissible concentration.**)

Tidal movement   Volume of air inspired of expired during each respiratory cycle.

Time weighted average exposure   Average exposure for an individual over a given working period, as determined by sampling at given times during the period.

Toxic agent   Substance potentially or actually poisonous to the human body.

Toxicologic effect   Harmful or poisonous effect of a chemical agent.

Toxicologist   Specialist in the science that deals with poisons and their effects.

Toxicology   Scientific study of poisons, their actions, their detection, and the treatment of conditions produced by them.

Toxic reaction   Alteration of a biologic system or organ due to the action of toxic agents.

Toxic Substances List   Annual compilation of known toxic substances prepared by the National Institute for Occupational Safety and Health and containing about 25,000 names representing some 11,000 different chemical compounds.

UEL   Upper explosive limit.

UL   Underwriters' Laboratories, Inc.

Ultraviolet radiation   Wavelengths of the electromagnetic spectrum that are shorter than those of visible light and longer than X rays; wavelengths measure 10^{-5} to 10^{-6} cm.

UV   Ultraviolet.

Vapor   Gaseous phase of a substance ordinarily liquid or solid at 25°C and 760 mm Hg.

Volatile   Readily convertible to a vapor or gaseous state.

VP   Vapor pressure.

Wavelength   In a periodic wave, the distance between two points of corresponding phase in consecutive cycles.

Working fluids   Materials whose height indicates pressure in a barometer or a manometer. The most commonly used working fluid for a barometer is mercury; other fluids can be used but are not as convenient as Hg. There are many working fluids used in manometers.

Workplace Environmental Exposure Limit (WEEL)   From AIHA.

Appendix

1. MISCELLANEOUS CONVERSION FACTORS

Mass:

$$453.59 \text{ gram (g)} = \text{pound (lb)}$$

$$\text{pound mass (lb}_M) = 16 \text{ ounces (oz)}$$

$$1 \text{ gram} = 15.43 \text{ grains}$$

Volume:

$$28.316\,85 \text{ liters (l)} = \text{cubic foot (ft}^3)$$

$$\text{gallon (gal)} = 3.785329 \text{ liters(l)}$$

Length:

$$2.540\,000 \text{ centimeter (cm)} = \text{inch (in)}$$

Force:

$$\text{kilogram force} = 9.8066 \text{ Newtons (N)}$$

$$\text{pound force (lb)} = 4.448 \text{ Newton (N)}$$

$$\text{dyne} = 1.00 \times 10^{-5} \text{ Newtons (N)}$$

Pressure:

Pascal (Pa) = 1 Newton per square meter (N/m^2)

$P_{ATM} = 14.659 \text{ lb}/\text{ft}^3$ (77°F)   (atmospheric pressure in the English system)

2. MISCELLANEOUS PHYSICAL CONSTANTS

Avogadro's constant = 6.022×10^{23} molecules/mole
Planck's constant = 6.626×10^{-34} Joule · second
Velocity of light = 186 283 miles per second
Velocity of light = 2.997×10^8 meters per second
Boltzmann's constant = 1.380×10^{-23} J/K deg
Molar volume of ideal gas = 22.414 liters (1 atmosphere and 0°C)
This book uses a molar volume of 24.45 liters (1 atmosphere and 25°C) (NTP).

Ice-point = 273.1500 ± 0.0002 K
Density of water, at 25°C = $0.99797 \text{ g}/\text{cm}^3$
Density of mercury, at 25°C = $13.5340 \text{ g}/\text{cm}^3$
Velocity of sound in air, at 25°C = 346.2 m/sec

3. GRAVITATIONAL ACCELERATION AS A FUNCTION OF LATITUDE

TABLE A-1.

Latitude	ft/sec^2	m/sec^2
0°	32.0878	9.78039
10°	32.0929	9.78195
20°	32.1076	9.79641
30°	32.1302	9.79329
40°	32.1578	9.80171
50°	32.1873	9.81071
60°	32.2151	9.81918
70°	32.2377	9.82608
80°	32.2525	9.83059
90°	32.2577	9.83217

Note: Latitude is degrees north.

4. GRAVITATIONAL ACCELERATION AS A FUNCTION OF ALTITUDE

TABLE A-2.

Altitude (ft)	ft/sec^2	Altitude (m)	m/sec^2
0	32.1578	0	9.80171
500	32.1563	500	9.80017
1000	32.1547	1000	9.79864
1500		1500	
2000	32.1516	2000	9.79554
4000	32.1454	4000	9.78937
8000	32.1331	8000	9.77702
10000		10000	
20000		20000	
32000	32.0608	32000	9.70296

5. CALCULATED PRESSURE CORRECTION FACTORS FOR ALTITUDES TO 10 000 METERS (32 808 FEET)

Altitude		Exponential Calculated				ASHRAE Calculated			
(Meters)	(Feet)	F_P	P_{ATM} (mm Hg)	P_{ATM} (in Hg)	Pa (Pascals)	F_P	P_{ATM} (mm Hg)	P_{ATM} (in Hg)	Pa (Pascals)
−500	−1640	1.06	805.6	31.72	107405	1.056	802.6	31.60	106999
	−1000	1.04	790.4	31.12	105378	1.034	785.8	30.94	104770
0	0	1.00	760.0	29.92	101325	1.00	760.0	29.92	101325
	1000	0.97	737.2	29.02	98285	0.966	734.2	28.90	97880
500	1640	0.95	722.0	28.42					
	2000	0.93	706.8	27.83	94232	0.94	714.4	28.13	95246
	3000	0.90	684.0	26.93	91193	0.897	681.7	26.84	90889
1000	3281	0.89	676.4	26.63	90179	0.90	684.0	26.93	91193
	4000	0.87	661.2	26.03	88153	0.863	655.9	25.82	87443
	5000	0.84	638.4	25.13	85113	0.83	630.8	24.83	84100
	6000	0.81	615.6	24.24	82073	0.79	600.4	23.64	80047
2000	6562					0.80	608.0	23.94	81060
	7000	0.78	592.8	23.34	79034	0.772	586.7	23.10	78223
	8000	0.76	577.6	22.74	77007	0.73	554.8	21.84	73967
	9000	0.73	554.8	21.84	73976				
3000	9843					0.72	547.2	21.54	72954
	10000	0.71	539.6	21.24	71941	0.682	518.3	20.41	69104
4000	13123	0.65	494.0	19.45	65861	—	—	—	—
5000	16404	0.58	440.8	17.35	58769	—	—	—	—
6000	19685	0.52	395.2	15.56	52689	—	—	—	—
7000	22966	0.47	357.2	14.06	47623	—	—	—	—
8000	26247	0.42	319.2	12.57	42557	—	—	—	—
9000	29528	0.37	281.2	11.07	37490	—	—	—	—
10000	32808	0.34	258.4	10.17	34451	—	—	—	—

Source: ASHRAE, *Handbook of Fundamentals* (1981), p. 5.1.
ACGIH, *Industrial Ventilation: A Manual of Recommended Practice*, 21st Edition (1992), p. 5-44.

6. VAPOR PRESSURE OF MERCURY (mm Hg)

TABLE A-4.

Temperature °C	0	2	4	6	8
0	0.000185	0.000228	0.000276	0.000335	0.000406
10	0.000490	0.000588	0.000706	0.000846	0.001009
20	0.001201	0.001426	0.001691	0.002000	0.002359
30	0.002777	0.003261	0.003823	0.004471	0.005219
40	0.006079	0.007067	0.008200	0.009497	0.01098
50	0.01267	0.01459	0.01677	0.01925	0.02206
60	0.02524	0.02883	0.03287	0.03740	0.04251
70	0.04825	0.05469	0.06189	0.06993	0.07889
80	0.08880	0.1000	0.1124	0.1261	0.1413
90	0.1582	0.1769	0.1976	0.2202	0.2453

How to use this table: Vapor pressure at 44°C is 0.008200 mm Hg, by direct reading. Vapor pressure at 13°C is 0.000647 mm Hg, by interpolation. Vapor pressure at 25°C is 0.001846 mm Hg, by interpolation.

Source: *Handbook of Chemistry and Physics*, ed. Weast, R. C., 46th Edition. CRC Press, Cleveland, OH (1965), pp. D-96.

7. ABSOLUTE DENSITY OF MERCURY (15°C TO 35°C)

TABLE A-5.

Temperature (°C)	Density (g/ml)	Temperature (°C)	Density (g/ml)
15	13.5585	25	13.5340
16	13.5561	26	13.5315
17	13.5536	27	13.5291
18	13.5512	28	13.5266
19	13.5487	29	13.5242
20	13.5462	30	13.5217
21	13.5438	31	13.5193
22	13.5413	32	13.5168
23	13.5389	33	13.5144
24	13.5364	34	13.5119

The values presented are numerically equal to the absolute density of mercury in grams per milliliter (g/ml).

Source: *Handbook of Chemistry and Physics*, ed. Weast, R. C., 70th Edition. CRC Press, Boca Raton, FL (1989), p. F-6.

8. DENSITY AND VAPOR PRESSURE OF WATER

TABLE A-6.

Temperature (°C)	Density (g/ml)	Vapor pressure (mm Hg)	Temperature (°C)	Density (g/ml)	Vapor pressure (mm Hg)
15	0.99913	12.788	25	0.99707	23.756
16	0.99897	13.634	26	0.99681	25.209
17	0.99880	14.530	27	0.99654	26.739
18	0.99862	15.477	28	0.99626	28.349
19	0.99843	16.477	29	0.99597	30.043
20	0.99823	17.535	30	0.99567	31.824
21	0.99802	18.650	31	0.99537	33.695
22	0.99780	19.827	32	0.99505	35.663
23	0.99756	21.068	33	0.99473	37.729
24	0.99732	22.377	34	0.99440	39.898

The values presented are numerically equal to the absolute density of H_2O in grams per milliliter (g/ml). These data are linear with respect to temperature; the density and the vapor pressure may be determined for intermediate temperatures using linear extrapolation techniques.

Source: *Handbook of Chemistry and Physics*, ed. Weast, R. C., 70th Edition. CRC Press, Boca Raton, FL (1989), pp. F-10, D-192.

Index